ICOSANOIDS AND CANCER

Icosanoids and Cancer

Editors

Hélène Thaler-Dao, M.D.
Chargée de Recherche
INSERM U58
Montpellier, France

André Crastes de Paulet, M.D.
Professor and Director
INSERM U58
Montpellier, France

Rodolfo Paoletti, M.D.
Professor and Director
Institute of Pharmacology
and Pharmacognosy
University of Milan
Milan, Italy

Raven Press ■ New York

Raven Press, 1140 Avenue of the Americas, New York, New York 10036

Made in the United States of America

Library of Congress Cataloging in Publication Data
Main entry under title:

Icosanoids and cancer.

"Proceedings of the Icosanoids and Cancer Symposium, a
satellite of the 2nd International Congress on Hormones
and Cancer, held in Ile de Bendor, September 1983"—
Acknowledgments.
   Includes bibliographical references and index.
   1. Carcinogenesis—Congresses.   2. Arachidic acid—
Analogs—Physiological effect—Congresses.   3. Cancer cells
—Congresses.   4. Cell transformation—Congresses.
5. Lipids—Metabolism—Congresses.   6. Active oxygen in
the body—Congresses.   I. Thaler-Dao, H.
II. Crastes de Paulet, A.   III. Paoletti, Rodolfo.
IV. Icosanoids and Cancer Symposium (1983 : Bendor, France)
V. International Congress on Hormones and Cancer (2nd :
1983 : Bendor, France)   [DNLM: 1. Cell Transformation,
Neoplastic—congresses.   2. Fatty Acids, Unsaturated—
physiology—congresses.   3. Lipid Peroxides—physiology—
congresses.   4. Neoplasms—etiology—congresses.
QZ 202 I17 1983]
RC268.5.I28   1984   616.99′4071   84-8410
ISBN 0-88167-019-7

Preface

The purpose of this volume is to clarify the state of a subject undergoing tremendous evolution: the relationships between cancer and icosanoids.

These compounds are now considered intracellular lipidic mediators or microenvironmental hormones, synthesized by cells in extremely small quantities in response to diverse membrane stimuli. Gradually emerging from a tremendous body of work published during the last decade is the idea that some icosanoids could participate in the control of cell proliferation and differentiation. At the same time, a number of observations have given rise to the idea that some relationships may exist between the same icosanoids and the apparition and development of tumors. In fact, the problem is incredibly complex. Indeed, it is probable that the icosanoids and, more particularly, the hydroperoxides from which they are derived as well as the enzymatic or nonenzymatic processes that give rise to them, are suggestive in the early stages of carcinogenesis. Consequently, the first section of this volume is concerned with the up-to-date data on the relationships between lipid peroxides and cancer.

This volume brings together specialists in the chemistry of the active forms of oxygen and specialists in icosanoid biology. The chapters are organized in a sequence defined in part by the up-to-date concepts in carcinogenesis: free radicals, lipid peroxidation and cancer; polyunsaturated fatty acids as substrates for active oxygen (oxygenases and proximate carcinogen formation); icosanoids and carcinogenesis promotion; icosanoids and the control of cell proliferation and cell differentiation; icosanoids and tumor metastasis; and icosanoids and host tumor interactions.

The confrontation of two subjects as large as those of icosanoids and cancer cannot, at the present time, lead to a definitive explanation of precisely what their relationship is. The ambition of the editors is much more modest; it is to focus on the following points: What is the state of the research at present? What are we certain of? What are the false hypotheses? What are the most recent results?

This volume will be of interest to researchers, clinical specialists, medical students, and people interested in cancer research.

The Editors

Acknowledgment

This volume presents the proceedings of the Icosanoids and Cancer Symposium, a Satellite of the 2nd International Congress on Hormones and Cancer held in Ile de Bendor, September 1983.

Contents

Free Radicals, Lipid Peroxidation and Cancer

Polyunsaturated Fatty Acids as Substrates for Active Oxygen (Oxygenases and Proximate Carcinogen Formation)

Icosanoids and Carcinogenesis Promotion

Free Communications

Active Oxygen

Icosanoids and Cell Division and Differentiation

Host Tumor Interactions

Contributors

J. C. Aldigier
Immunology and Biochemistry Research Unit-
Medical School
2, Rue du Dr. Marcland
87032 Limoges, Cédex, France

M. Barbero
Istituto di Ginecologia e Ostetricia
Cattedra A
Via Ventimiglia 3
10126 Torino, Italy

H. Bartsch
International Agency for Research on Cancer
150, Cours Albert Thomas
F-69372 Lyon, Cédex 08, France

R. Becker
Institut für Gynäkologische Endokrinologie
Sterilitat und Familienplanung Klinikum
  Steglitz
Freie Universität Berlin
Berlin, Federal Republic of Germany

A. Bellin
Memorial Sloan-Kettering Cancer Center
1275 York Avenue
New York, New York 10021

Chiara Benedetto
Istituto di Ginecologia e Ostetricia
Cattedra A
Via Ventimiglia 3
10126 Torino, Italy

Alan Bennett
Department of Surgery
King's College Hospital Medical School
Rayne Institute
123 Coldharbour Lane
London, SE5 9NU United Kingdom

J.-C. Béréziat
International Agency for Research on Cancer
150, Cours Albert Thomas
F-69372 Lyon, Cédex 08, France

R. Bockman
Memorial Sloan-Kettering Cancer Center
1275 York Avenue
New York, New York 10021

J. A. Boyd
National Institute of Environmental Health
  Sciences
Laboratory of Molecular Biophysics
Prostaglandin Group
P.O. Box 12233
Research Triangle Park,
  North Carolina 27709

P. Braquet
Institut H. Beaufour
17 Avenue Descartes
92350 Le Plessis Robinson, France

G. W. Burton
Division of Chemistry
National Research Council of Ottawa
Ontario, K1A 0R6 Canada

Enrique Cadenas
Institut für Physiologische Chemie I
Universität Düsseldorf
Moorenstrasse 5
D-4000 Düsseldorf 1, Federal Republic
  of Germany

P. Cerutti
Institut Biomédical des Cordeliers
15, Rue de l'Ecole de Médecine
Paris 6, France; and
Department of Carcinogenesis
Swiss Institute for Experimental Cancer
  Research
CH-1066 Epalinges/Lausanne, Switzerland

K. W. Cheeseman
Department of Biochemistry
Brunel University
Uxbridge
Middlesex, UB8 3PH United Kingdom

N. Christeff
U.224 INSERM
CNRS ERA 881
Faculté Xavier Bichat
75018 Paris, France

Samuel M. Cohen
Department of Pathology and Laboratory
   Medicine, and the Eppley Institute for
   Research in Cancer
University of Nebraska Medical Center
42nd and Dewey Avenue
Omaha, Nebraska 68105

David G. Cornwell
Department of Physiological Chemistry
The Ohio State University
Columbus, Ohio 43210

M. Corrias
Istituto di Ginecologia e Ostetricia
Cattedra A
Via Ventimiglia 3
10126 Torino, Italy

J. R. F. Corvalan
Lilly Research Centre Limited
Erl Wood Manor
Windlesham, Surrey,
   GU20 6PH United Kingdom

Bernard B. Davis
Geriatric Research
Education and Clinical Center
VA Medical Center, and
Departments of Medicine and Biochemistry
St. Louis University School of Medicine
St. Louis, Missouri 63125

W. Dawson
Lilly Research Centre Limited
Erl Wood Manor
Windlesham, Surrey,
   GU20 6PH United Kingdom

Luis Jimenez de Asua
Friedrich Miescher-Institut
P.O. Box 2543
CH-4002 Basel, Switzerland

C. Deby
Laboratoire de Biochimie Appliquée
32, Boulevard de la Constitution
4020 Liège, Belgium

G. Deby-Dupont
Laboratoire de Biochimie Appliquée
32, Boulevard de la Constitution
4020 Liège, Belgium

Alan H. Drummond
Department of Pharmacology
University of Glasgow
Glasgow, G12 8QQ Scotland

D. Duval
U7 INSERM
Hôpital Necker
161 rue de Sèvres
75015 Paris, France

Martha M. Eibl
2nd Department of Medicine
Vienna Medical Hospital and Institute of
   Immunology
University of Vienna
A-1090 Vienna, Austria

T. E. Eling
National Institute of Enviromental Health
   Sciences
Laboratory of Molecular Biophysics
Prostaglandin Group
P.O. Box 12233
Research Triangle Park,
   North Carolina 27709

I. Emerit
Institut Biomédical des Cordeliers
15, Rue de l'Ecole de Médecine
Paris 6, France, and
Department of Carcinogenesis
Swiss Institute for Experimental Cancer
   Research
CH-1066 Epalinges/Lausanne, Switzerland

Susan M. Fischer
The University of Texas System Cancer Center
Science Park-Research Division
Smithville, Texas 78957

Masanori Fukushima
Aichi Cancer Center
Department of Internal Medicine and
   Laboratory of Chemotherapy
Chikusa-ku, Nagoya 464, Japan

G. Fürstenberger
Institute of Biochemistry
German Cancer Research Center
D-6900 Heidelberg, Federal Republic
  of Germany

Lyne Gagnon
Laboratoires d' Immunologie
Département de Pédiatrie
Faculté de Médecine
Université de Sherbrooke
Sherbrooke, Quebec J1H 5N4 Canada

S. Gauthier-Rahman
U.20 INSERM
CNRS LA 143
Hôpital Broussais
75014 Paris, France

Christoph Gisinger
2nd Department of Medicine
Vienna Medical Hospital and Institute of
  Immunology
University of Vienna
A-1090 Vienna, Austria

S. M. Goldstein
Department of Biochemistry
Brandeis University
Waltham, Massachusetts 02254

J. S. Goodwin
University of New Mexico Medical School
Albuquerque, New Mexico

R. Goutier
Laboratoire de Biochimie Appliquée
32, Boulevard de la Constitution
4020 Liège, Belgium

M. Gross
Institute of Biochemistry
German Cancer Research Center
D-6900 Heidelberg, Federal Republic
  of Germany

N. Gualde
Immunology and Biochemistry Research Unit-
  Medical School
2, Rue du Dr. Marcland
87032 Limoges, Cédex, France

J. Hammerstein
Institut für Gynäkologische Endokrinologie
Sterilitat und Familenplanung Klinikum
  Steglitz
Freie Universität Berlin
Berlin, Federal Republic of Germany

Sven Hammarström
Department of Physiological Chemistry
Karolinska Institutet
P.O. Box 60400
S-104 01, Stockholm, Sweden

T. Heinonen
International Agency for Research on Cancer
150, Cours Albert Thomas
F-69372 Lyon, Cédex 08, France

N. Hickok
Memorial Sloan-Kettering Cancer Center
1275 York Avenue
New York, New York 10021

E. Hietanen
International Agency for Research on Cancer
150, Cours Albert Thomas
F-69372 Lyon, Cédex 08, France

F. Homo-Delarche
U7 INSERM
Hôpital Necker
161 rue de Sèvres
75015 Paris, France

K. U. Ingold
Division of Chemistry
National Research Council of Ottawa
Ontario, K1A 0R6 Canada

Ryuichi Kato
Department of Pharmacology
School of Medicine
Keio University
Tokyo 160, Japan

Taketoshi Kato
Aichi Cancer Center
Department of Internal Medicine and
  Laboratory of Chemotherapy
Chikusa-ku, Nagoya 464, Japan

A. Kauppila
Departments of Obstetrics and Gynecology
University of Oulu
SF-90220 Oulu 22, Finland

E. Ann Kitchen
Lilly Research Centre Limited
Erl Wood Manor
Windlesham, Surrey,
* GU20 6PH United Kingdom*

H. Korpela
Department of Clinical Chemistry
University of Oulu
SF-90220 Oulu 22, Finland

R. S. Krauss
National Institute of Environmental Health
* Sciences*
Laboratory of Molecular Biophysics
Prostaglandin Group
P.O. Box 12233
Research Triangle Park,
* North Carolina 27709*

William E. M. Lands
Department of Biological Chemistry
University of Illinois at Chicago
1853 West Polk Street
Chicago, Illinois 60612

L. Levine
Department of Biochemistry
Brandeis University
Waltham, Massachusetts 02254

M. Liacopoulos-Briot
U.20 INSERM
CNRS LA 143
Hôpital Broussais
75014 Paris, France

Jenifer A. Lindsey
Department of Physiological Chemistry
The Ohio State University
Columbus, Ohio 43210

Colin Macphee
Department of Pharmacology
University of Glasgow
Glasgow, G12 8QQ Scotland

F. Marks
Institute of Biochemistry
German Cancer Research Center
D-6900 Heidelberg, Federal Republic
* of Germany*

Wayne Marshall
Department of Biochemistry
Memorial University of Newfoundland
St. John's, Newfoundland, A1B 3X9 Canada

R. P. Mason
National Institute of Environmental Health
* Sciences*
Laboratory of Molecular Biophysics
Prostaglandin Group
P.O. Box 12233
Research Triangle Park,
* North Carolina 27709*

M. Massobrio
Istituto di Ginecologia e Ostetricia
Cattedra A
Via Ventimiglia 3
10126 Torino, Italy

Michael B. Mattammal
Geriatric Research
Education and Clinical Center
VA Medical Center, and
Departments of Medicine and Biochemistry
St. Louis University School of Medicine
St. Louis, Missouri 63125

I. Mavelli
Institute of Applied Biochemistry and CNR
* Center of Molecular Biology*
University of Rome
00185 Rome, Italy

S. Mexmain
Immunology and Biochemistry Research Unit-
* Medical School*
2, rue du Dr. Marcland
87032 Limoges, Cédex, France

Nobuhiro Morisaki
Department of Physiological Chemistry
The Ohio State University
Columbus, Ohio 43210

Teruo Nakadate
Department of Pharmacology
School of Medicine
Keio University
Tokyo 160, Japan

W. Nastainczyk
Physiological Chemistry
University of Saarland
D-6650 Homburg/Saar, Federal Republic
* of Germany*

S. Nigam
Institut für Gynäkologische Endokrinologie
Sterilitat und Familienplanung Klinikum
  Steglitz
Freie Universität Berlin
Berlin, Federal Republic of Germany

J. T. Nodes
Department of Biochemistry
Brunel University
Uxbridge
Middlesex, UB8 3PH United Kingdom

E. A. Nunez
U.224 INSERM
CNRS ERA 881
Faculté Xavier Bichat
75018 Paris, France

Peter J. O'Brien
Department of Biochemistry
Memorial University of Newfoundland
St. John's, Newfoundland A1B 3X9 Canada

Angela M. Otto
Friedrich Miescher-Institut
P.O. Box 2534
CH-4002 Basel, Switzerland

Mark O. Palmier
Geriatric Research
Education and Clinical Center
VA Medical Center, and
Departments of Medicine and Biochemistry
St. Louis University School of Medicine
St. Louis, Missouri 63125

M. Papiernik
U.25 INSERM
Hôpital Necker
161 rue de Sèvres
75015 Paris, France

J. Parlebas
U.20 INSERM
CNRS LA 143
Hôpital Broussais
75014 Paris, France

M. G. Parry
Lilly Research Centre Limited
Erl Wood Manor
Windlesham, Surrey,
  GU20 6PH United Kingdom

Louis M. Pelus
Department of Developmental Hematopoiesis
Sloan Kettering Institute
1250 First Avenue
New York, New York 10021

E. Petitti
Istituto di Ginecologia e Ostetricia
Cattedra A
Via Ventimiglia 3
10126 Torino, Italy

J. Pincemail
Laboratoire de Biochimie Appliquée
32, Boulevard de la Constitution
4020 Liège, Belgium

G. A. Reed
National Institute of Environmental Health
  Sciences
Laboratory of Molecular Biophysics
Prostaglandin Group
P.O. Box 12233
Research Triangle Park,
  North Carolina 27709

A. Rigas
Department of Biochemistry
Brandeis University
Waltham, Massachusetts 02254

M. Rigaud
Immunology and Biochemistry Research Unit-
  Medical School
2, rue du Dr. Marcland
87032 Limoges, Cédex, France

Marek Rola-Pleszczynski
Laboratoires d'Immunologie
Département de Pédiatrie
Faculté de Médecine
Université de Sherbrooke
Sherbrooke, Quebec, J1H 5N4 Canada

G. Rotilio
Department of Biology
Second University of Rome
00173 Rome, Italy

H. H. Ruf
Physiological Chemistry
University of Saarland
D-6650 Homburg/Saar, Federal Republic
  of Germany

D. Schuhn
Physiological Chemistry
University of Saarland
D-6650 Homburg/Saar, Federal Republic
of Germany

Helmut Sies
Institut für Physiologische Chemie I
Universität Düsseldorf
Moorenstrasse 5
D-4000 Düsseldorf 1, Federal Republic
of Germany

Pierre Sirois
Laboratoire de Pharmacologie
Département de Pédiatrie
Faculté de Médecine
Université de Sherbrooke
Sherbrooke, Quebec J1H 5N4 Canada

T. F. Slater
Department of Biochemistry
Brunel University
Uxbridge
Middlesex, UB8 3PH United Kingdom

G. T. Snoek
Department of Biochemistry
Brandeis University
Waltham, Massachusetts 02254

C. Stiffel
U.125 INSERM
CNRS ER 70
Institut Curie
75005 Paris, France

H. Sundström
Departments of Obstetrics and Gynecology
University of Oulu
SF-90220 Oulu 22, Finland

G. Vallette
U.224 INSERM
CNRS ERA 881
Faculté Xavier Bichat
75018 Paris, France

L. Viinikka
Department of Clinical Chemistry
University of Oulu
SF-90220 Oulu 22, Finland

Heribert Wefers
Institut für Physiologische Chemie I
Universität Düsseldorf
Moorenstrasse 5
D-4000 Düsseldorf 1, Federal Republic
of Germany

Ronald W. Wise
Geriatric Research
Education and Clinical Center
VA Medical Center, and
Departments of Medicine and Biochemistry
St. Louis University School of Medicine
St. Louis, Missouri 63125

Satoshi Yamamoto
Department of Pharmacology
School of Medicine
Keio University
Tokyo 160, Japan

E. Yrjänheikki
Oulu Regional Institute of Occupational
Health
SF-90150 Oulu 15, Finland

Terry V. Zenser
Geriatric Research
Education and Clinical Center
VA Medical Center, and
Departments of Medicine and Biochemistry
St. Louis University School of Medicine
St. Louis, Missouri 63125

Christoph C. Zielinski
2nd Department of Medicine
Vienna Medical Hospital and Institute of
Immunology
University of Vienna
A-1090 Vienna, Austria

Hanfang Zhang
Department of Physiological Chemistry
The Ohio State University
Columbus, Ohio 43210

ICOSANOIDS AND CANCER

Icosanoids and Cancer, edited by H. Thaler-Dao, et al. Raven Press, New York © 1984.

Oxygen Free Radicals, and Tumor Cells

*I. Mavelli and **G. Rotilio

*Institute of Applied Biochemistry and CNR Center of Molecular Biology, University of Rome, 00185 Rome; and **Department of Biology, Second University of Rome, 00173 Rome, Italy*

The interactions between oxygen free radicals and tumor cells can be studied from different points of view with regard to both cancer prevention and cancer treatment. Several studies are in progress to investigate the role of oxygen radicals in the processes of mutagenicity and carcinogenesis. On the other hand, a number of different treatments of cancer therapy are based on recent knowledge concerning production of oxy-radicals and relative lack of antioxidative defences in tumor cells. In fact a great deal of evidence supports the hypothesis that tumor cells may be a selective target for oxygen free radicals.

The denomination "oxygen free radical " is properly referred to superoxide anion (O_2^-), the first product of monovalent reduction of oxygen, and to the hydroxyl radical ($OH^\cdot$), but it can be conveniently extended to hydrogen peroxide (H_2O_2) which is a product and/or a source of the other "oxygen radicals". There has been a great interest in the biological production of "oxygen free radicals", and in their consequences, after the discovery of enzymatic catalysis of O_2^- dismutation (reaction 1) by McCord and Fridovich (40) about 15 years ago.

$$O_2^- + O_2^- + 2H^+ \xrightarrow{\text{(SOD)}} H_2O_2 + O_2 \qquad \text{(react. 1)}$$

Spontaneous O_2^- dismutation is most rapid at acidic pH values, near to the pK of O_2^-/HO_2 (pH 4.8) and it is much slower at physiological pH. A family of superoxide dismutases was discovered in living organism, with either copper and zinc, or manganese or iron at the active site. These enzymes scavenge O_2^- with very high catalytic efficiency: the catalytic constant of Cu-Zn superoxide dismutase is in the order of $10^9 M^{-1} sec^{-1}$. The Mn-enzyme is less efficient, and in eucaryotic cells seems to be typical of the mitochondrial matrix . There is substantial evidence that superoxide dismutases are necessary for survival in all oxygen-metabolizing cells and that their physiological function is to provide a defence against potentially damaging effects of O_2^- (22, 23, 41).

1

Systems generating O_2^- in aqueous solution have been reported to kill bacteria and animal cells, inactivate enzymes, degrade DNA and polysaccharides and induce lipid peroxidation (11, 20, 33, 43).

Mechanisms of oxygen free radical production in biological systems.

Oxygen free radicals can be produced in aqueous solutions by physical agents such as high energy radiation (6). The interaction between ionizing radiation and biological systems can be understood in terms of the nature of ions and free radicals formed in irradiated water and their reactions with a number of solutes of biological relevance. The "primary" radicals formed in irradiated water are atomic hydrogen ($H\cdot$), the hydroxyl radical ($OH\cdot$) and the hydrated electron (e_{aq}^-). They can react with each other producing stable molecular products, namely H_2, H_2O_2, OH^-, and H_2O. $H\cdot$ and e_{aq}^- are strong reducing agents, whereas $OH\cdot$ is the most important oxidizing agent which forms in irradiated water. Primary radicals can also react, producing unstable secondary radicals, with inorganic ions and organic compounds of biological occurrence among which molecular oxygen is particularly important. In fact it is a very effective scavenger of the primary reducing radicals, and therefore in irradiated biological systems the reducing radicals are normally converted to O_2^- (6). The involvement of O_2^- in the oxygen enhancement of radiation damage in bacterial cells is suggested by protective effects ascribed to superoxide dismutase (47). Moreover evidence has been presented that damage of rat pulmonary macrophages by ionizing radiation may be due to $OH\cdot$ generated from O_2^-, H_2O_2 and iron (42).

Oxy-radicals can be produced in biological systems also by photooxidation (21). The absorption of light by endogenous or exogenous photosensitizers in the presence of oxygen causes the oxidation of a number of biological molecules that are able to bind the light absorbing species. Photosensitizers of this sort are dyes (e.g. methylene blue), pigments (e.g. porphyrins or flavins) and aromatic hydrocarbons. Their more stable electronically excited state is usually the triplet state. Triplet sensitizers can draw electrons from reducing molecules, and the resulting radicals can react further with oxygen and produce O_2^-. Otherwise the triplet sensitizers can transfer the excitation to molecular oxygen, thus producing an electronically excited singlet oxygen ($^1O_2$) which is a much easier oxidizing agent than the ordinary triplet state. In a broader meaning, also singlet oxygen can be included among "oxygen free radicals". Target molecules of photosensitized oxidation can be amino acids, nucleosides, lipids and other cell constituents such as tocopherols. The reaction of α-tocopherol, in particular, involves both reaction with and quenching of singlet oxygen (21). The latter mechanism may be, at least in part, responsible for the protective action of α-tocopherols against lipid photooxidation. Another possible biological defence against singlet oxygen is β-carotene,which quenches singlet oxygen very efficiently, essentially with no reaction (21).

Besides these physical agents, the biological production of oxy-radicals is associated with a number of <u>enzymes</u>, located in plasma membranes, mitochondria, endoplasmic reticulum, peroxisomes and cytosol, which have been recognized as effective H_2O_2 generators. Beside the well-known case of plasma membranes of activated phagocytes (13), NAD(P)H dependent redox chains associated with microsomal, mitochondrial and nuclear membranes, either from normal (13) or tumor (4, 48,50) cells, have been shown to generate O_2^- and H_2O_2. The monovalent reduction of molecular oxygen is believed to involve autoxidation of flavoproteins or hemoproteins: NADPH-cytochrome c reductase, cytochrome b_5 and cytochrome P_{450} in microsomal and nuclear membranes, NADH-ubiquinone reductase and ubiquinol cytochrome c reductase in the mitochondrial membranes are well characterized examples. Ubisemiquinone and ubiquinol are also capable to generate H_2O_2 in mitochondria via a non enzymatic reaction with oxygen (13). Furthermore quinone-like drugs, such as naphtoquinone, menadione, and anthracyclin antibiotics, can interact with electron-transport chains and divert the electron flux to univalent oxygen reduction (2). In this way these drugs increase the generation of O_2^- and H_2O_2 by either microsomes (29) and microsomal enzymes (24) or by submitochondrial particles (60). As far as H_2O_2 is concerned, it is formed in considerable amounts also in peroxisomes as demonstrated by the detection of a specific H_2O_2-catalase complex (13). In this case, however, there is no evidence for the production of other "oxygen radicals".

<u>Mechanisms of cellular damage by oxygen free radicals.</u>

Since O_2^- is poorly reactive in aqueous solution, being mainly a reducing agent, deleterious effects of O_2^--generating systems are presumably caused by hydroxyl radicals (OH·), or by other species, such as ferryl or perferryl radicals, which show similar reactivity to OH· (28). OH· is formed <u>in vitro</u> (27) by the redox metal-catalyzed Haber-Weiss cycle (reaction 2).

$$Me^{n+1} + O_2^- \longrightarrow O_2^- + Me^n$$

$$\underline{Me^n + H_2O_2 \longrightarrow Me^{n+1} + OH· + OH^-} \quad (react. \ 2)$$

$$\overset{Me^{n+1}}{O_2^- + H_2O_2 \longrightarrow O_2 + OH· + OH^-}$$

It is likely that Haber-Weiss-like reactions occur <u>in vivo</u>(52) since redox-active transition metal ions,especially iron, are

present in significant amounts in living systems (25). Although iron in animal tissues is mainly bound to proteins,
iron-nucleotides complexes have been isolated from erythrocytes (3) and non-protein-bound iron has been detected in
many biological systems (25, 51, 59). Such forms of non-protein-bound iron would be most suitable candidates to catalyze $OH^{\cdot}$ production, however evidence has recently been reported that indicates the involvment of non-heme iron proteins,
such as lactoferrin or transferrin, in $OH^{\cdot}$ formation from
iron catalyzed reduction of H_2O_2 (1, 45, 67). Iron-dependent
formation of $OH^{\cdot}$ from H_2O_2 (Fenton's reaction) could also
involve, in the iron reduction step, some physiological reducing agents such as glutathione (GSH), NADH, NADPH and
ascorbic acid (66). There is also evidence (65,69) that $OH^{\cdot}$,
or $OH^{\cdot}$ complexes with very similar reactivity, are produced
by the reaction of H_2O_2 with various organic radicals, such
as those derived from adriamycin, paraquat, nitrofurantoin,
and plumbagin.

Mechanisms of enzymatic defence and their role in tumor cells

Enzymatic defence against H_2O_2-mediated cytotoxicity,is
provided mainly by catalase and peroxidases. In animal cells
glutathione peroxidase appears to be the predominant peroxidase active in H_2O_2 detoxification. The action of these enzymes is complementary to that of superoxide dismutase in order
to provide an optimal control of the intracellular concentration of oxy-radicals. In fact superoxide dismutase catalyzes
the O_2^--mediated production of H_2O_2, while catalase and peroxidases remove H_2O_2. The ratio between superoxide dismutase
activity and that of the enzymes decomposing H_2O_2 appears to
be crucial in maintaining the steady-state concentration of
H_2O_2 at non toxic levels (38, 39).
In this respect some tumor cells may offer an interesting experimental model, and also provide a guideline for
tumor therapy by treatment more or less directly associated
with production of reactive oxygen species (e.g. hyperbaric
oxygen, ionizing radiations, photosensitization, quinone-like
drugs, etc.). It has been found that the activity of antioxidative enzymes in some tumors is less than normal, in particular catalase and Mn superoxide dismutase (5, 7, 8, 48).
Furthermore we have shown that some experimental ascites
tumors of rodents contain no catalase and specific activities
of superoxide dismutase and glutathione peroxidase lower
than hepathocytes or red blood cells (8). Specifically in
Ehrlich ascites cells the decrease of glutathione peroxidase
is greater than that of superoxide dismutase with reference
to the values found in normal control cells.
Ehrlich ascites cells were found to be more sensitive to
O_2^--generating systems than either normal controls or other
tumor cells with lower superoxide dismutase/glutathione peroxidase ratio (e.g. Yoshida ascites cells). Ehrlich and Yoshi-

da ascites cells were treated with either illuminated FMN-EDTA under aerobic conditions (9), which produces O_2^- and H_2O_2 outside the cells, or quinone drugs, namely daunomycin, streptonigrin, and naphtoquinone, which stimulate intracellular O_2^- production by interacting with mitochondrial and microsomal respiratory chains (10, 53). In both cases the Ehrlich cells resulted to be sensitive, whereas Yoshida cells were almost as resistant as liver cells. In the photochemical treatment (9) H_2O_2 was shown to be the most relevant oxygen derivative responsible for cell damage, since catalase was the only externally added agent that protected sensitive cells and addition of H_2O_2 produced the same effects as the FMN-EDTA treatment. In the other experimental approach, evidence for the mechanism of activation of the quinone drugs, and for the role of oxygen in this process was obtained from e.p.r. experiments on intact cells (10, 53). A free radical e.p.r. signal appeared upon anaerobiotic incubation of the tumor cells in the presence of either daunomycin or streptonigrin or naphtoquinone. The signal, that is due to the semiquinone forms of the drugs, disappeared when the cell suspensions were oxygenated, suggesting that oxygen is the main cellular scavenger of the drug radicals and that the products of the reaction are primarily O_2^- and H_2O_2. GSH was oxidized during the treatments in either Ehrlich or Yoshida cells, but to much lesser extent in Ehrlich than in Yoshida cells. Therefore the differential response of the two tumor cell types to this oxidative treatment is related to the efficiency of GSH-mediated H_2O_2 detoxifying system, in a cell model that is lacking of catalase. It seems reasonable to correlate these results with a higher H_2O_2 concentration in the sensitive cells due to relative lack of H_2O_2-destroying enzyme activities.

Mutagenicity and carcinogenicity.

Concerning the role of oxygen free radicals in mutagenicity and carcinogenesis, it has been reported that dioxygen is mutagenic (12) and ionizing radiations are both mutagenic and carcinogenic (61). Furthermore mutagenic effects have been shown for activated phagocytes (64), which are known to produce O_2^- and other partially reduced oxygen species. Also the mutagenicity of paraquat can be related to its ability to increase the intracellular production of O_2^- (44). Moreover recent in vitro studies have shown that O_2^--generating systems cause single-strand scissions in DNA and that superoxide dismutase, catalase or scavengers of $OH^\cdot$ protect against this damage (11, 35). Oxygen free radicals could contribute to DNA damage either by chemical reaction with it, directly or via induction of lipoperoxidation, either by interfering with DNA repair enzymes (32). The mutagenic species of oxygen and the exact mechanism of oxygen mutagenicity are yet to be identified.

Tumor promotion.

     Involvement of reactive oxygen has recently been sugge-
sted also in the second stage of carcinogenesis, i.e. tumor
promotion. It has been found that phorbol esters, which are
among the most potent tumor promoters, produce a rapid and
sustained decrease of murine epidermal superoxide dismutase
and catalase activities (57). This suggests that the increased steady-state concentration of oxygen free radicals, resulting from lowered levels of superoxide dismutase and catalase activities, can induce the neoplastic progression that
occurs in phorbol ester-treated mouse skin. Other studies
(19), on the other hand, have shown that phorbol esters induce in human lymphocytes chromosomal aberrations, whose extent
was found to be correlated to the degree of promoting efficiency of various phorbol esters and which were inhibited by
superoxide dismutase, thus supporting the role of O_2^--induced
lesions in tumor promotion. Moreover phorbol esters of varying tumor-promoting and pro-inflammatory efficacy have been
reported to induce O_2^- production by human granulocytes to an
extent which correlates with their tumor promoting activity
better than with their inflammatory action (68). Also the
recent finding (30) that a low molecular weight copper chela-
te with superoxide dismutase activity can inhibit some effects of phorbol esters is in line with these previous results.

Oxidative killing of tumor cells.

     Several studies are presently being carried out in the
field of oxidative killing of tumor cells. In particular, the
following examples may give an idea of current lines of research.

A. Intracellular production of oxy-radicals in tumor cells
by treatment with bleomycin-iron or quinone derivatives.

     Bleomycin, a glycopeptide antibiotic,induces DNA cleava-
ge only in the presence of Fe(II) (54) and this process has
been reported to be inhibited by superoxide dismutase or catalase or free radical scavengers (37). The mechanism seems
to involve a site-specific OH· release (49) because of preferential binding of Fe(II)-bleomycin to DNA.
     As regards quinone-type anticancer drugs, it has been
shown (29) that addition of mitomycin-C, daunomycin or carba-
zilquinone to microsomes from AH-109A hepatoma cells or from
Ehrlich ascites cells in the presence of NADPH markedly enhances sulfite oxidation. The mechanism proposed is the reduction
of the drugs to their semiquinone forms which can then reduce
molecular oxygen to yield O_2^-. O_2^- is known to specifically initiate sulfite oxidation. O_2^- and OH· seem also to participate
in the mechanism of DNA degradation by NADH-reduced streptonigrin, an antitumor antibiotic which contains an aminoquino-
ne moiety (16), because this process is completely inhibited

by superoxide dismutase and by catalase, while it is stimulated by cupric ions. The toxic effects of β-lapachone, an antimicrobial and antitrypanosomal o-naphtoquinone, on sarcoma 180 ascites tumor cells have been interpreted in terms of an increase of the intracellular flow of O_2^- and H_2O_2, mediated by the reduction of β-lapachone to its semiquinone radical (18).

B. Inhibition of antioxidative enzymes in cancer cells.

An increase of cytotoxicity of bleomycin has been reported in Chinese hamster cells (V79) treated in vitro with diethyldithiocarbamate (DDC), a copper chelator which is known to inactivate superoxide dismutase (15). It has been suggested (36) that combination of DDC and bleomycin in tumor therapy might be useful in order to increase the efficiency of bleomycin. In fact, besides sequestering free copper ions, which lower bleomycin toxicity (55), DDC would enhance the steady-state concentration of O_2^-, that has been shown to stimulate DNA degradation by bleomycin (31, 55).

C. Addition of compounds with superoxide dismutase-like activity, to either stimulate differentiation of tumor cells or to cause a cytotoxic build up of H_2O_2.

An antitumor effect has been observed with Cu(II) (3, 5 diisopropylsalicylate)$_2$ (Cu-DIPS) (34), a low molecular weight copper complex, which exhibits superoxide dismutase activity (17, 58) is lipid-soluble and can penetrate cell membranes. Growth of Ehrlich carcinomas in CBA mice has been reported to be retarded by administration of Cu-DIPS. Reduction in tumor size, delay of metastasis and a significant increase in host survival has been also observed. Although an increased immunological response of the host to the tumor may also be involved, the strong antitumor effect exerted by Cu-DIPS may be associated with its superoxide dismutase activity in this tumor; in fact, this type of tumor has been shown to be deficient in both Cu,Zn and Mn superoxide dismutase (34), and uptake of a superoxide dismuting compound in such cells could result in the inhibition of cell proliferation either by scavenging O_2^- (a likely tumor-promoter, see above),or increasing intracellular H_2O_2. Unfortunately, these authors do not present data on the H_2O_2-scavenging enzymes. A relative lack of them would be in favor of the idea (see above) that increase of H_2O_2 production occurs inside cells when the ratio between the activity of superoxide dismutase and that of the enzymes catabolizing H_2O_2 is increased.

D. Killing of cancer cells by immune mechanisms related to superoxide.

It has been reported (26, 46, 56, 62) that activated macrophages, granulocytes or monocytes induce extracellular cytolysis of erythrocytes and of different types of tumor cells, which is very likely to involve O_2^- and H_2O_2 release by killer cells. On the other hand, more recent studies have suggested

a role of the H_2O_2-myeloperoxidase-chloride system in tumor
cell destruction by activated human granulocytes and monocytes, which typically have a high myeloperoxidase content. In
this hypothesis peroxidative chlorination of cell components
is the mediator of cell damage with hypochlorous acid, or
species of similar reactivity, as the actual chlorinating
agent (14, 63).

REFERENCES

1. Ambruso, D.R. and Johnston, R.B. (1981): J. Clin. Invest.
   67:352-360.
2. Bachur, N.R., Gordon, S.L. and Gee, M.V. (1978): Cancer
   Res., 38:1745-1750.
3. Barlett, G.R. (1976): Biochem. Biophys. Res. Commun., 70:
   1063-1070.
4. Bartoli, G.M., Galeotti, T. and Azzi, A. (1977): Biochim.
   Biophys. Acta, 497:622-626.
5. Bartkowiak, A. and Bartkowiak, J. (1981): Comp. Biochem.
   Physiol., 70B:819-820.
6. Bielski, B.H.J. and Gebicki, J.M. (1977): In: Free Radicals in Biology, vol. III, edited by W.A. Pryor, pp. 1-
   51. Academic Press, New York, San Francisco, London.
7. Bize, I.B., Oberley, L.W. and Morris, H.P. (1980): Cancer
   Res., 40:3686-3693.
8. Bozzi, A., Mavelli, I., Finazzi-Agrò, A., Strom, R., Wolf
   A.M., Mondovì, B. and Rotilio, G. (1976): Mol. Cell.
   Biochem., 10:11-16.
9. Bozzi, A., Mavelli, I., Mondovì, B., Strom, R., and Rotilio, G. (1979): Cancer Biochem. Biophys., 3:135-141.
10. Bozzi, A., Mavelli, I., Mondovì, B., Strom, R. and Roti-
    lio, G. (1981): Biochem. J., 194:369-372.
11. Brawn, K. and Fridovich, I. (1981): Arch. Biochem. Bio-
    phys., 206:414-419.
12. Bruyninckx, W.J., Mason, H.S. and Morse, S.A. (1978):
    Nature, 274:606-607.
13. Chance, B., Sies, H. and Boveris, A. (1979): Physiol.Rev.
    59:527-605.
14. Clark, R.A., Szot, S. (1981): J. Immunol., 126:1295-1301.
15. Cocco, C., Calabrese, L., Rigo, A., Argese, E. and Roti-
    lio, G. (1981): J. Biol. Chem., 256:8983-8986.
16. Cone, R., Hasan, S.K., Lown, J.W. and Morgan, A.R. (1976):
    Can. J. Biochem., 54:219-223.
17. De Alvare, L.R., Goda, K. and Kimura, T. (1976): Biochem.
    Biophys. Res. Commun., 69:687-694.
18. Docampo, R., Cruz, F.S., Boveris, A., Muniz, R.P. and
    Esquivel, D.M. (1979): Biochem. Pharmacol., 28:723-728.
19. Emerit, I. and Cerutti, P.A. (1981): Nature, 293:144-146.
20. Fong, K., McCay, P.B., Poyer, J.L., Keel, B.B. and Misra,
    H. (1973): J. Biol. Chem. 248: 7792-7797.
21. Foote, C.S. (1976): In: Free Radicals in Biology vol. II,
    edited by W.A. Pryor, pp. 38-133. Academic Press, New
    York, San Francisco, London.

22. Fridovich, I. (1975): Ann. Rev. Biochem., 44:147-159.
23. Fridovich, I. (1978): Science, 201:875-880.
24. Goodman, J. and Hochstein, P. (1977): Biochem. Biophys. Res. Commun., 77:793-803.
25. Gutteridge, J.M.C., Rowley, D.A. and Halliwell,B. (1981): Biochem. J., 199:263-265.
26. Hafeman, D.G. and Lucas, Z.J. (1979): J. Immunol., 123: 55-62.
27. Halliwell,B. (1978): FEBS Lett., 92:321-326.
28. Halliwell,B. (1981): Bull. Eur. Physiopathol., Respir., 17:21-28.
29. Handa, K. and Sato, S. (1975): Gann, 66:43-47.
30. Kensler, T.W., Bush, D.M. and Kozumbo, W.J. (1983): Science, 221:75-77.
31. Ishida, R. and Takahashi, T. (1975): Biochem. Biophys. Res. Commun., 66: 1432-1438.
32. Joenje, H., Arwert, F., Eriksson, A.W., de Koning, H. and Oostra, A.B. (1981): Nature, 290:142-143.
33. Lavelle, F., Michelson, A.M. and Dimitrijevich, L. (1973): Biochem. Biophys. Res. Commun., 55:350-357.
34. Leuthauser, S.W., Oberley, L.W.,Oberley, T.D., Sorenson, J.R. and Ramakrishna, K. (1981): J. Natl. Canc. Inst.,66: 1077-1081.
35. Lesko, S.A., Lorentzen, R.J. and Tso P.O.P. (1980): Biochemistry, 19:3023-3028.
36. Lin, P.S., Kwock, L. and Goodchild, N.T. (1980): Cancer, 46:2360-2364.
37. Lown, J.W. and Sim, S.K. (1977): Biochem. Biophys. Res. Commun., 77:1150-1157.
38. Mavelli, I., Rigo, A., Federico, R., Ciriolo, M.R. and Rotilio, G. (1982): Biochem. J., 204:535-540.
39. Mavelli, I., Ciriolo, M.R., De Sole, P., Castorino, M., Stabile, A. (1982): Biochem. Biophys. Res. Commun., 106: 286-290.
40. McCord, J.M. and Fridovich, I. (1969): J. Biol. Chem., 244:6049-6055.
41. McCord, J.M., Keele, B.B. and Fridovich, I. (1971): Proc. Natl. Acad. Sci., 68:1024-1027.
42. McLennan, G., Oberley, L.W. and Autor, A.P. (1980):Radiat. Res., 84:122-132.
43. Michelson, A.M. and Buckingham, M.E. (1974): Biochem. Biophys. Res. Commun., 58: 1079-1086.
44. Moody, C.S. and Hassan, H.M. (1982): Proc. Natl. Acad. Sci. USA, 79: 2855-2859.
45. Motohashi, N. and Mori, I. (1983): FEBS Lett., 157:197-193.
46. Nathan, C.F., Silverstein, S.C., Bruknar, L.H. and Cohn, Z.A. (1979): J. Exp. Med., 149:100-113.
47. Oberley, L.W., Baker, S.A., Lindgren, A.L. and Stevens, R.H. (1976): Radiat. Res., 67: 535-541.
48. Oberley, L.W. and Buettner, G.R. (1979): Cancer Res., 39: 1141-1149.
49. Oberley, L.W. and Buettner, C.R. (1979): FEBS Lett., 97: 47-49.
50. Pskin, A.V., Zbarsky, I.B. and Konstantinov, A.A. (1980):

FEBS Lett., 117:44-48.

51. Pollack, S. and Campana, T. (1981): Biochim. Biophys. Acta, 673:366-373.

52. Repine, J.E., Fox, R.B. and Berger, E.M. (1981): J. Biol. Chem., 256:7094-7096.

53. Rotilio, G., Bozzi, A., Mavelli, I., Mondovì, B. and Strom, R. (1980): In: Biological and Clinical Aspects of Superoxide and Superoxide Dismutase, edited by W.H. Bannister and J.V. Bannister, pp. 118-126. Elsevier, North-Holland, New York, Amsterdam, Oxford.

54. Sausville, E.A., Peisach, J. and Horwitz, S.B. (1976): Biochem. Biophys. Res. Commun., 73:814-822.

55. Sausville, E.A., Peisach, J. and Horwitz, S.B. (1978): Biochemistry, 17:2740-2745.

56. Slivka, A. and Weiss, S.J. (1979): Clin. Res., 27: 640A.

57. Solanki, V., Rana, R.S. and Slaga, T.J. (1981): Carcinogenesis, 2:1141-1146.

58. Sorenson, J.R. (1976): J. Med. Chem., 19: 135-148.

59. Tangeras, A., Flatmark, T., Backstrom, D. and Ehrenberg, A. (1980): Biochim. Biophys. Acta, 589:162-175.

60. Thayer, W.S. (1977): Chem. Biol. Interact., 19:265-278.

61. Ward, J.F. (1975): Adv. Rad. Biol., 5: 182-239.

62. Weiss, S.J. (1980): J. Biol. Chem., 255:9912-9917.

63. Weiss, S.J. and Slivka, A. (1982): J. Clin. Invest., 69: 255-262.

64. Weitzman, S.A. and Stossel, T.P. (1981): Science, 212: 546-547.

65. Winterbourn, C.C. (1981): FEBS Lett., 136: 89-94.

66. Winterbourn, C.C. (1981): Biochem. J., 198:125-131.

67. Winterbourn, C.C. (1983): Biochem. J., 210:15-19.

68. Witz, G., Goldstein, B.D., Amoruso, M., Stone, D.S. and Troll, W. (1980): Proc. Am. Assoc. Cancer Res., 21:112.

69. Youngman, R.J., Osswald, W.F. and Elstnern, E.F. (1982): Biochem. Pharmacol., 31:603-606.

Icosanoids and Cancer, edited by H. Thaler-Dao, et al. Raven Press, New York © 1984.

Photoemission in Lipid Peroxidation and Prostaglandin G$_2$ Reduction and During Quinone Redox Cycling: Involvement of Singlet Oxygen

Helmut Sies, Heribert Wefers, and Enrique Cadenas

Institut für Physiologische Chemie I, Universität Düsseldorf, D-4000 Düsseldorf 1, Federal Republic of Germany

Aggressive oxygen species are implicated in a variety of physiological and pathological processes, and biological systems are equipped with detoxication devices, both enzymatic and nonenzymatic (27,41). Singlet molecular oxygen has come recently into focus with regard to damage of membranes and proteins, and possibly also nucleic acids. Krinsky (31) has reviewed the biological roles of singlet oxygen, and it may be fair to state at this stage that the identity of singlet oxygen in biological materials is still under debate. Due to the very low concentration of this excited species, there is only physical-chemical evidence for its occurrence, while attemps to directly demonstrate this species by chemical trapping [e.g. with detection of 5-α-hydroperoxy-cholesterol (40)] have been fruitless, perhaps due to the fact that cholesterol is not an efficient singlet oxygen trap (19).

PHOTOEMISSION: METHODOLOGICAL COMMENTS

Low-level (or ultraweak) chemiluminescence of biological samples can be detected by a single-photon-counting apparatus such as the one used by Tarusov et al. (44) or as improved to be applicable in a wider range of objects and towards higher efficiency by Boveris et al. (3), Deneke and Krinsky (15), and Inaba et al. (22). The technical problems and a description of a suitable set-up incorporating a light-tight box have been recently described (11). The apparatus used for the present study is the one described in (11). Spectral analysis was performed by employing different interference filters or cut-off gelatin filters as indicated in (3,11).

RED PHOTOEMISSION: INDICATION OF SINGLET OXYGEN

Spectral analysis of emitted light has been most fruitful in identifying singlet oxygen. Khan and Kasha (28) showed that in contrast to more broad bands of other emitters, singlet oxygen emits in the dimol reaction at 634 and 703 nm. Thus, it is highly useful to detect at these two wavelengths in comparison to another one in between, e.g., 668 nm. This

criterion for singlet oxygen identification has been applied to some of
the biological systems to be discussed below, and also there has been
spectral resolution. Fig. 1 compares spectral analysis of chemiluminescence of oxene donor-supplemented ram seminal vesicle microsomes with
photoemission from a known singlet oxygen source, the H_2O_2/OCl^- system.
In addition, the latter spectrum detected by the described photon counting apparatus (11) conforms to that expected for singlet oxygen dimol
emission. The photoemission arising from the arachidonate-supplemented
isolated prostaglandin-endoperoxide synthase as purified from ram
seminal vesicles exhibits peaks in the wavelength range illustrated in
Fig. 1. The biochemical aspects of this reaction will be discussed
below.

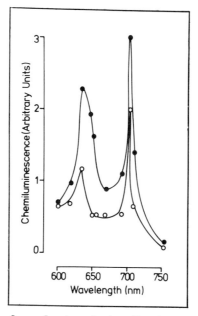

Fig. 1. Spectral analysis of chemiluminescence from the
H_2O_2/OCl^- reaction [(●), ref. 33] and iodosobenzene-
supplemented ram seminal vesicles microsomes [(o), ref.
37].

    The 1270 nm emission band characteristic of the singlet oxygen mono-
mol emission (29) has often been quoted as being diagnostic of singlet
oxygen. However, the current technology of detecting energies at this
wavelength range, based mainly on germanium diodes, appears not yet
suitable for application to the cellular or microsomal systems we are
studying. In a recent comparative study between the single-photon counting apparatus [red-sensitive photomultiplier EMI type 9658A; EMI-Gencom
Plainview, NY, USA (11)] and the germanium diode system (type J-16,
Judson Infrared Inc., USA), using the H_2O_2/OCl^- reactions as a source of
singlet oxygen, a factor of 1,000 in the detection limits in favor of
the former was observed (33). Interestingly, a recent report by Kanofsky
(25) on photoemission from lactoperoxidase/halide/H_2O_2 system gave a
1270 nm signal attributed to singlet oxygen monomol emission. Further,

D_2O enhanced the signal substantially, in agreement with earlier reports (36).

LIPID PEROXIDATION

Peroxidation of microsomal unsaturated fatty acids is apparently initiated and supported by a redox cycling process, which proceeds at the expense of NADPH using the NADPH-cytochrome P-450 reductase activity, having as an intermediate redox carrier an iron-chelate complex, and yielding $O_2^{\cdot-}$ upon interaction of the latter with oxygen. Secondary and more oxidizing oxygen radicals might be formed at its expense, to account for the oxidation of membrane lipids. Alkoxy and peroxy radicals are formed in the decomposition of lipid hydroperoxides and are important in the maintainance of radical chain reactions. In the generation of the former oxygen-containing radicals metal ions would play a significant role.

Based on different evidence, the generation of singlet oxygen during lipid peroxidation is attributed to the free radical breakdown of lipid hydroperoxides (43,48). Therefore, singlet oxygen is regarded as a consequence of lipid peroxidation rather than an initiator of the process. This hypothesis is based on Russell's mechanism (21,39) and assumes the self-reaction of lipid peroxy radicals (ROO·) with formation of a cyclic intermediate. This intermediate may decompose into either a triplet state carbonyl compound or else yield singlet molecular oxygen. Thus, singlet oxygen formed during lipid peroxidation is considered to be a side-reaction channeled through peroxy radical decay.

Monitoring of low-level chemiluminescence during ongoing lipid peroxidation has also been shown with isolated rat hepatocytes (7); a good correlation between photoemission and accumulation of thiobarbiturate-reactive material has been often reported (7,42,51). Further, there is a good correlation also with alkanes produced (26,42). Thus, with a given type of membrane, there appears to be a constant relation between different pathways of oxidative breakdown of the polyunsaturated fatty acids, and any one of the parameters just mentioned above could be used.

Experimental models for microsomal lipid peroxidation rest on a general pattern involving two systems: on the one side, an oxygen free radical-generating system (either enzymatic, at expense of NADPH using the NADPH-cytochrome P-450 reductase activity, or non-enzymatic, generally using a reductant such as ascorbic acid) and, on the other side, a target system, the membrane unsaturated fatty acids. Peroxidation of fatty acids (detected either as malondialdehyde accumulation, or diene conjugate formation, or chemiluminescence, or alkane production) does not start immediately, but it is preceded by an induction period, the duration of which under standardized conditions could be related to the time necessary to overcome internal antioxidant activities, such as that of vitamin E (5). This induction period can be prolonged by different thiol-containing molecules and other compounds, ie, GSH (4,14), diethyldithiocarbamate, diethioerythritol (1,14), etc. Although a tentative explanation for this temporary protection exerted by different thiols and other molecules might rely on a regeneration of vitamin E, a direct free radical scavenging activity by the thiols (20,23,30) or detoxication by reduction of lipid hydroperoxides through an enzymatic activity (4) cannot be excluded. When hepatocytes isolated from livers of rats fed a diet deficient in vitamin E are exposed to oxidative stress, there is a larger response in lipid peroxidation and its dependent parameters.

Another aspect related to lipid peroxidation is the generation of
toxic products of non-radical nature which can exert cytotoxic effects
at a distance from the lipid peroxidation loci. Thus, in the last years
attention was focussed on the formation of alkenals, mainly 4-hydroxy-
2,3-trans-nonenal, during oxidation of membrane lipids (18). These
alkenals show a high affinity for SH groups and their incubation with
hepatocytes results in a rapid depletion of GSH in the form of a GS-
conjugate with nonenal (10). Although depletion of intrahepatic glutathione seems to be a deciding factor to increase the oxidative damage
of the cells [as detected by low-level chemiluminescence (7)], it seems
not to play a role in the 4-hydroxynonenal-enhanced chemiluminescence
and alkane formation (10). Furthermore, the enhanced chemiluminescence
and alkane formation by 4-hydroxynonenal-supplemented hepatocytes (Fig.
2) can be further augmented in vitamin E-deficient hepatocytes. These
observations were made analogously also with ethane instead of chemiluminescence (10). This enhanced light emission does not correlate with
an augmentation in malondialdehyde or diene conjugate formation. It
seems that side reactions from a minor oxidative pathway triggered during incubation of hepatocytes with the aldehyde could be responsible
for the enhanced photoemission observed.

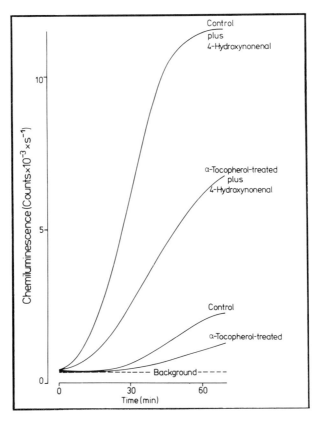

Fig. 2. Effect of vitamin E pretreatment of rats on 4-hydroxynonenal-
enhanced chemiluminescence of isolated hepatocytes. From ref. 10.

REDOX CYCLING

Redox cycling is quoted as the molecular mechanism of action of different xenobiotics, such as toxic or chemotherapeutic agents (16,27). In addition to the different oxygen radicals formed during redox cycling, photoemission might also occur. The chemiluminescence observed during redox cycling seems not to be associated with malondialdehyde formation; a reason might be found in a diversion of electrons from the NADPH-cytochrome P-450 reductase towards the xenobiotic instead of cytochrome P-450. Fig. 3A shows microsomes undergoing lipid peroxidation as indicated by an accumulation of malondialdehyde and an increase in chemiluminescence. When a substance capable of redox cycling, such as paraquat, is added to microsomes already undergoing lipid peroxidation (Fig. 3B), chemiluminescence is abruptly enhanced, whereas malondialdehyde formation is inhibited. Paraquat added at the beginning of the reaction (Fig. 3C) exerts a total inhibition of lipid peroxidation and yields light emission with a time course pattern different of that from microsomes during lipid peroxidation.

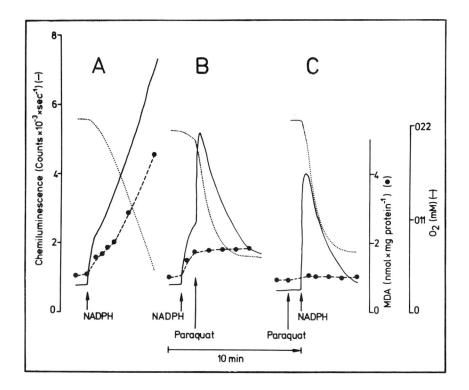

Fig. 3. Chemiluminescence, O_2 uptake, and malondialdehyde accumulation, of microsomal fractions in the absence and presence of paraquat. (A) Reaction started upon addition of $NADP^+$. (B) Paraquat added during an ongoing lipid peroxidation reaction. (C) Paraquat was present prior to the addition of $NADP^+$. From ref. (9).

The formation of paraquat radical will intercept lipid radicals and thus will arrest further malondialdehyde accumulation (9). This is not due to the reactions of peroxy radicals as outlined above but rather to the reactions of oxygen metabolites stemming from the initial formation of the O_2^-, formed as a product of redox cycling of paraquat. Similar observations are applicable to redox cyling of menadione and glutathione-conjugate of menadione in perfused liver, isolated hepatocytes, micro-somal membranes, and model systems (49).

PROSTAGLANDIN G_2 TO H_2 REDUCTION: A DISMUTATION REACTION GENERATING SINGLET OXYGEN

The oxidation of arachidonate by prostaglandin endoperoxide synthase involves cyclooxygenase and hydroperoxidase activities in a single protein (38,47), associated with the formation of a potent oxidant produced during the reduction of PGG_2 to PGH_2 (34). With respect to the nature of this oxidant, sometimes denoted as O_x (32), earlier attempts to identify it as being singlet molecular oxygen were inconclusive (34, 35). However, the lack of chemical adduct formation in the form of a 5-α-hydroperoxide of cholesterol could be due to problems in the indicat-or reaction and in itself is no positive argument against the occurrence of singlet oxygen. Using the spectral analysis as one criterion (Fig. 1), a mechanism for the generation of an active oxygen species during reduc-tion of PGG_2 to PGH_2 was recently proposed (13). The reaction does not involve an external hydrogen donor and formally follows the sequence of a dismutation (reactions 1-3):

$$PGG_2 + Fe^{3+} \rightarrow PGH_2 + [FeO]^{3+} \qquad (1)$$
$$PGG_2 + [FeO]^{3+} \rightarrow PGH_2 + Fe^{3+} + {}^1O_2 \qquad (2)$$

Sume (1) + (2)
$$PGG_2 + PGG_2 \rightarrow 2\ PGH_2 + {}^1O_2 \qquad (3)$$

The product of the dioxygenase reaction, PGG_2, gives rise to chemilumin-escence in the presence of isolated PG synthase under anaerobic condi-tions (Table 1). This indicates that the hydroperoxidase reaction of PG synthase is responsible for the formation of excited species, as singlet oxygen.

In this reaction sequence, there is an intermediate formation of an active $[FeO]^{3+}$ complex that can be formed with several oxene donors (37). The known heme requirement of the prostaglandin endoperoxide synthase thus would find its explanation. Such a mechanism relies on the similar characteristics of thromboxane and prostaglandin synthase to cytochrome P-450, the former being able to catalyze the heterolytic cleavage of the 9,11-endoperoxide of 15-hydroxy-arachidonic acid (45).

The formation of this oxidant during PGG_2 reduction leads to a des-truction of the enzyme; also it participates in the cooxidation of a large number of xenobiotics which might develop potent toxic and/or carcinogenic compounds. The possibility exists, therefore, that PG synthase, like the cytochrome P-450-dependent monooxygenase might be involved in the oxidative activation of xenobiotics. We have found that arachidonate-induced photoemission of ram seminal vesicle microsomes is effectively quenched by GSH as well as quinol and phenol (13). This inhibition of chemiluminescence and similar observed decreases in esr signals arising from this reaction (17) are associated with an enhance-ment of PG biosynthesis (possibly protecting cyclooxygenase from the oxidant generated). These empirical observations cannot unequivocally point to a mechanism for cooxidations during prostaglandin biosynthesis; various hypotheses could apply to this, among them, a direct reaction with the enzyme as a hydrogen donor for peroxidase activities, a free radical scavenging activity of the cooxidizing substance, a possible reaction of phenol-like molecules with singlet oxygen, etc.

TABLE 1.   Effect of Oxygen on Low-Level Chemiluminescence from Arachidonate of Prostaglandin G_2.
Ram vesicular gland microsomes or purified PG-endoperoxide synthase in O_2- or N_2-saturated 0.1 M Tris/HCl buffer, pH 8.1, were supplemented with 50 µM arachidonic acid or 17 µM PGG_2.

	Chemiluminescence (counts/s)			
	Aerobiosis		Anaerobiosis	
	Arachidonate	PGG_2	Arachidonate	PGG_2
Microsomes (1.1 mg/ml)	46,000	20,000	5,900	19,500
PG-endoperoxide synthase (58 µg/ml)	38,000	26,000	3,400	25,000

From ref. 13.

In fact, the oxene-transferase activity of cytochrome P-450 -under formation of a transient $[FeO]^{3+}$ species and implying a heterolytic cleavage of the O-O bond of hydroperoxides (46)- has been shown to be associated with chemiluminescence (12). Different oxene donors (iodoso-benezene, t-butyl hydroperoxide, cumene hydroperoxide, H_2O_2) are effective in reacting with cytochrome P-450 yielding light emission. In this case, photoemission is independent of oxygen, the oxygen atom being provided by the selected oxene donor. Furthermore, optimal conditions to observe light emission rely on the oxidized state of the cytochrome; in the presence of reducing equivalents to cytochrome P-450, a reductive type of peroxidase activity is supported with reduction of the hydroperoxide to the corresponding alcohol (2). In the presence of hydroxylatable substrates for the monooxygenase system, oxygen atom transfer to the substrate (46) will result in quenching of photoemission (12). Both previous conditions decrease significantly the destruction of cytochrome P-450 which occurs during the development of chemiluminescence (12).

Homolytic scission of hydroperoxides (50) could also be used as a tentative model for the generation of excited species by organic hydroperoxide-supplemented microsomal fractions (8). Formation of excited species in such a reaction would not be a primary consequence of cytochrome P-450 activity, but rather it might be attributed to further free radical interactions (8). Previous observations in model systems have shown that oxidized hemoproteins could catalyze hydroperoxide breakdown with formation of oxygen in the activated state (6) or peroxyl free radicals (24).

Acknowledgements

This work was supported by Deutsche Forschungsgemeinschaft, Schwerpunkt "Mechanismen toxischer Wirkungen von Fremdstoffen", Grant Si 255/5-4 and by Ministerium für Wissenschaft und Forschung, Nordrhein-Westfalen. Fruitful discussion and experimental cooperation, regarding various aspects, is gratefully acknowledged to G. Bartoli, Rome, H. Esterbauer, Graz, H. Kappus, Berlin, W. Nastainczyk, Homburg, and V. Ullrich, Konstanz.

REFERENCES

1. Bartoli, G.M., Müller, A., Cadenas, E., and Sies, H. (1983): FEBS Lett. submitted.
2. Bidlack, W.R. (1980): Biochem. Pharmacol. 29:1605-1608.
3. Boveris, A., Cadenas, E., and Chance, B. (1981): Fed. Proc. 40:195-198.
4. Burk, R.F. (1983): Biochim. Biophys. Acta 757:21-28.
5. Burton, G.W. and Ingold, K.U. (1983): In: Protective Agents in Cancer, edited by D.C.H. McBrien and T.F. Slater, pp. 81-100. Academic Press, New York.
6. Cadenas, E., Boveris, E., and Chance, B. (1980):Biochem. J., 187:131-140.
7. Cadenas, E., Wefers, H., and Sies, H. (1981): Eur. J. Biochem., 119:531-536.
8. Cadenas, E. and Sies, H. (1982):Eur. J. Biochem., 124:349-356.
9. Cadenas, E., Brigelius, R., and Sies, H. (1983): Biochem. Pharmacol., 32:147-150.
10. Cadenas, E., Müller, A., Brigelius, R., Esterbauer, H., and Sies, H. (1983): Biochem. J., 214:479-484.
11. Cadenas, E. and Sies, H. (1983): Methods Enzymol., 105, in press.
12. Cadenas, E., Sies, H., Graf, H., and Ullrich, V. (1983): Eur. J. Biochem.,130:117-121.
13. Cadenas, E., Sies, H., Nastainczyk, W., and Ullrich, V. (1983): Hoppe-Seÿler's Z. Physiol. Chem. 364:519-528.
14. Christophersen, B.O. (1968): Biochem. J., 106:515-532.
15. Deneke, C.F. and Krinsky, N.I. (1979): Photochem. Photobiol., 25:299-304.
16. Doroshow, J. and Hochstein, P. (1982): In: Pathology of Oxygen, edited by A.P. Autor, pp. 245-260. Academic Press, New York.
17. Egan, R.W., Gale, P.H., and Kuehl, F.A., Jr. (1979): J. Biol. Chem., 254:3295-3302.
18. Esterbauer, H. (1982): In: Free Radicals and Cancer, edited by D.C.H. McBrien and T.F. Slater, pp. 102-108. Academic Press, New York.
19. Foote, C.S. (1979):   In: Oxygen: Biochemical and Clinical Aspects, edited by W.S. Caughey, pp. 603-626. Academic Press, New York.
20. Forni L.G. and Willson, R.L. (1983): In: Protective Agents in Cancer, edited by D.C.H. McBrien and T.F. Slater, pp. 159-173. Academic Press, New York.
21. Howard, J.A. and Ingold, K.U. (1968): J. Am. Chem. Soc., 90:1056-1058.
22. Inaba, H., Shimizu, Y., Tsuji, Y. and Yamagishi, A. (1979):Photochem. Photobiol., 30:169-175.
23. Jocelyn, P.C. (1972): Biochemistry of the SH Group. Academic Press, New York.
24. Kalyanamaran, B., Mottley, C., and Mason, R.P. (1983): J. Biol. Chem.,

in press.

25. Kanofsky, J.R. (1983): J. Biol. Chem., 258:5991-5993.
26. Kappus, H. and Muliawan, M. (1982): Biochem. Pharmacol., 31:597-600.
27. Kappus, H. and Sies, H. (1981): Experientia 37:1233-1241.
28. Khan, A.U. and Kasha, M. (1970): J. Am. Chem. Soc., 92:3293-3300.
29. Khan, A.U. and Kasha, M. (1979): Proc. Natl. Acad. Sci. U.S.A., 76: 6047-6049.
30. Kosower, N.S. and Kosower, E.W. (1978): Intern. Rev. Cytol., 54:109-160.
31. Krinsky, N.I. (1979): In: Singlet Oxygen, edited by H.H. Wasserman and W.A. Murray, pp. 597-641. Academic Press, New York.
32. Kuehl, F.A., Jr., Humes, J.L., Ham, E.A., Egan, R.W. and Dougherty, H.W. (1980): In: Prostaglandin and Thromboxane Research, edited by B. Samuelsson, P.W. Ramwell, and R. Paleotti, pp. 77-84. Raven Press, New York.
33. Lengfelder, E., Cadenas, E., and Sies, H. (1983): FEBS Lett., submitted.
34. Marnett, L.J., Wlodawer, P. and Samuelsson, B. (1974): Biochem. Biophys. Res. Commun., 60:1286-1294.
35. Marnett, L.J., Wlodawer, P., and Samuelsson, B. (1975): J. Biol. Chem., 250:8510-8517.
36. Merkel, P.B., Nilsson, R., and Kearns, D.R. (1972): J. Am. Chem. Soc., 94:1030-1031.
37. Nastainczyk, W., Ullrich, V., Cadenas, E., and Sies, H. (1983): In: Third Internationl Conference on Oxygen Radicals in Chemistry and Biology, edited by W. Bors, M. Saran, and D. Tait. Walter de Gruyter, Berlin, in press.
38. Roth, G.J., Siok, Ch.J., and Ozols, J. (1980): J. Biol. Chem., 255: 1301-1304.
39. Russell, G.A. (1957): J. Am. Chem. Soc., 79:3871-3877.
40. Schenck, G.O., Gollnick, K., and Neumüller, O.A. (1957): Justus Liebigs. Ann. Chem., 603:46-59.
41. Sies, H. and Cadenas, E. (1983): In: Biological Basis of Detoxication, edited by J. Caldwell and W.B. Jakoby, pp. 181-211. Academic Press, New York.
42. Smith, M.T., Thor, H., Hartzell, P. and Orrenius, S. (1982): Biochem. Pharmacol., 31:19-26.
43. Sugioka, K. and Nakano, M. (1976): Biochim. Biophys. Acta 423:203-216.
44. Tarusov, B.N., Polidova, A.I., Yhuravlev, A.I. and Sekamova, E. (1962): Tsitologiya 4:696-699.
45. Ullrich V., Castle, L. and Weber, P. (1981): Biochem. Pharmacol., 30:2033-2036.
46. Ullrich, V. (1977): In: Microsomes and Drug Oxidations, edited by V. Ullrich, I. Roots, A. Hildebrandt, R.O. Estabrook, and A.H. Conney, pp. 192-201. Plenum Press, New York.
47. Van der Ouderaa, F.J., Buytenhek, M., Nugteren, D.H., and van Dorp, D.A. (1980): Eur. J. Biochem., 109:1-8.
48. Vladimirov, Yu.A., Korchagina, M.U., and Olenev, V.I. (1971): Biophysics (Moscow), 16:994-997.
49. Wefers, H. and Sies, H. (1983): Arch. Biochem. Biophys., 224:568-578.
50. White, R.E. and Coon, M.J. (1980): Annu. Rev. Biochem., 49:315-356.
51. Wright, J.R., Rumbaugh, R.C., Colby, H.D., and Miles, P.R. (1979): Arch. Biochem. Biophys., 192:344-351.

Icosanoids and Cancer, edited by H. Thaler-Dao, et al. Raven Press, New York © 1984.

Lipid Peroxidation in Animal Tumours: A Disturbance in the Control of Cell Division?

*T. F. Slater, **Chiara Benedetto, †G. W. Burton, *K. H. Cheeseman, †K. U. Ingold, and *J. T. Nodes

*Department of Biochemistry, Brunel University, Uxbridge, Middlesex, UB8 3PH United Kingdom; **Istituto di Ginecologia e Ostetricia, Cattedra A, Torino 10126, Italy; and †Division of Chemistry, National Research Council of Ottawa, Ontario, K1A 0R6 Canada*

The electron transport chain of the endoplasmic reticulum of liver cells that is dependent upon NADPH as the reducing source is associated with a number of important reactions including oxygen activation, cholesterol metabolism, and the transformation ('detoxification') of many exogenous drugs and other materials (for reviews see 6,11). Major components of the electron transport chain are an NADPH-linked flavoprotein (the enzymic activity of which is usually measured by coupling it to the reduction of cytochrome P_{450}, cytochrome c or ferricyanide), cytochrome P_{450} and phospholipid (see 34).

Significant activities of the NADPH-linked flavoprotein can be found in many tissues of the rat, whereas cytochrome P_{450} is rather strongly associated with the endoplasmic reticulum of liver cells. Data illustrating these points are given in Table 1.

Although the content of cytochrome P_{450} in particular tissues (see Table 1) may be small compared to liver on a wet weight basis, or when expressed per mg microsomal protein, it is important to note that this component of the drug metabolising system may be selectively distributed in certain regions or in particular cells of a tissue thereby creating locally high concentrations and activity. For example: cytochrome P_{450} is preferentially concentrated in the centrilobular zones of rat liver lobules (19) and in the Clara cells of lung (5). Moreover, a number of isozyme forms of cytochrome P_{450} occur that have different substrate specificities and different responses to inducing agents (see 27): such factors need to be carefully evaluated in making judgements on the qualitative and quantitative aspects of the metabolism of a substance under study.

Although the metabolism of many drugs and other substances by the NADPH-cytochrome P_{450} system results in a more hydrophilic and less toxic product, there is an increasing number of examples where this metabolism results in the formation of a more toxic species; such events are called metabolic activation (see 43). A variety of mutagens and/or carcinogens are metabolically activated in this way to free radical intermediates

(Table 2), but the free radical species may not be the only or even the major reactive intermediate formed by metabolic activation in the endoplasmic reticulum. Polycyclic hydrocarbons, for instance, are converted also to the epoxydihydrodiols that are known to bind strongly to DNA (37).

TABLE 1   The distributions of NADPH-cytochrome c reductase, NADPH-ferricyanide reductase, and cytochrome P_{450} in normal tissue of the rat.[a]

Rat tissue	NADPH-cyt.c reductase[b]	NADPH-ferricyanide reductase	Cytochrome P_{450}
Liver - adult	100	100	100
- foetal (20 d)	8	-[c]	nd[d]
- newborn (2-4 d)	41	-	23
- young (14 d)	59	-	48
Kidney	46	57	13
Lung	39	86	8
Brain	19	121	9
Spleen	12	85	1
Testis	17	82	9
Adrenal	90	420	76
Stomach	24	-	-

[a]Data from Benedetto et al (4); [b]Activities and contents shown are percentages of the adult liver values; [c]a dash indicates not measured; [d]nd, not detectable.

TABLE 2   Mutagenic and/or carcinogenic substances converted to free radical intermediates by the NADPH-cytochrome P_{450} system.[a]

Carbon tetrachloride	(38)
Various aromatic amines	(44)
Polycyclic hydrocarbons	(32)
Hydrazines	(28)
Dibromoethane	(45)
Some quinones	(28,31)
Some nitro-compounds	(29)

[a]the number in parenthesis is to an appropriate reference.

The production and identification of reactive free radical intermediates is often difficult to study directly as their high chemical reactivity results in corresponding short half-lives; this combined with a normally small rate of production usually results in very low concentrations. In consequence a direct evaluation by electron spin resonance (e.s.r.) spectroscopy is often not possible, but considerable advances and information have been achieved by the technique of e.s.r. spin trapping (3,23).

Another major property of the NADPH-cytochrome P_{450} system, at least in vitro, is the ability to catalyse lipid peroxidation whereby a free radical intermediate ($R^\bullet$) initiates the peroxidative degradation of polyunsaturated fatty acids (PUFA's), especially $C_{20:4}$ and $C_{22:6}$, in biomembranes. Lipid peroxidation can result in a complex variety of products (Table 3).

TABLE 3 Products of lipid peroxidation and lipoxygenase

Leukotrienes	Alkanals
Lipid hydroperoxides	Alkenals
Hydroxy fatty acids	4-hydroxy-alkenals
Epoxy-fatty acids	Ketones
	Alkanes

Lipid peroxidising systems that have been studied extensively with microsomal suspensions include those dependent on added (i) NADPH; (ii) NADP/ADP/Fe^{2+}; (iii) NADPH/CCl_4; (iv) ascorbate $\pm Fe^2$; (v) cumene hydroperoxide. For reviews of lipid peroxidation of the above types see references 14, 30, 39, 40.

Several studies have reported that various animal tumours peroxidise more slowly than corresponding normal tissue (1,7,25,33,46,47); related observations have been made in dividing normal cells where generally a decreased rate of lipid peroxidation and of the activity of the cytochrome P_{450} system have been found associated with an increased rate of cell division (2, 22). A hypothesis has been formulated that lipid peroxidation is in some way a regulator of cell division (see 7), perhaps through the metabolic effects of aldehydic products of lipid peroxidation (41).

Some experimental data concerning the depressed rate of lipid peroxidation in some animal tumours are shown in Tables 4 and 5.

TABLE 4 Lipid peroxidation[a] in ethionine-induced liver tumours compared to normal rat liver[b]

Microsomal fraction	Time (min)	Change in $C_{20:4}/C_{16:0}$ Ascorbate/ADP/Fe^{2+}	NADPH/CCl_4
Normal	0	100%	100%
	15	36%	79%
	30	25%	78%
Apparently Normal;	0	100%	97%
Hepatoma bearing rat	15	36%	86%
	30	28%	77%
Hepatoma	0	48%	47%
	15	44%	47%
	30	44%	44%

[a]measured by change in the $C_{20:4}$ content relative to $C_{16:0}$; two methods of stimulating microsomal peroxidation are shown: ascorbate/ADP/Fe^{2+} and NADPH in the presence of CCl_4. [b,]data from reference 1.

TABLE 5   <u>Lipid peroxidation[a] in aflatoxin-induced rat liver</u>
<u>tumours transplanted into nude mice [b]</u>

Measurement	Conditions	$\dfrac{\text{Tumour value}}{\text{Normal value}}$ x 100
Oxygen uptake	NADPH	0
	$NADPH/ADP/Fe^{2+}$	3
	$Ascorbate/ADP/Fe^{2+}$	9
Thiobarbituric acid	NADPH	38
reactive material	$NADPH + CCl_4$	14
	stimulation due to CCl_4	< 1

[a]Lipid peroxidation measured as oxygen consumption or by the thiobarbituric acid reaction for malonaldehyde-like materials.   [b], data from reference 1.

Additional data concerning possible mechanisms for such a decreased rate of lipid peroxidation in tumour cells are given in Table 6 for the Novikoff hepatoma.

TABLE 6   <u>Polyunsaturated fatty acid, cholesterol and antioxidant</u>
<u>content of Novikoff tumour cells compared to normal</u>
<u>rat hepatocytes [a]</u>

Substance measured	$\dfrac{\text{Tumour value}}{\text{Normal value}}$ x 100
$C_{20:4}$ [b]	61
$C_{22:6}$	26
Cholesterol	216
Total antioxidant[c]/Total Lipid	742
α-Tocopherol[c]/Total Lipid	724

[a], unpublished data of Burton, G.W., Cheeseman, K.H., Ingold, K.U. and Slater, T.F.
[b], fatty acid contents expressed as % total PUFA.
[c], for methods see reference 8.

It can be seen that there is a striking decrease in the $C_{20:4}$ and $C_{22:6}$ contents of Novikoff cells compared to isolated normal hepatocytes, and an increased cholesterol content. Moreover, the tumour cells have a large content of lipophilic chain breaking antioxidant (mainly α-tocopherol) in comparison to normal liver. Similar changes occur in the microsomal fractions (data not included) as in whole cells. Since the NADPH-cytochrome P_{450} system is also greatly decreased in the Novikoff cells compared to normal (Table 7) one can see that the substrate (PUFA), a catalytic propagating system (NADPH / cytochrome P_{450} system), and lipophilic chain breaking antioxidant (α-tocopherol) are all changed in a direction that favours reduced lipid peroxidation under conditions <u>in vitro</u>. An additional feature <u>in vivo</u> can be the generally decreased content of NADPH in many tumours (18).

TABLE 7   Levels of various measures of CCl_4 metabolism and lipid
peroxidation in Novikoff hepatoma microsomes relative
to normal liver microsomes. Mean ± standard deviation;
number of determinations in parenthesis.

Parameter	Percent value relative to liver microsomes
Cytochrome P_{450} level	n.d.[b] (4)
NADPH:cytochrome c reductase	10 ± 2 (4)
Covalent binding of ^{14}C-CCl_4	n.d. (4)
CCl_4-dependent MDA production	n.d. (4)
NADPH/ADP/Fe-dependent oxygen uptake	n.d. (2)
NADPH/ADP/Fe-dependent MDA production	9 ± 1 (2)
Ascorbate/Fe-dependent MDA production	5 ± 7 (6)

[a,]data from Cheeseman (9)   [b,]n.d. = not detectable

A decreased rate of lipid peroxidation has been reported for a wide
range of animal tumours as already mentioned. However, recently, an
homogenate of a cultured line of hepatoma cells has been reported to
peroxidise normally (15). A possible explanation for this seeming
anomaly is that the cell line has undergone at least one additional
mutation during its repeated passages in vitro, and has thereby lost its
ability to maintain a high lipophilic antioxidant level.

A consequence of the generally low rate of lipid peroxidation in
animal tumours is a decreased formation of products of lipid peroxidation,
the variety of which has been mentioned in Table 3. Among the products
are aldehydes that have been studied extensively by Schauenstein,
Esterbauer and coworkers (35). The complex spectra of aldehydic products
of lipid peroxidation of rat liver microsomes in the presence of NADPH,
NADPH/ADP/Fe^{2+}, NADPH/CCl_4 and Ascorbate/Fe^{2+} have been reported by
Esterbauer et al (16,17) using high pressure liquid chromatographic
techniques. In particular, the group of 4-hydroxy-alkenals have
specially interesting biological effects at very low concentrations
(for example, on chemotaxis (12) and adenyl cyclase (13)), and are major
products of rat liver microsomal peroxidation carried out in the
presence of NADPH/ADP/Fe^{2+} (17). The 4-hydroxy-alkenals have been shown
to have inhibitory effects on cell division in a number of animal tumour
models (10,35) in vitro, but their administration and use in vivo has
been found to be restricted by a combination of toxicity and short
biological half-life.

The effects of 4-hydroxy-alkenals (e.g. 4-hydroxy-pentenal or 4-
hydroxy-nonenal) on tumour cell division is probably via their facile
interaction with thiol groups (35). In fact, it has been known for a
long time that cell division is related to the content of thiols in
proteins and in low molecular weight components (24,36). The synthesis
of DNA is also known to be dependent on the presence of SH-groups, so
that the inhibitory action of 4-hydroxy-alkenals on DNA synthesis in
various animal tumour cells (Table 8) is not unexpected.

The above discussion has indicated that one result of a decreased
lipid peroxidation in tumour cells could be a decreased production
of 4-hydroxy-alkenals, which normally may exert a coarse inhibition
on DNA-synthesis and, hence, on cell division.   However, at present
we have no data as to the extent of lipid peroxidation under normal
conditions in vivo, or of the physiological significance of

TABLE 8   Effects of 4-hydroxy-pentenal (HPE) on ³H-thymidine
           incorporation into DNA of animal tumours.[a]

Tumour	Pre-incubation time with HPE (min)	HPE (μM)	Incubation time with ³H-thymidine	% of control incorporation
Walker-256	60	100	20	20
	60	200	20	5
	–	100	20	85
		200	20	45
Gardner lympho-sarcoma	30	40	30	85
	30	80	30	35
	30	160	30	10
	30	320	30	8
Ehrlich	30	40	30	85
	30	80	30	65
	30	160	30	25
	30	320	30	6
Sarcoma-180	30	40	30	81
	30	80	30	42
	30	160	30	8

[a,]Data from unpublished experiments of Conroy, P.J., Nodes, J.T. and
    Slater, T.F.

products of lipid peroxidation such as the 4-hydroxy-alkenals. Since
some aspects of the prostaglandin cascade involve or require SH-groups
(20) and are affected by lipid hydroperoxides (21) it is also possible
that this important pathway of metabolism, which is known to be dis-
turbed in many tumour systems (26), is closely linked to lipid peroxidation in a complex pattern of interactions and feedbacks (see 42). A
simple diagrammatic view is presented in Figure 1; such possibilities
are under active investigation.

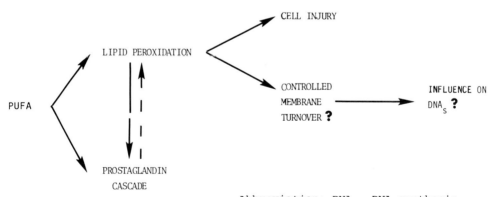

Abbreviation: DNA$_s$, DNA synthesis

FIGURE 1

ACKNOWLEDGEMENTS

We are grateful to the National Foundation for Cancer Research for generous financial help, and to our colleagues Professor M.U.Dianzani and Professor H.Esterbauer, for helpful advice.

REFERENCES

1. Ahmed, S.M. and Slater, T.F. (1981): In: Recent Advances in Lipid Peroxidation and Tissue Injury, edited by T.F.Slater and A.Garner, pp.177-194. Brunel University Printing Services, Biochemistry Department, Uxbridge, U.K.

2. Alasenko, A.V. and Burlakova, E.B. (1972): Doklady Akademi Nauk, U.S.S.R., 207:1471-1474.

3. Albano, E., Lott, K.A.K., Slater, T.F., Stier, A., Symons, M.C.R. and Tomasi, A. (1982): Biochem. J, 204:593-603.

4. Benedetto, C., Dianzani, M.U., Ahmed, M., Cheeseman, K., Connelly, C. and Slater, T.F. (1981): Biochim. biophys. Acta, 677:363-372.

5. Boyd, M.R. (1977): Nature, Lond., 269:713-715.

6. Briggs, M. and Briggs, M. (1974): The Chemistry and Metabolism of Drugs and Toxins. William Heinemann Medical Books Ltd., London.

7. Burlakova, E.B. (1975): Russian Chemical Reviews, 44:871-880.

8. Burton, G.W., Joyce, A. and Ingold, K.U. (1983): Archs. Biochem. Biophys., 221:281-290.

9. Cheeseman, K.H. (1982): Ph.D. thesis, Department of Biochemistry, Brunel University, Uxbridge, U.K.

10. Conroy, P.J., Nodes, J.T., Slater, T.F. and White, G.W. (1975): Eur. J. Cancer, 11:231-240.

11. Coon, M.J., Conney, A.H., Estabrook, R.W., Gelboin, H.V., Gillette, J.R. and O'Brien, P.J. editors (1980): Microsomes, Drug Oxidations, and Chemical Carcinogenesis. Academic Press, New York.

12. Curzio, M., Roch-Arveiller, Negro, F., Giroud, J.P., Esterbauer, H., Torrielli, M.V. and Dianzani, M.U. (1981): Boll. Soc. Ital. Biol. Sper., 57: 2479-2485.

13. Dianzani, M.U. (1982): In: Free Radicals, Lipid Peroxidation and Cancer, edited by D.C.H.McBrien and T.F.Slater, pp.129-151. Academic Press, London.

14. Dianzani, M.U. and Ugazio, G. (1978): In: Biochemical Mechanisms of Liver Injury, edited by T.F.Slater, pp.669-707. Academic Press, London.

15. Dianzani, M.U. and Rossi, M.A. (1982): In: Recent Trends in Chemical Carcinogenesis, edited by P.Pani, F.Feo and A.Columbano, pp.243-257. ESA, Cagliari, Italy.

16. Esterbauer, H. (1982): In: Free Radicals, Lipid Peroxidation and Cancer, edited by D.C.H.McBrien and T.F.Slater, pp.101-122. Academic Press, London.

17. Esterbauer, H., Cheeseman, K.H., Dianzani, M.U., Poli, G. and Slater, T.F. (1982): Biochem. J., 208:129-140.

18. Glock, G.E. and McLean, P. (1957): Biochem. J., 65:413-416.

19. Gooding, P.E., Chayen, J., Sawyer, B.C. and Slater, T.F. (1978): Chem. Biol. Int., 20:299-310.

20. Grundfest, C.C., Chang, J. and Newcombe, D. (1982): Biochim. biophys. Acta, 713:149-159.

21. Hemler, M.E. and Lands, W.E.M. (1980): J.biol.Chem., 255:6253-6261.

22. Henderson, P.T. and Kersten, K.J. (1970): Biochem. Pharmacol., 19: 2343-2351.
23. Janzen, E.G. (1980): In: Free Radicals in Biology, volume 4, edited by W.A.Pryor, pp.115-154. Academic Press, New York.
24. Jocelyn, P.C. (1972): Biochemistry of the SH-Group. Academic Press, London.
25. Lash, E.D. (1966): Archs. Biochem. Biophys., 115:332-336.
26. Levine, L. (1981): Advances in Cancer Research, 35:49-79.
27. Lu, A.Y.H. and West, S.B. (1980): Pharmacol. Revs., 31:277-295.
28. Mason, R.P. (1982): In: Free Radicals in Biology, volume 5, edited by W.A.Pryor, pp.161-221. Academic Press, New York.
29. Mason, R.P. and Chignell, C.F. (1982): Pharmacol. Revs., 33:189-211.
30. Mead, J.F. (1976): In: Free Radicals in Biology, volume 1, edited by W.A.Pryor, pp.51-68. Academic Press, New York.
31. Mimnaugh, E.G., Trush, M.A., Ginsburg, E. and Gram, T.E. (1982): Cancer Res., 42: 3574-3582.
32. Nagata, C., Tagashira, Y. and Kodama, M. (1974): In: Chemical Carcinogenesis, edited by P.O.P.Ts'o and J.A.Di Paolo, pp.87-111. Marcel Dekker Inc., New York.
33. Player, T.J. (1982): In: Free Radicals, Lipid Peroxidation and Cancer, edited by D.C.H.McBrien and T.F.Slater, pp.173-192. Academic Press, London.
34. Sato, R. and Omura, T., editors (1978): Cytochrome P_{450}. Kodansha Ltd., Tokyo.
35. Schauenstein, E., Esterbauer, H. and Zollner, H. (1977): Aldehydes in Biological Systems. Pion Ltd., London.
36. Schauenstein, E., Gölles, J., Waltersdorfer, H. and Schaur, R.J. (1978): Z. Naturforsch., 33c:79-83.
37. Sims, P. (1982): In: Biological Reactive Intermediates-II, edited by R.Snyder, D.J.Jollow, D.V.Parke, C.G.Gibson, J.J.Kocsis, and C.M.Witmer, pp.487-500. Plenum Press, New York.
38. Slater, T.F. (1972): Free Radical Mechanisms in Tissue Injury. Pion Ltd., London.
39. Slater, T.F. (1975): In: Pathogenesis and Mechanisms of Liver Cell Necrosis, edited by D.Keppler, pp.209-223. MTP Press, Lancaster, U.K.
40. Slater, T.F. (1982): Biochem. Soc. Trans., 10:70-71.
41. Slater, T.F., Conroy, P., Fraval, H., Jose, P.J., McBrien, D.C.H., Nodes, J.T., Sawyer, B. and White, G.W. (1973): Eur.Assoc.Cancer Res., 2nd Meeting, Abstract 2.2-3.1.2. Deutsches Krebsforschungszentrum, Heidelberg.
42. Slater, T.F. and Benedetto, C. (1981): In: The Prostaglandin System, edited by F.Berti and G.P.Velo, pp.109-126. Plenum Publishing Corp., New York.
43. Slater, T.F., Cheeseman, K. and Benedetto, C. (1982): In: Recent Trends in Chemical Carcinogenesis, edited by P.Pani, F.Feo and A.Columbano, pp.261-268. ESA, Cagliari, Italy.
44. Stier, A., Clauss, R., Lücke, A. and Reitz, I. (1982): In: Free Radicals, Lipid Peroxidation and Cancer, edited by D.C.H.McBrien and T.F.Slater, pp.329-343. Academic Press, London.
45. Tomasi, A., Albano, E., Dianzani, M.U., Slater, T.F. and Vannini, V. (1983): FEBS Letters, 160:191-194.

46. Ugazio, G., Gabriel, L. and Burdino, E. (1968): Bull. Soc. Ital.
    Sper., 44:30-33.
47. Utsumi, K., Yamamoto, G. and Inaba, K. (1965): Biochem. biophys.
    Acta, 105:368-371.

Icosanoids and Cancer, edited by H. Thaler-Dao, et al. Raven Press, New York © 1984.

Secondary Chemical Reactions Mediated by Cyclooxygenase

*C. Deby, *J. Pincemail, *G. Deby-Dupont, **P. Braquet, and *R. Goutier

*Laboratoire de Biochimie Appliquée, 4020 Liège, Belguim; and **Institut H. Beaufour, Le Plessis Robinson, France

1. ACTIVATED OXYGEN SPECIES AND CYAC

The mechanism of cyclooxygenase activity (CYAC), leading to the biosynthesis of prostaglandins and related compounds of biological interest, was elucidated in the same year by Van Dorp's team (41), in the Netherlands, and by Bergström's team (2), in Sweden. Cyclooxygenase substrates are polyunsaturated fatty acids with 20 carbons chain; arachidonic acid (AA) is the main substrate, producing the prostanoids of the serie 2. Cyclooxygenase requires a heme as a cofactor and displays two activities (fig. 1) :

1) It incorporates 2 oxygen molecules on the polyunsaturated chain, playing the role of a dioxygenase. So are generated the endoperoxides G, with a hydroperoxy function -OOH.

2) It reduces the hydroperoxy function of the endoperoxides G into a hydroxy function, forming endoperoxides H. By this way, cyclooxygenase exerts a peroxidasic role (34).

As soon as 1966, Nugteren demonstrated that CYAC is accompanied by an ESR signal, proving that a free radical is generated during the enzyme activity (32). In 1980, Mason found that an obligatory intermediate in the formation of PGG_2 is a carbon-centered free radical (30). In 1976, Egan et al. described a free radical ESR signal, attributed to an oxygen-centered species, which could arise from the cleavage of endoperoxide G_2, and which could be the hydroxyl radical (18). This finding can be explained as follows.

An hydrogen donor is required for every peroxidasic reaction, in order to permit the following reaction :

$$X\text{-OOH} + RH_2 \longrightarrow HROH + X\text{-OH}$$

In some cases, a free radical can be generated :

$$RO\text{:}OH + 2\,D\text{:}H \longrightarrow RO\text{:}H + H\text{:}OH + 2\,D^{\bullet}$$

which is at the origin of a cascade of radicalar reactions.

DH is generally an aromatic hydrogen donor, becoming radicalar by H$^{\bullet}$ abs-

traction. Generation of ·OH radical during the peroxidasic phase of CYAC
was first proposed (18,35), but further studies could not precise the
exact chemical nature of this involved oxidant released from PGG hydroperoxy group, during the peroxidasic reduction (22,19).

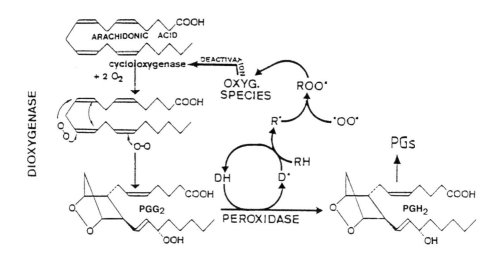

Fig. 1 : The two enzymatic activities displayed by cyclooxygenase :
a. AA ⟶ PGG$_2$ (dioxygenasic activity). b. PGG$_2$ ⟶ PGH$_2$ (peroxidasic
activity). Hypothetic mechanism of activated oxygen species.

Bors et al. excellently reviewed the problem of ·OH generation in biological medium (4). Recent experiments lead to the hypothesis that ·OH
cannot appear in living tissues; alkoxy radicals RO·, arising from lipo-
peroxides reduction, could be more likely generated than the ·OH.
On the other hand, an other oxygenated species, singlet oxygen, has been
implicated in cyclooxygenase activity, more particularly by the studies
of Rahimtula and O'Brien (37). However, in a first time, this statement
was only supported by the use of unspecific scavengers, and the singlet
oxygen hypothesis was abandoned until the recent paper of Cadenas and
Sies (6), which evidenced spectrophotometrically the presence of singlet
oxygen, during the reduction of PGG$_2$ to PGH$_2$.
The hypothesis of a small oxygen radical generated by CYAC, firstly evoked by Egan et al. (18), was sustained by the demonstration of the cyclooxygenase self-inactivation. Early investigations on cyclooxygenase kinetics, by Smith and Lands (39), have demonstrated that this enzyme is a
"suicide enzyme", irreversibly self-deactivated during its own functioning (fig. 1). This finding was confirmed by Duvivier et al. (17), who
observed that the overstepping of an optimal arachidonate concentration,
during CYAC assays, leads to a fall in prostanoids production.
Egan and Kuehl (18,22) hypothesized that the reduction of the hydropero-

xy function of PGG_2 into hydroxy function was accompanied by the release
of an activated oxygen species, which destroys the cyclooxygenase active
site. The lenghtening of the enzyme life time, obtained by use of free
radical scavengers, such as methional and phenol, confirmed this hypothesis.

Our own experiences evidenced an $^{\cdot}OH$ production during CYAC activity but
only when H_2O_2 was added to the bull seminal vesicles microsomes in a mo-
larity higher than 10^{-6} M (fig. 2). Technical details are given in ref.
9. We used the same $^{\cdot}OH$ detection technique as O'Brien and Hawco (35) :
measurement, by gas liquid chromatography, of ethylene formed during the
reaction between 2-keto-methylthiobutyric acid and $^{\cdot}OH$ radical. O'Brien
and Hawco (35) found ethylene emission during CYAC, even in the absence
of H_2O_2. However, there are some differences between the methods of
these two groups : we used glutathion as a cofactor, while the canadian
team employed haemin. We observed also that the higher the ethylene escape, the smaller the PG biosynthesis rate by seminal microsomes (fig.2).

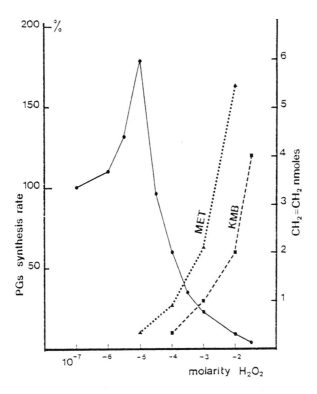

Fig. 2 : Ethylene production (evidencing $^{\cdot}OH$ generation), during CYAC,
in the presence of H_2O_2. MET : results obtained with methional. KMB :
results obtained with 2-keto-4-methylbutyric acid.

2. MECHANISMS OF COOXYGENATION

Marnett et al. (25-29) found that the microsomal fraction of seminal vesicle tissue was able to oxygenate various organic substances (luminol,
methional, benzopyrene, diphenylisobenzofurane), during incubation with
arachidonic acid. Radical scavengers, used to extend the life time of
cyclooxygenase (see above), are oxidated by CYAC. All these reactions
are called cooxygenation reactions, and seem to be extended to a broad
variety of substrates (20). The peroxidasic activity linked to CYAC can
modify some aromatic compounds, which play the role of hydrogen donors,
and form free radicals able to bind proteins and DNA (33). O'Brien
found that diethylstilboestrol and dimethylazobenzen can be attacked by
the peroxidasic activity of cyclooxygenase (33). Paracetamol can also
be cooxidated by CYAC (31). Cooxidation of organic sulfides was reported by Egan et al. (20). Thus, CYAC could generate oxidized by-products,
some of which are noxious.

3. URIC ACID COOXYGENATION

We have demonstrated that uric acid acts as a potent cofactor for CYAC
(14), enhancing more than three times the prostanoids production. Uric
acid acts here as an efficient $^{\cdot}$OH scavenger (10), but it is also recognized by Bors (3) to be a good alkoxy radical scavenger.
An important biological question is to know how uric acid chemically
acts during CYAC enhancement and what it is becoming ? It is well known
that oxidation products of uric acid, such as alloxan and dialuric acid,
can be highly toxic (7), inducing particularly diabetes mellitus by pan-
creatic islets necrosis. Data given in the literature plead for a first
oxidized step of uric acid which could be alloxan (40,36,23).
A lot of research were carried out during the years fifty and sixty, in
order to detect alloxan in mammalian tissues. Alloxan was discovered in
the liver of fasting man and animals (24); hyperglycaemia following uric
acid injection was observed in animals maintained on a diet poor in sulf-
hydrilated amino acids (21). It was also reported that 20% of labelled
uric acid parenterally administered to man is catabolized; this fact was
opposed to the classical concept, that, by absence of uricase, uric acid
is the ultimate step of the purine catabolism, in man. Soberon and Cohen found that uric acid is catabolized in several products by leucocytes (40); one out of these products is probably alloxan. Peroxidasic activities of leucocytes were involved in this phenomenon.
It then seems logical to suppose that uric acid, which deeply modifies
CYAC, is transformed by the oxidant species generated during PGG_2 reduction.
Uric acid oxidation by CYAC has been evidenced by us in several experiments detailed elsewhere (16). Let us resume our studies as follows :
a) The direct attack of uric acid by $^{\cdot}$OH radical generated during a Fenton reaction ($H_2O_2 + Fe^{2+} \longrightarrow Fe^{3+} + {\cdot}OH + OH^-$) produces derivatives, of which some present the same Rf as alloxan, when chromato-
   graphed on polyethylene-imine cellulose plates. The mixture used for

these chromatographies was NaCl 0.15 M / 95% ethanol (4 : 1). We suppose that an intermediary compound is formed, by addition of two 'OH on uric acid (fig. 3).

b) $2-{}^{14}C$-uric acid was incubated at 37° C with bull seminal vesicles microsomes, in the presence of glutathion, according to a previously described method (14,10). Reactions were started by the addition of arachidonic acid (10^{-5} M) and were stopped by acidification after 10 minutes. Fluorometric detection of alloxan (1) was positive in the reaction mixture.

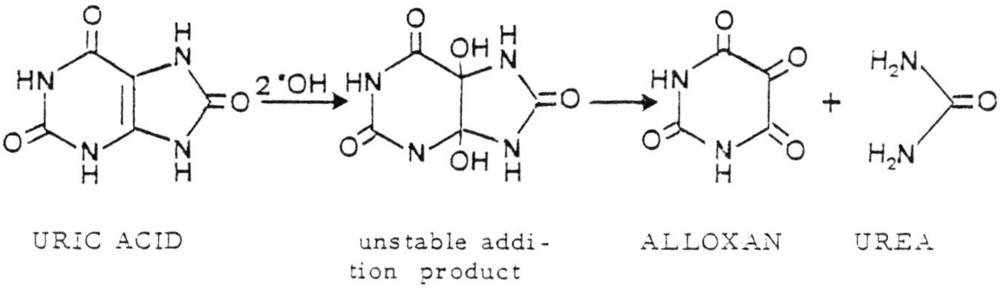

URIC ACID   unstable addition product   ALLOXAN   UREA

Fig. 3 : Proposed mechanism for the reaction between uric acid and 'OH forming alloxan.

The reaction mixtures were ultrafiltrated on CF25 conic filters; the ultrafiltrates were chromatographied on cellulose plates, in the mixture water/pyridine/isobutanol (1 : 1 : 1), or on polyethylene-imine-cellulose plates, in the mixture NaCl 0.15 M / 95% ethanol (4 : 1).
$2-{}^{14}C$-uric acid derivatives were detected on the TLC plates by autoradiography. Besides the uric acid, another compound was regularly observed, presenting an Rf quite different from the Rf of uric acid, alloxan, allantoin and parabanic acid, when uric acid was incubated with active microsomes. However, a compound having the Rf of alloxan appeared when heat inactivated microsomes were allowed to incubate with uric acid. It seems to be admitted, from these experiments, that uric acid can be transformed into alloxan by the sole presence of a heme (for instance, the cyclooxygenase heme). When uric acid is incubated with active microsomes, alloxan could be itself metabolized into another compound; dialuric acid and alloxantine were suspected to be this unknown metabolite, the reactions being explained on fig. 4.
The proof that uric acid is catabolized by CYAC was given :
a) by the presence of a derivative chromatographically different of uric acid itself;
b) by the inability of uric acid to be metabolized into allantoin by uricasic activity, after incubation with microsomes presenting suitable CYAC.

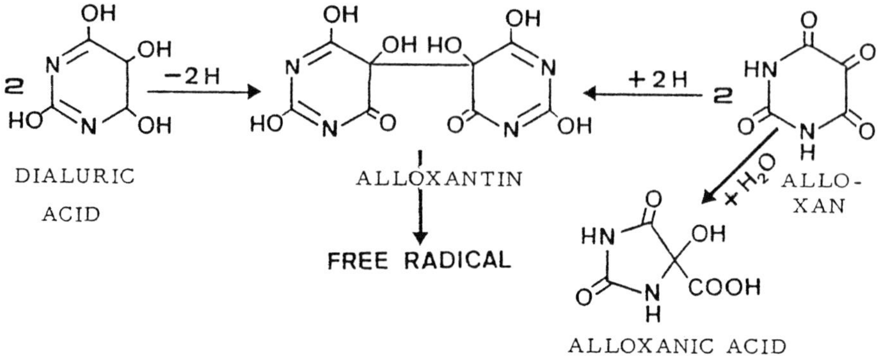

Fig. 4 : Alloxan is very unstable in biological conditions. A possible reaction to explain free radical generation (23).

From these experiments, it may be concluded that :
a) the purine catabolism in man could overstep the classical uric acid end point. Hypouricemia may thus arise from an accelerated CYAC, and hyperuricemia from an inhibition of this CYAC.
It could be supposed that aspirin and other non-steroidal anti-inflammatory (NSAI) compounds will enhance the uricemia, by uric acid catabolism inhibition. But it is well known that, even at high NSAI doses, the cyclooxygenase renewall takes only thirty minutes in tissues; thus, the NSAI do not significantly modify the uricemia;
b) uric acid can be converted into a lot of products which can be noxious, under the activity of several oxidizing biological processes, such as CYAC. Like myeloperoxidase, cyclooxygenase appears thus as an enzyme able to catabolize uric acid (40).

4. CYCLOOXYGENASE REGULATION

a) In vivo PGs biosynthesis stimulation and inhibition : a rabbit in vivo model was realized, convenient for studying various agents which can modify in vivo cyclooxygenase activity. Intraveinously injected arachidonate induces a fall of the arterial blood pressure by conversion into prostanoids, mainly prostacyclin. The efficiency of exogenous AA can be considerably enhanced by the combined effects of high doses of heparin and by perfusion of autologous hemolyzed blood (12). In this manner, the AA-induced hypotension can be obtained with AA doses twentyfold lower than before this treatment. Other parameters can be monitored, such as venous pressure and EKG, and also plasma levels of prostacyclin and thromboxane.
AA_{50} is the intraveinous AA dose necessary to produce a hypotension representing 50% of the initial blood pressure. Before the above treatment, the AA_{50} was comprised between 400 and 600 µg/kg, the lethal dose being higher than 1 mg/kg. After the sensitizing treatment,

the AA_{50} fell below 30 µg/kg, and death often survened after only 100-150 µg/kg (fig. 5).

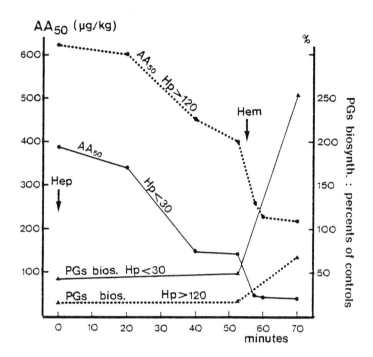

Fig. 5 : a) Values of AA_{50} (dose of i.v. injected AA needed to induce a fall of the arterial blood pressure equal to 50% of its initial value), lowered by heparin (Hep) and hemolyzed blood (Hem) i.v. injections in normal (—————) and resistant (··········) rabbits.

b) Direct relationship between "acute phase" proteins plasma levels (indexed by haptoglobin measurements : Hp in mg%) and increases of AA_{50} (demonstrating an inhibition of PG synthesis).

c) Evolution of the inhibiting property of plasma, on PG in vitro synthesis (expressed in % of controls : left ordinates), during the rabbit sensitization : at 10 ul/2 ml (microsomal suspension) and when taken after Hem, the plasma becomes stimulating for cyclooxygenase, if its Hp level is low.

However, from time to time, resistant rabbits were observed : they could not be sensitized, as usually, to the AA effects. These animals often presented chronic inflammation foci, or parasitical illness (coccidiosis). In spite of heparinization and hemolysis, the

AA_{50} remained higher than 150 µg/kg, and the lethal dose stayed higher than 800 µg/kg (13).

We have demonstrated (15) that plasma inhibitors, discovered by Saeed et al. (38), are significantly enhanced in these resistant rabbits, in the same time as the "acute phase" proteins which increase, during inflammation (C-reactive protein, ceruleoplasmin, orosomucoid, haptoglobin, fibrinogen, and α_1-antitrypsin). There is a good positive correlation between the haptoglobin level and the rabbit resistance to AA injection effects, as measured by increase of the AA   (11). The resistance to AA can be induced in most rabbits by muscular injections of turpentin oil, which enhances, in 36 hours, the acute phase proteins, and particularly haptoglobin (11).

If haptoglobin can be taken as an index for measuring the resistance to unesterified AA, nevertheless it is not the agent mediating this resistance, as claimed by Saeed et al. (38). Up to the present time, we have unsuccessfully tested the above cited acute proteins on CYAC. Plasma levels of acute phase proteins also rise after veinous administration of a leucocyte extract, LEM (leucocyte endogenous factor). The induction time for these proteins by LEM administration is shorter than for turpentin oil (24 hours against 36 hours) (5). After LEM injection, the animals became highly resistant to AA injection effects.

b) On the in vitro cyclooxygenase activity, the plasma samples of resistant rabbits (as well those treated by LEM, as those treated by turpentin oil) exert a strong inhibitory effect, proportional to the acute phase proteins level (measured for instance by the haptoglobin index). It is well known (38) that albumin exerts its own inhibitory effect on CYAC, but the albumin level does not change during inflammation, or after LEM treatment. Another factor must thus appear or increase during acute phase of inflammation. There are thus new factors which impair the utilization of free arachidonate by cyclooxygenase. These regulating factots are as important as phospholipase modulating agents, for the control of cyclooxygenase activity.

c) GSH peroxydase, in vitro inhibitor of cyclooxygenase (8), is another regulating factor, which should be more investigated in vivo.

5. CONCLUSIONS

A new example is given of the cyclooxygenase ability to co-oxygenate organic substrates. Uric acid, which enhances CYAC, is catabolized in several derivatives, some of which are noxious (alloxan, dialuric acid and derivative free radical). There are thus additive medical reasons to slow CYAC : the use of NSAI is of short duration. It is to be desired that more investigations can be devoted to the natural cyclooxygenase inhibitors. Phospholipase inhibitors are actually actively studied, but few attention was accorded, these late years, to the direct inhibition of cyclooxygenase. On the other hand, the rabbit model described in this paper shows us an example of CYAC enhancement, by natural agents. New research are needed in this field.

REFERENCES

1. Archibald, R.M. (1945) : J. Biol. Chem., 158:347.
2. Bergström, S., Danielsson, H., and Samuelsson, B. (1964) : Biochem. Biophys. Acta, 90:207-210.
3. Bors, W. (1981) : personal communication.
4. Bors, W., Saran, M., and Czapsky, G. (1980) : In : Biological and Clinical Aspects of Superoxide and Superoxide Dismutase, edited by W.H. Bannister and J.V. Bannister, pp. 1-31. Elsevier/North-Holland, New York.
5. Bornstein, D.L., and Walsh, E.C. (1978) : J. Lab. Clin. Med., 91:236-246.
6. Cadenas, E., and Sies, H. (1983) : Hoppe-Seyler's Z. Physiol. Chem., 364:519-528.
7. Cohen, G., and Heikkila, R.E. (1974) : J. Biol. Chem., 249:2247-2452.
8. Cook, H.W., and Lands, W.E.M. (1976) : Nature, 260:630-632.
9. Deby, C., and Deby-Dupont, G. (1980) : In : Biological and Clinical Aspects of Superoxide and Superoxide Dismutase, edited by W.H. Bannister and J.V. Bannister, pp. 84-97. Elsevier/North-Holland, New York.
10. Deby, C., and Deby-Dupont, G. (1981) : Clin. Res. Physiol., 17 (sup): 129-139.
11. Deby, C., Van Caneghem, P., and Bacq, Z.M. (1978) : Biochem. Pharmacol., 27:613-615.
12. Deby, C., Deby-Dupont, G., and Bacq, Z.M. (1979) : Arch. Int. Physiol. 87:149-155.
13. Deby, C., Deby-Dupont, G., Bacq, Z.M., and Van Caneghem, P. (1978) : Arch. Intern. Physiol. Bioch., 87:149-152.
14. Deby, C., Deby-Dupont, G., Noël, F.X., and Lavergne, L. (1981) : Biochem. Pharmacol., 30:2243-2249.
15. Deby, C., Deby-Dupont, G., Noël, F.X., Goutier, R., and Bacq, Z.M. (1979) : Bull. Acad. Roy. Méd. Belg., 134:315-329.
16. Deby, C. et al. (1983) : Submitted to Biochem. Pharmacol.
17. Duvivier, J., Wolf, D., and Heusghem, C. (1975) : Biochimie, 57:521-528.
18. Egan, R.W., Paxton, J., and Kuehl, F.A. (1976) : J. Biol. Chem., 251: 7329-7335.
19. Egan, R.W., Gale, P.H., and Kuehl, F.A. (1979) : J. Biol. Chem., 254: 3295-3302.
20. Egan, R.W., Gale, P.H., Baptista, E.M., and Kuehl, F.A. (1981) : Progr. Lipid Res., 20:173-178.
21. Griffiths, M. (1945) : J. Biol. Chem., 172:853.
22. Kuehl, F.A., and Egan, R.W. (1980) : Science, 210:918-984.
23. Lagercrantz, C., and Yhland, M. (1963) : Acta Chem. Scan., 17:1677-1682.
24. Loubatieres, A., and Bouiard, P. (1951) : C.R. Soc. Biol. (Paris), 145:344-351.
25. Marnett, L.J., and Reed, G.A. (1979) : Biochemistry, 18 : 2925-2928.
26. Marnett, L.J., Wlodawer, P., and Samuelsson, B. (1975) : J. Biol. Chem., 250:8510-8517.
27. Marnett, L.J., Reed, G.A., and Johnson, J.T. (1977) : Biochem. Biophys. Res. Commun., 79:569-576.

28. Marnett, L.J., Reed, G.A., and Dennison, D.J. (1978) : Biochem. Bio-
        phys. Res. Commun., 82:210-216.
29. Marnett, L.J., Bienkowski, M.J., and Pagels, W.R. (1979) : J. Biol.
        Chem., 254:5077-5082.
30. Mason, R.P., Kalyanaraman, B., Tainer, B.E., and Elings, T.E. (1980):
        J. Biol. Chem.,255:5019-5022.
31. Moldeus, P. (1981) : ESPB Confer. on Peroxides in biological sys-
        tems, Otzenhausen/Saar.
32. Nugteren, D.H., Beerthuis, R.K., and Van Dorp, D.A. (1966) : Rec.
        Trav. Chim. Pays-Bas, 85:405-419.
33. O'Brien, P.J. (1981) : ESPB Confer. on Peroxides in biological sys-
        tems, Otzenhausen/Saar.
34. O'Brien, P.J., and Rahimtula, A. (1976) : Biochem. Biophys. Res.
        Commun., 70:832-839.
35. O'Brien, P.J., and Hawco, F.J. (1978) : Biochem. Soc. Trans., 6:
        1169-1171.
36. Poje, M., Paulus, E.F., and Rocic, B. (1980) : J. Org. Chem., 45:
        65-68.
37. Rahimtula, A., and O'Brien, P.J. (1976) : Biochem. Biophys. Res.
        Commun., 70:833-899.
38. Saaed, S.A., Mc Donald-Gibson, W.J., Cuthbert, J., Copas, J.L.,
        Schneider, C., Gardiner, P.J., Butt, N.M., and Collier, H.O.J.
        (1977) : Nature, 270:32-36.
39. Smith, W.L., and Lands, W.E.M. (1972) : Biochemistry, 11:3276-3285.
40. Soberon, G., and Cohen, P.P. (1963) : Arch. Biochem. Biophys., 103:
        331-337.
41. Van Dorp, D.A., Beerthuis, R.K., Nugteren, D.H., and Vonkeman, H.
        (1964) : Nature, 203:839-841.

Icosanoids and Cancer, edited by H. Thaler-Dao, et al. Raven Press, New York © 1984.

Radicals and Peroxides Modulate the Enzymic Synthesis of Eicosanoids from Polyunsaturated Fatty Acids

William E. M. Lands

Department of Biological Chemistry, University of Illinois at Chicago, Chicago, Illinois 60612

In considering the relationships between eicosanoids and cancer, several examples in the literature indicate that sometimes tumors lead to an increased production of eicosanoids (12,13). Also, there are data suggesting that sometimes eicosanoids may increase tumor proliferation. The latter interpretation is primarily derived from results with inhibitors of eicosanoid biosynthesis that tended to inhibit tumor growth (e.g., Bennett et al, (2). The thrust of this presentation is to examine how lipid peroxides and radicals are involved in the proliferation of both eicosanoids and tumors.

One of the major features that we shall examine is that related to oxygen. Many investigators, particular those in the area of toxicology, have pointed out that the appearance of superoxide and hydrogen peroxide can be related to a wide range of tissue pathologies which include inflammation, arthritis, thrombosis and stroke, aging, and of course, cancer. In our laboratory, research on eicosanoid biosynthesis has allow us to reinterpret the ways that reduced forms of oxygen could influence cell pathophysiology. I want to show you results that let us now reinterpret the possible mechanisms whereby superoxide and hydrogen peroxide could contribute to cellular pathology by promoting eicosanoid formation.

The eicosanoids are 20–carbon autacoids derived from arachidonic acid. They are a widely diverse family of compounds that can be categorized in terms of enzymatic origins. We recognize two major families: those derived from lipooxygenase action and those derived from cyclooxygenase action. The lipoxygenase and cyclooxygenase activities are fatty acid oxygenases which convert the arachidonic acid into oxidized forms. These intermediates are then subsequently converted into the highly potent autacoids that affect cell physiology when they are present in concentrations of 10^{-10} to 10^{-7} M. The fatty acid oxygenases are somewhat unusual in that they introduce molecular oxygen into the polyunsaturated fatty acids without requiring any other evident cosubstrate. Our experiments with these oxygenases have led us to recognize that three components are necessary for enzymatic function. The dioxygenation reaction require molecular oxygen, nonesterified polyunsaturated fatty acid, and in addition, have a requirement for lipid hydroperoxide as an activator (9). Because of this requirement, the rate of oxygenation of arachidonate through these pathways may be suppressed by a decreased (or inadequate) availability of either oxygen, nonesterified substrate acid, or hydroperoxide activator. The type of evidence that indicates the need for hydroperoxide comes from adding glutathione peroxidase to a fatty acid oxygenase reaction system that had begun to proceed towards full velocity. When glutathione peroxidase was added to the system, the oxygenation reaction ceased rapidly, and no further reaction occurred. Glutathione is a needed cosubstrate for the glutathione peroxidase, and when it was removed by adding N-ethylmaleimide to the reaction mixture, a release of the oxygenating enzyme from the inhibition was observed (8) as the oxygenation reaction proceeded further. If glutathione peroxidase was added initially, then no detectable oxygenation occurred, and when glutathione peroxidase was added at different stages during the reaction (4), the rapid cessation indicated that there was a continual need for the hydroperoxide activator. Thus, one cannot merely activate the enzyme and expect it to proceed without a continued supply of peroxide activator.

The purified PGH synthase has very complex kinetic features, and it contains two separate forms of catalytic activity: the cyclooxygenase activity which forms the 9,11-endoperoxide-15-hydroperoxide derivative (PGG), and a peroxidase activity which converts that intermediate to the 15-hydroxy derivative, (PGH). These two catalytic activities copurify during isolation of the prostaglandin H synthase, and both activities require heme. They appear to be inseparable features of a single protein. Thus the synthase has a somewhat paradoxical behavior in that one of its activities amplifies the presence of small amounts of lipid hydroperoxide by generating more and more lipid hydroperoxide, whereas at the same time the peroxidase activity is removing lipid hydroperoxide and preventing high concentrations of hydroperoxide from accumulating in the reaction mixture. Careful quantitation of the level of lipid hydroperoxide needed for the two PGH synthase activities (6) indicated that the cyclooxygenase activity which proliferates lipid

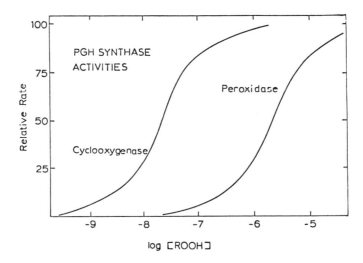

FIG. 1. Different Requirements for the Proliferation and Removal of
Lipid Hydroperoxides

peroxide is half-activated at 2 x 10^{-8} M lipid peroxide whereas the peroxidase activity which removes the hydroperoxide is not very active until the hydroperoxide concentration reaches 10^{-6} M. The consequence of the two separate values for catalytic effectiveness with hydroperoxide is that the cyclooxygenase is stimulated to proliferate lipid peroxides at a rapid rate even when the initial lipid peroxide concentration is 10^{-9} M, a concentration at which the peroxidase is essentially unable to consume peroxide effectively. However, once the peroxide concentration approaches 10^{-7} M, then the peroxidase activity becomes increasingly effective, and at 10^{-6} or 10^{-5} M concentrations of peroxides, the peroxidase operates near its maximum velocity. The difference in the two Km values has important physiologic and pathophysiologic significance to us, and it will be examined in more detail later as we look at mechanisms by which lipid peroxides may influence tumor initiation and proliferation.

Important to tumor initiation is the ability of the PGH synthase peroxidase activity to generate oxidants and organic radicals while removing the lipid hydroperoxides. These products may damage DNA and lead to malignant cell forms. Glutathione peroxidase (an enzyme that

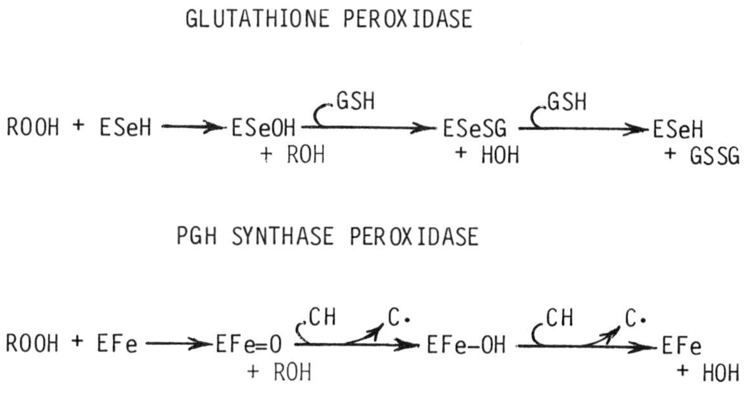

GLUTATHIONE PEROXIDASE

$$ROOH + ESeH \longrightarrow ESeOH \xrightarrow{\overset{GSH}{\frown}} ESeSG \xrightarrow{\overset{GSH}{\frown}} ESeH$$
$$\quad\quad\quad\quad\quad\quad + ROH \quad\quad\quad + HOH \quad\quad\quad + GSSG$$

PGH SYNTHASE PEROXIDASE

$$ROOH + EFe \longrightarrow EFe=0 \xrightarrow[\quad]{\overset{CH}{\frown}\ \overset{C\cdot}{\nearrow}} EFe-OH \xrightarrow[\quad]{\overset{CH}{\frown}\ \overset{C\cdot}{\nearrow}} EFe$$
$$\quad\quad\quad\quad\quad\quad + ROH \quad\quad\quad\quad\quad\quad\quad\quad\quad + HOH$$

FIG. 2. Mechanisms for Removal of Lipid Hydroperoxides

is abundant in many tissues) can also remove lipid hydroperoxides, but it converts them to alcohols without generating any recognized radical intermediates. Thus although both peroxidase enzymes can decrease the level of lipid hydroperoxides in a cell, only the heme-containing PGH synthase peroxidase may generate carcinogenic materals if the cellular peroxide content becomes high enough.

We can summarize eicosanoid biosynthesis in terms of the introduction of activator hydroperoxides at 10^{-9} to 10^{-10} M concentrations and the removal of lipid hydroperoxides at 10^{-6} to 10^{-7} M ranges. Proliferation of hydroperoxides by the fatty acid oxygenases appears to dominate in the concentration range of 10^{-9} to 10^{-7} molar. We hypothesize that a physiologically normal level of hydroperoxide in cells is in the range of 10^{-9} M, and that physiologic stimuli which lead to normal levels of eicosanoid production may generate 10^{-8} to 10^{-7} M hydroperoxide. The occurrence of 10^{-6} M superoxide and/or hydrogen peroxide in tissues seems easily capable of generating 10^{-8} M lipid hydroperoxide which could appreciably activate the fatty acid oxygenases and lead to a further proliferation of cellular hydroperoxides by those enzymes. The proliferation of hydroperoxides to a level of 10^{-7} molar may permit the physiologic expression of the customarily recognized eicosanoids, whereas an accumulation of peroxides above 10^{-7} molar would represent a pathological level of generation. This higher level could also be associated with a rapid functioning of the heme-containing peroxidase activities and an elevated steady state level of radicals or epoxides that could lead to further tissue pathology. As long as cellular peroxidases prevent the accumulation of peroxides above 10^{-7} M, there will be only a low probability of significantly elevated mutagens.

The cellular events associated with carcinogenesis have concepts analogous to those of the enzymatic events noted above : initiation, propagation and termination. When DNA is damaged, we introduce a potential future error in the DNA transcription. However, DNA repair enzymes quite often can remove the damaged section and replace it with the appropriately repaired part before replication of the DNA occurs. As long as the DNA repair is successfully completed prior to the replication, there will be no subsequent proliferation of the error. If, however, the repair is slow relative to the rate of replication, errors in the DNA will be retained in the erroneous replicated derivatives, and subsequent daughters cells may proliferate the mutation which in some cases could be the bases for malignancy. Thus a "threshold" phenomenon that occurs in these cellular events depends on the relative rate of DNA repair versus replication.

Lipid peroxides and radicals have been implicated in the initiation of tumors, and an illustration of peroxide-mediated DNA damage occurs in the recent report by Weitberg et. al. (15) showing the influence of promoter-stimulated white blood cells upon the frequency of sister-chromatid exchanges in CHO cells in culture. Normal white cells when stimulated with the promoter, caused a several-fold increase in the number of sister-chromatid exchanges, whereas cells from subjects with chronic granulomatosis disease gave no significant elevation in sister-chromatid exchange of the cultured CHO cells. These results also illustrate how adding a tumor promoter may also cause an increased initiation of tumors cells. Somewhat similar initiation was obtained with a cell-free superoxide generating system that led to a several-fold increase in sister-chromatid exchanges. Since the added promoter alone produced no increase in the apparent mutation of the cells, the results were interpreted to indicate a primary role for oxygen metabolites in the generation of sister-chromatid exchanges. The observation may help explain the relationship between cancer and chronic inflammatory conditions in vivo. Our growing knowledge of physiological cellular peroxide levels suggests that the rate of PG synthase peroxidase-mediated breaks in DNA may be very low so that normal repair might occur prior to normal replication. This would mean that the low level of tissue lipid peroxides might play a less significant role in the initiation of tumors than in the eicosanoid-facilitated promotion of tumor proliferation. We need to carefully examine the experimental systems used to study carcinogenesis to resolve these aspects of initiation and proliferation.

Although organic radicals and oxygen-based radicals are widely discussed as potential agents for the initiation of malignant tumors, the proliferative phases may be much more serious in the development of fatal tumors since a single tumor cell that does not proliferate is not likely to cause harm. From one point of view, we may already be carrying thousands of initiated cancer cells, but some threshold phenomenon may be preventing them from being converted into large-scale clinically detectable malignancies. This phenomenon would depend upon factors mediating proliferative, metastatic events such as mitogen levels, tissue invasiveness, vascularization and immune surveillance. It seems likely that most tumor cells that get into the circulation are killed before they establish a new focus in another tissue. To exit the blood stream, cells must disturb the vascular endothelium while attaching to the walls, migrating beneath the endothelial cells, degrading the surrounding matrix and thereby invading the tissue.

PEROXIDES, ARACHIDONATE AUTACOIDS AND CANCER

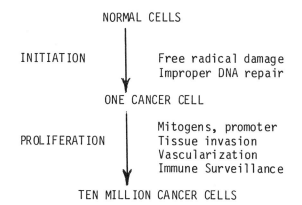

FIG. 3. Cellular Events Related to Peroxides and Eicosanoids

The conditions for these events resemble those that favor thrombosis and atherosclerosis, and they are facilitated by local inflammatory actions of platelets and neutrophils. We now recognize a significant role for eicosanoids in these local inflammatory actions.

The protumor role of peroxides and eicosanoids in facilitating tumor invasion of tissues may be enhanced by an inhibition of the immune surveillance process. At the present time there is a confusing set of actions for eicosanoids in the immune response system and no clear overall function can be definitely described. In the early phases of antibody formation, prostaglandins and eicosanoids may facilitate immune responses by aiding the macrophage presentation of antigen to the antibody-forming cells, whereas prostaglandins may also interfere with immune responses by facilitating the function of T-suppressor cells in inhibiting the proliferation of antibody-forming cells. On the other hand, eicosanoids may play an important role in facilitating chemotaxis of immune effector cells, moving them to the locus of antigen-antibody complex formation. A further complication is that the excessive generation of prostaglandins associated with overactive effector cell action may also be associated with suppression of the immune response (11). The partially isolated models and experimental systems used to study the immune system are slowly yielding useful information, but at this time they do not definitely ascribe either an overall positive or negative role to eicosanoids.

An interesting approach to the role of eicosanoids in immune surveillance may be derived from some epidemiological studies of individuals who have chronically altered dietary levels of polyunsaturated fatty acids. To interpret the significance of that situation, it's important to recall that the eicosanoids are derived from arachidonic acid, an essential fatty acid. This type of fatty acid cannot be synthesized from carbohydrates or amino acids in our tissues, and it must be derived from a dietary precursor such as linoleic acid. Linoleic acid is a polyunsaturated acid with a terminal double bond that is six carbons from the methyl end. This arrangement is the principal chemical feature of an essential fatty acid (14), and although we have enzymes that can elongate and desaturate these fatty acids to a wide range of longer chain polyunsaturated fatty acids, we cannot synthesized these compounds de novo. Another type of polyunsaturated fatty acid that we cannot synthesize is the n-3 type of fatty acid that is synthesized by plants and ingested in animal diets. The n-3 fatty acids can also be elongated and desaturated by the same enzymes that handle the n-6 isomers, but the subsequent elongated form (20:5n-3) that resembles arachidonic acid (20:4n-6) is not known to form an active autacoid under physiologic conditions in vivo (7). The n-3 and n-6 types of fatty acid are capable of esterification, elongation, and desaturation, and they both are capable of decreasing the levels of serum triglycerides and serum cholesterol, but the n-3 acids exhibit no essential fatty acid activity and no detectable biosynthesis of prostaglandin under conditions resembling in vivo conditions (10). This major difference between the two types of polyunsaturated fatty acid may be an important underlying basis for the

TABLE 1.   Diseases among Eskimos/Danes[†]

Infections	---	(30-34%)[*]
Malignancies	46/53	(21-26%)[*]
Cerebral aneurisms	25/15	(10-6%)[*]
Myocardial infarctions	3/40	
Psoriasis	2/40	
Diabetes	1/ 9	
Bronchial asthma	1/25	
Thyrotoxicosis	0/ 7	
Multiple sclerosis	0/ 2	

[*]Causes of death; ref. 1
[†]Ref. 5

finding that Eskimos have no significant amount of myocardial infarction or cerebral thrombosis. The impact of dietary n-3 fatty acids in reducing platelet function has now also been demonstrated in a series of experiments with human volunteers, and an antithrombotic role seems definite. This role can help interpret the fact that the strokes that occur in Eskimos and Japanese are not thrombotic, but are predominantly aneurisms.

It now seems useful to look at other diseases among Eskimos

relative to the frequency of those diseases in corresponding age-matched group of Danes to see if other disorders could be attributed to a chronic overproduction of eicosanoids. A significantly lower incidence of bronchial asthma in Eskimos (5) may be due to a chronic decreased capacity for eicosanoid biosynthesis and it may also reflect a decreased immune response in either antibody forming cells or effector cells. This hypothesis also could pertain to the lack of detected cases of thyrotoxicosis or multiple sclerosis in a population that might be expected to have 7 and 2 cases respectively. These small bits of data provoke curiosity as to whether the chronic ingestion of n-3 fatty acids from birth to adulthood has led to some decreased immune responsiveness that parallels the lower platelet function in these subjects. A corresponding curiosity evolves with regard to whether the lower incidence of psoriasis and diabetes among these people may also reflect some decreased immune activity in these individuals. One corollary to that hypothesis anticipates the much greater incidence of deaths caused by infections that is reported among Eskimos (1). Thus we see the Eskimo population exhibiting a pattern for the frequency of causes of death that has infection>malignancies>myocardial infarction, whereas we find an opposite pattern in the typical western industrial society: cardiovascular death>maligancies>infections.

Another interesting correlation between dietary fat and cancer was provided recently by Caroll (3). The very clear, positive correlation between total dietary fat and the incidence of breast cancers requires some very careful analysis and interpretation. It is interesting to note that the population ingesting low amounts of total fat may also be ingesting a higher ratio of n-3 to n-6 fatty acids compared to those populations ingesting larger amounts of total fat. Thus some new stratification of the data could prove to be interesting in relation to eicosanoid biosynthesis. Diets rich in n-3 fatty acids might be regarded heuristically as somewhat "antiinflammatory" and therefore "antiinvasive" for tumors. If the fatal tumors studied could be classified in terms of their dependency upon inflammatory invasive processes, we might see some different frequencies of incidence among populations related to the dietary content of n-3 acids as noted earlier for the incidence of the two types of strokes.

We can summarize our overview of nutrition, eicosanoids and cancer by indicating that high dietary fat is related to more breast cancer; high dietary n-6 fat does elevate eicosanoids; and that a high dietary ratio of n-3 to n-6 fats is known to cut platelet function, and it may also decrease modulator release, tissue invasiveness and immune surveillance. Underlying all these cellular and enzymatic events is the obligatory action of lipid hydroperoxides in mediating eicosanoid formation. Thus, even when the peroxides do not reach levels sufficient to initiate tumors, they may easily reach levels that can promote eicosanoid formation that might aid proliferative, invasive events of tumors.

ACKNOWLEDGEMENT

The work described in this report was supported in part by research grants GM30509 and GM31494 from the United States Public Health Service.

REFERENCES

1. Arthaud, B. (1970) Arch. Path., 90:433–438.
2. Bennett, A., Houghton, J., Leaper, D.J. and Stamford, I.F. (1979) Prostaglandins, 17:179–191.
3. Carroll, K., Hopkins, G.J., Kennedy, T.G. and Davidson, M.B. (1982) Progress in Lipid Res., 20:685–690.
4. Hemler, M.E. and Lands, W.E.M. (1980) J. Biol. Chem., 255:6253–6261.
5. Kromann, N. and Green, A., (1980) Acta Med. Scand., 208:401–406.
6. Kulmacz, R.J., and Lands, W.E.M. (1983) Prostaglandins 25:531-540
7. Lands, W.E.M., and Byrnes, M.J. (1982) Prog. in Lipid Res., 20:287–290.
8. Lands, W.E.M., Cook, H.W., and Rome, L.H. (1976) Adv. Prost. and Thromboxane Res., 1:7–17.
9. Lands, W.E.M., Lee, R.E., and Smith, W.L. (1971) Am. N.Y. Acad. Sci., 180:107–122.
10. Lands, W.E.M., LeTellier, P.R., Rome, L.H., and Vanderhoek, J.Y. (1973) Adv. Biosci., 9:15–28.
11. Plescia, O.J., Smith, A.H., Grinwich, K. (1975) Proc. Nat Acad. Sci. USA, 72:1848–1851.
12. Seyberth, H.W., Hubbard, W.C., Oelz, O., Sweetman, B.J., Watson, J.T., and Oates, J.A. (1977) Prostaglandins, 14:319–331.
13. Tashjian, A.H. Jr., Voelkel, E.F., and Jevine, L. (1977) Prostaglandins, 14:309–317.
14. Thomassen, H.J., (1953) Int. Review Vitamin Res., 25:62– .
15. Weitberg, A.B., Weitzman, S.A., Destrempes, M., Latt, S.A., and Stossel, T.P. (1983) New Engl. J. Med., 308:26–30.

Icosanoids and Cancer, edited by H. Thaler-Dao,
et al. Raven Press, New York © 1984.

Multiple Mechanisms for the Activation of the Carcinogen Acetylaminofluorene

Wayne Marshall and Peter J. O'Brien

Department of Biochemistry, Memorial University of Newfoundland, St. John's, Newfoundland, A1B 3X9 Canada

One of the initiating events in the process of carcinogenicity is thought to be the covalent interaction of electrophilic intermediates of the carcinogens with DNA (39). A good correlation exists between the DNA binding in vivo and the carcinogenic potency of a carcinogen whereas no such relationship between the degree of carcinogenicity and binding to RNA and protein has been found (8).

Target tissues for chemical carcinogens often include tissues where -le oxidizing systems, such as peroxidase and prostaglandin synthetase activities, are high and -2e oxidizing systems, such as mixed function oxidase and amine oxidase, are low (44). In rats, these include the Zymbal gland, a sebaceous gland located in the external ear duct and the Harderian gland, a large gland located deep within the optical orbit with a single excretory duct opening at the base of the nictating membrane. The Zymbal gland is the main target tissue for the carcinogen trans-4-aminostilbene (15) and is also a target for acetylaminofluorene (22) or monomethylaminoazobenzene (9). The Harderian gland is a target for benzidine derivatives (19). Lactoperoxidase is present in high levels in these glands (41,45) but mixed function oxidase activity is low (28) and no arylamine-N-hydroxylase has yet been demonstrated. The uterus also contains peroxidase (5) and prostaglandin synthetase (12) but has no mixed function oxidase activity (5). It is also a target for the peroxidase substrate diethylstilbestrol and DNA binding occurs following activation by these -le oxidizing systems (38). The salivary gland and thyroid are also target organs in human cancer and contain high concentrations of peroxidases (57) and little mixed function oxidase activity (60).

Acetylaminofluorene (AAF), when fed in the diet at 0.01-0.05%, induces primarily liver tumors in male rats and mammary tumors in female rats; in addition some Zymbal gland and small intestine tumors appear in both sexes. There is convincing evidence that the first step of activation involves an initial N-hydroxylation by the liver mixed function oxidase. The acetylaminofluorene : DNA adducts isolated from the liver after in vivo administration have been attributed to DNA binding with the N-O-sulfate ester formed from the activation of the N-hydroxy-2-acetylaminofluorene by the sulfotransferase (11). However the mammary and the Zymbal gland contain no sulfotransferase activity (22). In the case of mammary gland, therefore, a one electron oxidation activation mechanism involving eicosanoids has been suggested in which

the oxidation of N-OH-AAF is catalyzed by lipoxygenase and peroxidase
(62). N-acetoxy-AAF and nitrosofluorene were first shown to be
dismutation products of the nitroxy radicals formed by a peroxidase
catalyzed oxidation by Bartsch et al (1, 2). N-Acetoxy-AAF also readily
forms AAF : DNA adducts with DNA (30). Floyd et al (62) have since
shown that incubating NOH-AAF with mammary gland epithelial cells or
platelets in the presence of arachidonic acid produces nitrosofluorene
and N-acetoxy-acetylaminofluorene (62,48). They suggested that a
lipoxygenase was the catalyst and that the oxidant involved was
12L-hydroperoxy 5,8,10,14-eicosatetraenoic acid. Previous experiments
showed that linolcic acid-13-hydroperoxide (formed with soybean
lipoxygenase) in the presence of a heme catalyst also oxidized NOH-AAF
to these dismutation products (15). Ram seminal vesicle microsomes
which have a high prostaglandin synthetase activity also readily carried
out this reaction with arachidonate and was inhibited by indomethacin.
In the absence of added arachidonate, there was no inhibition of
nitrosofluorene production by mammary gland epithelial cells by
indomethacin (a prostaglandin synthetase inhibitor), paraoxon (a
deacetylase inhibitor) and p-aminophenol (a N,O acyl-transferase
inhibitor) but 5,8,11,14-eicosatetraynoic acid (a lipoxygenase
inhibitor) was effective. They also suggested that mammary gland
peroxidase was the catalyst in the oxidation of the NOH-AAF by the 12L-
hydroperoxy-5,8,10,14-eicosatetraenoic acid but no evidence was given
(62).

   Deacetylated amino-fluorene : DNA adducts however form 80% of the DNA
adducts formed in vivo. They have been attributed to direct DNA binding
by NOH-aminofluorene formed by deacetylation of NOH-AAF or by N-acetoxy-
aminofluorene formed from NOH-AAF by a N,O acyltransferase (4).
However, little N,O-acyltransferase activity has been found in the
Zymbal gland, bladder or the nonlacting mammary gland of rats.
It is also not found in the dog or goat (25). In the following, a one
electron oxidation activation mechanism for acetylaminofluorene is
described for the first time which could result in the formation of
deacetylated aminofluorene : DNA adducts. The properties of the reactive
species involved in DNA binding by acetylaminofluorene following various
activation mechanisms are also compared.

                      EXPERIMENTAL PROCEDURES

   Chemicals. The following reagents were purchased from Sigma Chemical
Co. (St. Louis, MO); calf thymus DNA (type I), horseradish peroxidase
(type VI), porcine carboxyesterase (types I and II), diethyl-p-nitrophenyl phosphate (paraoxon), glutathione, NADPH, N-acetylcysteine, N-
acetyl methionine, N-acetyl-tyrosine, 2,6 dimethylphenol and butylated
hydroxyanisole. Hydrogen peroxide was obtained from British Drug Houses
Chemicals (Toronto, Canada). Cumene hydroperoxide was obtained from
Aldrich Chemicals (Montreal, Canada). N-(9-^{14}C)-Acetyl-2-aminofluorene
(AAF),(specific activity - 50 mCi/mmol) was purchased from New England
Nuclear (Boston, MA.). ^{14}C-N-hydroxy-acetylaminofluorene (NOH-AAF),
(specific activity - 25 mCi/mmol) was purchased from ICN Chemical and
Radioisotopes (Irvine, CA).

   DNA binding. The reaction mixture (2.0 ml) for determining
peroxidase-H_2O_2 catalyzed N-OH-AAF and AAF binding to macromolecules
contained 5 μM N-(C^{14})-acetylaminofluorene or N-OH-acetylaminofluorene,
0.1 M Tris-HCl (pH 7.4), horseradish peroxidase (10 μg), hydrogen
peroxide (0.5 mM) and calf thymus DNA (3 mg). Carboxyesterase II (0.1 mg)

or 1 mM diethyl-p-nitrophenyl phosphate was added where indicated. The
reaction was started by the addition of hydrogen peroxide and carried
out for 30 min at 37°C with shaking. The reaction was stopped by
extraction with ethyl acetate-acetone (2:1) (2.0 ml) and the organic
solvent was removed. The extraction was repeated 3 times. The residual
organic solvent in the aqueous layer was then removed by bubbling with
nitrogen. Following the removal of the residual organic solvent in the
aqueous layer by bubbling with nitrogen gas, sodium dodecyl sulfate
solution (10%, 200 μl) and protease (0.5 mg) were added and the mixture
allowed to incubate at 37°C for 30 min. After digestion of any possible
contaminating protein, the mixture was treated with water-saturated
phenol (1 ml) and water-saturated $CHCl_3$ (1 ml) and the mixture was
shaken vigorously. After centrifugation, the aqueous phase was
transferred to a new test tube. The macromolecules were subsequently
precipitated by the addition of NaCl (5 M, 100 μl) and ethanol (6 ml).
After centrifugation, the supernatant was discarded. The macromolecules
were dissolved in water (1 ml), reprecipitated with NaCl (5 M, 100 μl)
and ethanol (2.5 ml), washed with ethanol (1 ml) and ether (1 ml) and
dried under nitrogen. The isolated macromolecules were dissolved in
water (1.0 ml). An aliquot was used for the determination of
macromolecule concentration by UV absorption and the rest was used for
the measurement of the visible absorbance spectra and radioactivity of
bound AAF and N-OH-AAF. The radioactivity was measured with a Beckman
LS-330 scintillation counter.

 <u>Microsomal catalyzed binding</u>. Rat liver microsomes were prepared
from 200-250 g, overnight fasted Sprague-Dawley derived albino rats. A
microsomal protein concentration of approximately 1 mg/ml in Tris-HCl
buffer (pH 7.4) was used in the reaction mixture. Ram seminal vesicles
were obtained from a slaughter house and stored at -70°C until used. The
tissue was thawed and trimmed of excess fat and connective tissue and
microsomes were prepared as previously described (12). Protein
determination was made by the method of Lowry et al (33), using bovine
serum albumin as a standard. Microsomal prostaglandin endoperoxide
synthetase activity was determined by measuring oxygen incorporation
into arachidonic acid with a Clark-type oxygen electrode.

RESULTS

 N-acetoxy-AAF reacts with deoxyribonucleic acid to form 2 AAF-DNA
adducts: N-(deoxyguanosin-8-yl)-AAF and (deoxyguanosin-N^2-yl)-AAF (27).
Following the <u>in vivo</u> administration of AAF to rats these two adducts
could be isolated. The former adduct is rapidly excised from the liver
DNA, whereas the latter adduct persists much longer (27). The binding
of the bulky carcinogen AAF to nucleic acids leads to a marked distortion
of their conformation. The former adduct causes much more distortion
than the latter adduct (63). N-acetoxy-AAF is so reactive that adducts
can be formed with guanosine (29). Adducts are also formed with N-acetyl
methionine. Bartsch and Hecker (2) showed that a similar methionine
adduct was also formed following the activation of N-OH-AAF by a
peroxidase-H_2O_2 reaction mixture (3). N-Acetoxy-2-acetylaminofluorene
formation was demonstrated (2) and as nitrosofluorene and nitroxy
radicals were also formed, it was suggested that the N-acetoxy-AAF and
nitrosofluorene were formed by the dismutation of the nitroxy radicals.

 In Table 1, it can be seen that the peroxidase-H_2O_2 catalyzed
oxidation also results in the irreversible binding of ^{14}C-N-OH-AAF to

TABLE 1. A comparison of various activation mechanisms for acetylamino-
          fluorene binding to polyribonucleotides.

	^{14}C-AAF/esterase + H_2O_2/HRP	^{14}C-NOH-AAF + H_2O_2/HRP	^{14}C-NOH-AAF + esterase
DNA	158 (9%)	90 (5.7%)	212 (15%)
Denatured DNA	357 (21%)	128 (8.1%)	179 (12%)
Polyriboadenylic acid	186	75	19
Polyriboguanylic acid	389	221	175
Polyribouridylic acid	31	6	1
Polyribocytidylic acid	114	10	3

( ) = % trapped.

The reaction mixture (5 ml) contained 3 mg calf thymus DNA or poly-
ribonucleotide, 5 μM ^{14}C-acetylaminofluorene or ^{14}C-N-OH-acetylamino-
fluorene, 0.1 M Tris HCl buffer (pH 7.0) and 20 M H_2O_2, 20 μg horseradish peroxidase (type VI) and/or 10 μg carboxyesterase (type I). The
mixture was incubated for 30 mins at 37 C. DNA was isolated as
described in 'experimental procedures'. Denatured DNA was prepared by
heating DNA to 80°C for 5 minutes and rapidly cooling in an ice bath.

DNA. About 8% of the radioactivity was trapped by denatured DNA and a
binding level of 128 pmoles NOH- acetylaminofluorene per mg DNA was
found. Double stranded DNA was less effective. Guanine was the most
reactive nucleic acid base as polyriboguanylic acid was much more
effective in adduct formation than the other polyribonucleotides and
trapped 15% of the N-OH-AAF. Binding to polyriboadenylic acid was one-
third as effective as polyriboguanylic acid but little binding to
polyribouridylic acid or polyribocytidylic acid occurred. Similar
results were found for the binding of N-acetoxy-AAF to various polyribonucleotides ([30]). Guanosine was also more reactive than adenosine
by a factor of 35 ([51]). N-acetoxy-2-acetylaminofluorene however did
not react with adenine of deoxyribonucleic acid ([17]) and acetylaminofluorene administered _in vivo_ does not modify adenine in DNA ([27]).

Evidence that the product responsible for the DNA binding is N-
acetoxy-AAF is the substantial inhibition of DNA binding by N-acetyl-
methionine and guanosine monophosphate (Table 2) indicating that the
reactive species involved reacts with the adducts ([31]). Furthermore at
pH 7.4, the product was stable as DNA binding was only slightly
decreased by adding the DNA at 2 minutes after the reaction was started.
However at pH 5.0, the DNA binding was decreased 50% by adding the DNA
at 2 minutes. It has previously been reported that N-acetoxy-AAF is
much less stable at pH 5.0 than at pH 7.0 ([2]). Evidence that nitroxy
radicals are involved in the formation of the reactive species was the
drastic inhibition of DNA binding by the biological hydrogen donors
ascorbate, NADPH or glutathione (Table 2). In the absence of N-OH-AAF,
no oxidation of NADPH or glutathione was found indicating that at pH
7.4 they are not inhibiting by acting as competitive peroxidase donors.
However NADPH oxidation did occur in this system when N-OH-AAF was added
indicating that the nitroxy radicals or reactive species were reduced by
NADPH. N-Acetoxy-AAF is known to form adducts with glutathione which
have been identified as 1-,3-,4- and 7- (glutathion-S-yl)-N-acetyl-2-
aminofluorene respectively at a yield of 17% ([37]). However although

TABLE 2. Inhibitors of various acetylaminofluorene activation mechanisms

Inhibitor	% DNA binding		
	AAF/esterase + H_2O_2/HRP	N-OH-AAF + H_2O_2/HRP	N-OH-AAF + esterase
None	100[a]	100[b]	100[c]
Ascorbate (20 μM)	0	0	90
NADPH (20 μM)	4	25	92
Glutathione (20 μM)	31	74	77
N-acetylcysteine (20 μM)	18	73	65
N-acetylmethionine (1 mM)	70	26	24
Guanosine Monophosphate (1 mM)	77	65	36
N-acetyltyrosine (20 μM)	7	14	70
2,6-dimethylphenol (5 μM)	29	17	90
Butyl.hydroxyanisole (5 μM)	1	1	51
Paraoxon (0.2 mM)	3	98	3

a. corresponds to 158 pmoles/mg DNA
b. corresponds to 128 pmoles/mg DNA
c. corresponds to 212 pmoles/mg DNA
   The reaction conditions are described in Table 1.

methionine can trap up to 60% of N-acetoxy-AAF, only 17% is trapped by GSH (37). It is therefore likely that GSH and N-acetylcysteine protect the DNA by reducing the nitroxy radicals. Ascorbate has also been found to prevent nitroxy radical formation in this system and a lipid hydroperoxide-hematin system (14,15) suggesting that it acts by reducing the nitroxy radical. DNA binding was also prevented by the phenolic antioxidants, 2,6 dimethylphenol and butylated hydroxyanisole (Table 2).

Enzymatic deacetylation of N-OH-AAF by microsomal or cytosolic deacetylases is an important activation mechanism to explain the formation of deacetylated aminofluorene. The N-OH-AAF formed can bind to nuclear microsomal protein (49) or be autoxidized to the highly mutagenic nitrosofluorene which can add covalently to membrane lipids to form a 2-nitrosofluorene-lipid free radical adduct (53). Previously N-OH-AAF has been shown to form a N-(deoxyguanosin-8-yl)-2-aminofluorene adduct when reacted with calf thymus DNA (4). This reaction was much more effective at pH 5.0 than pH 7.5 and up to 8% of the N-OH-AAF was trapped (16). In Table 1, it can be seen that 15% of the N-OH-AAF can be trapped by calf thymus DNA in the presence of carboxyesterase. The esterase inhibitor paraoxon completely inhibited the binding and no binding occurred in the absence of esterase. Up to 15% of the N-OH-AAF was trapped by the DNA and a level of binding of 212 pmoles/mg DNA was obtained. Polyriboguanylic acid was also very effective in trapping the N-OH-AAF. Polyriboadenylic acid was much less effective and polyribocytidylic acid and polyuridylic acid were ineffective. In Table 2, it can be seen that N-acetylmethionine and guanosine monophosphate inhibit DNA binding, presumably as a result of adduct formation. In contrast to the free radical mediated peroxidase catalyzed activation, this mechanism was much more resistant to reduction by biological hydrogen donors and denatured DNA was less effective than double stranded DNA. Nuclear DNA binding by N-OH-AAF was readily inhibited by paraoxon but

TABLE 3. Microsomal catalyzed acetylaminofluorene activation

Activating system	DNA binding (pmol/mg)			
	^{14}C-N-OH-AAF		^{14}C-AAF	
		+ Paraoxon		+ Paraoxon
Microsomes	102.2	4.1	0.2	0.2
Microsomes + HRP + H_2O_2	110.1	14.2	107.5	0.4
H_2O_2 + HRP	145.5	143.4	0.2	0.2
Microsomes + NADPH	91.3	5.3	6.5	0.4
3MC-Microsomes + NADPH	34.7	2.7	32.6	0.4
3MC-Microsomes + NADPH + DPEA	30.2	2.3	0.6	0.4
3MC-Microsomes	35.8	2.1	0.2	0.2
SVG Microsomes + Arachidonate	25.4	15.9		
SVG Microsomes + Esterase + Arachidonate			20.2	0.4

The reaction conditions are as described for Table 1. The following were added where indicated: liver microsomes (2 mg) from normal or 3-methylcholanthrene (3MC) induced rats, 1 mM NADPH, 0.5 mM 2- (2,4 dichloro-6-phenyl)-phenoxy-ethylamine (DPEA) or 0.1 mM arachidonate and 2 mg sheep vesicular gland (SVG) microsomes. H_2O_2 was generated in the reaction mixture with 1 mM glucose and 10 u glucose oxidase.

not affected by high concentrations of cysteamine or ascorbate [49].

The binding of acetylaminofluorene to DNA catalyzed by rat liver microsomal mixed function oxidase was next investigated. However as shown in Table 3, the microsomal catalyzed binding of ^{14}C-N-OH-AAF to DNA was not affected by NADPH. The binding was inhibited 96% by paraoxon, a carboxyesterase inhibitor, suggesting that the binding is mediated by N-OH-AF formed by microsomal deacetylase. By contrast, the peroxidase-H_2O_2 catalyzed activation was not affected by paraoxon. Liver microsomes isolated from 3-methylcholanthrene (3MC) induced rats were less effective which may indicate decreased deacetylase activity.

Microsomal mixed function oxidase however catalyzed DNA binding by acetylaminofluorene. Liver microsomes from 3-methylcholanthrene injected rats were much more effective, presumably because of the induction of AAF N-hydroxylase activity [52]. The cytochrome P450 inhibitors, SKF 525A (0.2 mM) or 2-(2,4 dichloro-6-phenyl)-phenoxy-ethylamine (0.5 mM), inhibited the binding. Paraoxon also markedly inhibited the binding indicating that the mechanism of activation involves an N-hydroxylation followed by a deacetylation. Rat liver microsomes unlike microsomes from other species are low in deacetylase activity towards AAF although they are active with respect to N-OH-AAF [32]. However, this low activity is clearly enough to activate the AAF. By contrast, ^{14}C-acetylaminofluorene was not affected by peroxidase-H_2O_2 and the acetylaminofluorene (as measured by HPLC) was unaffected. The acetyl group presumably prevents the one electron oxidation of the amine group. However the addition of liver microsomes or carboxyesterase (type I) to the peroxidase system resulted in extensive DNA binding. This was prevented by paraoxon indicating that the mechanism involves a deacetylation to aminofluorene which can be readily oxidized and therefore activated by peroxidase-H_2O_2.

The properties of the reactive species involved in the peroxidase-H_2O_2 catalyzed activation of aminofluorene were next investigated. As shown in Table 1, polyriboguanylic acid was much more effective than polyriboadenylic acid and the other polyribonucleotides were ineffective. Denatured DNA was also much more effective than double stranded DNA. The biological hydrogen donors, ascorbate and NADPH, prevented the DNA binding presumably by reducing the free radicals and/or the oxidized species involved in DNA binding. NADPH was not oxidized by the peroxidase-H_2O_2 system unless aminofluorene was present. N-acetyl-methionine was much less effective as an inhibitor in this system than the other mechanisms of activation shown in Table 1. This could indicate that the species involved in DNA binding does not form adducts with N-acetyl methionine. Guanosine monophosphate was also less effective as an inhibitor. However, the remarkable inhibition of DNA binding by phenolic antioxidants at concentrations much less than that of H_2O_2 clearly indicates adduct formation with the reactive oxidized aminofluorene species. We have recently shown that phenolic anti-oxidants and N-acetyltyrosine inhibit peroxidase-H_2O_2 catalyzed benzidine binding to DNA as a result of adduct formation (56). Boyd et al (7) have recently reported a butylated hydroxyanisole adduct with aminofluorene formed during oxidation by horseradish peroxidase or prostaglandin endoperoxide synthetase. The inhibition by glutathione or N-acetyl-cysteine is more likely to be due to the reduction of the reactive species than adduct formation but remains to be determined.

As shown in Table 3, DNA binding by N-OH-AAF could be catalyzed by vesicular gland microsomes and arachidonate. Previously Floyd et al (62) have demonstrated nitrosofluorene formation. The poor inhibition by paraoxon indicates that deacetylase was not responsible for the activation. Indomethacin (1 mM) markedly inhibited the activation indicating that prostaglandin synthetase catalyzed the activation. DNA binding by aminofluorene was also catalyzed by the vesicular gland microsome-arachidonate system and inhibited by indomethacin. Presumably aminofluorene and N-OH-AAF are activated by the prostaglandin G_2 and the prostaglandin synthetase peroxidase. A similar level of DNA binding by ^{14}C-aminofluorene in this prostaglandin synthetase system has been previously reported ([24]). In Table 4, it can be seen that microsomal protein is much more effective than DNA in trapping ^{14}C-aminofluorene when oxidized by prostaglandin synthetase. However microsomal lipid peroxidation catalyzed by lipoxygenase or the NADPH-ADP/Fe^{3+} system ([20]) resulted in extensive protein binding by acetyl-aminofluorene. The degree of protein binding correlated with the amount of lipid peroxidation as determined by malonaldehyde formation. Paraoxon markedly inhibited the protein binding without affecting lipid peroxidation indicating that a deacetylation to aminofluorene was involved. Asbestos has previously been shown to catalyze microsomal lipid peroxidation ([18]) and also catalyzed microsomal protein binding by aminofluorene. EDTA only partially inhibited this indicating that the surface charges of the asbestos as well as its iron content were involved in catalyzing microsomal lipid peroxidation.

TABLE 4. ^{14}C-Acetylaminofluorene activation by liver microsomal lipid peroxidation.

Prooxidant	Lipid Peroxidation nmol MDA/20'	Microsomal protein binding (pmol/mg)
None	2.3	14
+ Lipoxygenase	17.1	345
+ Lipoxygenase + Paraoxon	17.4	12
+ NADPH + ADP/Fe^{3+}	31.2	1,362
+ NADPH + ADP/Fe^{3+} + Paraoxon	29.3	40
+ NADPH + EDTA	2.5	40
+ NADPH + EDTA + Paraoxon	2.8	30
+ Blue Asbestos	14.5	128
+ Blue Asbestos +EDTA	6.2	61
+ SVG Microsomes + Arachidonate + Esterase	102.3	2,460
+ SVG Microsomes + Arachidonate + Paraoxon + Esterase	104.1	14

The reaction mixture (3 ml) contained 0.1 M Tris-HCl buffer (pH 8.0) and where indicated 1 mg rat liver microsomes, 1 mM NADPH, 15 μM FeCl$_3$, 4 mM ADP, 1 mg soybean lipoxygenase, 0.1 mM paraoxon,3 mg blue crocidolite asbestos, 1 mM ethylenediaminetetraacetic acid (EDTA), 1 mg sheep vesicular gland microsomes and 0.1 mM arachidonate. Malonaldehyde was determined (6) after incubation at 37°C for 1 hour. Microsomal protein binding (7) was determined with 5 μM ^{14}C-acetylaminofluorene in the reaction mixture.

DISCUSSION

It is therefore clear that many mechanisms can activate acetylamino-fluorene to DNA reactive species. These mechanisms are summarized in Figure 1. The acetylated DNA adducts are believed to be formed in vivo by N-hydroxylation of AAF by a cytochrome P448 dependent monoxygenase followed by activation by cytosolic sulfotransferases or seryl-transferases (26). However 80% of the adducts formed in vivo are deacetylated. For this the NOH-AAF is believed to be activated by microsomal or cytosolic deacetylases or N,O acyltransferase (4). The experiments reported here suggest that microsomal deacetylases may be a more important activation mechanism than was realized. The N-OH-amino-fluorene formed probably reacts via the nitrenium ion with nucleophilic sites on the DNA (27). In Figure 1, the numbers in parenthesis reflect the enzyme rates reported (21,47).

In Table 5, it can be seen that whilst the liver contains high levels of mixed function oxidase, sulfotransferase, N,O acyltransferase and deacetylase, a different situation exists for the other target tissues. The lack of sulfotransferase and N,O acyltransferase in the Zymbal gland makes it likely that a peroxidase mediated activation exists. The high levels of deacetylase and peroxidase should readily catalyze aminofluorene : DNA adduct formation by a -1e oxidation mechanism. The high deacetylase activity and low mixed function oxidase activity make

Figure 1. <u>Metabolic Activation of Acetylaminofluorene by Different</u>
<u>Target Tissues</u>

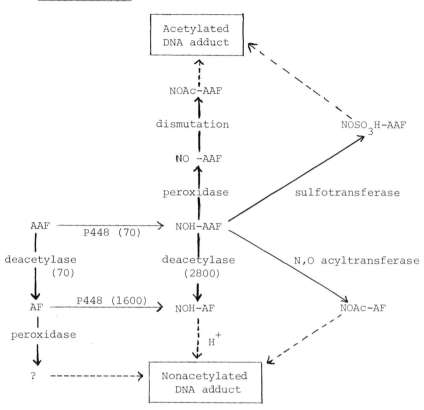

it unlikely that acetylated DNA adducts will be formed. In the case of
the mammary gland and small intestine, the absence of sulfotransferase
argues against acetylated DNA adduct formation but the low levels of all
the other enzymes make it difficult to ascertain what is the mechanism
for aminofluorene : DNA adduct formation. The -1e oxidation mechanisms
available for NOH-AAF activity in the mammary gland include peroxidase
and lipoxygenase (62). The induction of mammary tumors by AAF required
ovarian hormones (36) which also induce mammary gland peroxidase (55)
and AAF-N-hydroxylase activity (36). Estrogen also induces uterine
peroxidase activity (34) and uterine mixed function oxidase activity
(5). AAF-N-hydroxylase activity is absent in microsomes from uninduced
non-lactating mammary gland (36) and the liver is the principal site
for N-hydroxylation. The inhibition of hepatic N-hydroxylation of AAF
by disulfiram <u>in</u> <u>vivo</u> reduced its tumorigenicity in the mammary gland
(35).
   A comparison of the properties of the reactive species involved in
DNA binding by three AAF activation mechanisms indicate that different
species seem to be involved. The -1e oxidation activation mechanisms
are particularly sensitive to reduction by biological hydrogen donors
or adduct formation by phenolic antioxidants. The latter effect could
be an explanation for the inhibition of <u>in</u> <u>vivo</u> chemical carcinogenesis

TABLE 5. Enzymes involved in multiple mechanisms of acetylaminofluorene
          activation

Target tissue	(a)	(b)	(c)	(d)	(e)
Liver	++++	+++	----	++++	+++
Mammary Gland	(+)	----	+	±	(+)
Zymbal gland	(+)	----	+	±	++++
Small Intestine	(+)	----	+	+	+
Bladder (Other Arylamines)	(+)	----	+	----	?

(a) Mixed function oxidase (60)
(b) Cytosolic sulfotransferase (22)
(c) Peroxidase (44)
(d) Acyltransferase (N-OH-AAF) (25)
(e) Deacetylase (N-OH-AAF) (32)

by phenolic antioxidants. The N-acetoxy-AAF and N-OH-AAF are clearly
more reactive than the aminofluorene peroxidase product with regards to
forming adducts with N-acetylmethionine and GMP. Recently evidence has
been presented that aminofluorene is oxidized by prostaglandin
synthetase-arachidonate systems to azoaminofluorene (37%) and nitrofluorene (20%) (7). The formation of nitrofluorene may prove to be
due to the formation of N-OH-AF and its subsequent oxidation to 2-
nitrosofluorene and 2-nitrofluorene. The DNA reactive species could be
N-OH-AAF. However in the case of oxidation by peroxidase-H_2O_2, 82% of
the product was a nonorganic extractable polymeric material, with the
rest being 7% azoaminofluorene and 3% 2-nitrofluorene. The results
described here show that up to 24% of the aminofluorene can be trapped
by polyriboguanylic acid, so that clearly the DNA reactive species is
not N-OH-AAF and is presumably an intermediate involved in the formation
of the polymeric material.

Carcinogenic arylamines, hydrazines and polycyclic aromatic hydrocarbons inhibit lipid autoxidation (43) and some were formerly used as
antioxidants before their carcinogenic properties were discovered.
These carcinogens are thus oxidized by autoxidizing lipids as a result
of their antioxidant function (43). In the case of aminofluorene, this
oxidation clearly produces DNA and protein reactive species as shown by
the activation of aminofluorene by microsomal lipid peroxidation.
Enhanced in vivo lipid peroxidation is associated with carcinogenesis
induced by chlorined hydrocarbons (52, 54), hydrazines (23) and metals
(46). Furthermore enhanced in vivo lipid peroxidation following choline
deficiency results in carcinogenesis (50). The induction of peroxisomes
by hypolipidemic dugs in rats also increases in vivo lipid
peroxidation and carcinogenesis (58) although the drugs are not
activated to mutagens or products which bind to DNA (10). Most
antioxidants and selenium protect against chemical carcinogenesis and
selenium deficiency potentiates chemical carcinogenesis (59). Antioxidants and selenium have similar effects on in vivo lipid peroxidation
(61).

Microsomal lipid peroxidation catalyzed by ascorbate has recently
been shown to oxidize benzopyrene to quinones (40). Furthermore
microsomal lipid peroxidation induced by NADPH/ADP/Fe^{3+} or ascorbate

oxidizes benzopyrene 7,8 diol to the highly mutagenic and carcinogenic diol epoxide**s**(13). In contrast to the mixed function oxidase, the 7S, 8S(+) enantiomer of benzopyrene diol was oxidized to the (-)-anti diol epoxide rather than the (+)-syn diol epoxide. The enhanced lipid peroxidation by asbestos leading to carcinogen activation could be relevant to our understanding of the remarkable potentiating effects of exposure to asbestos and cigarette smoking on the development of brochogenic carcinoma as shown by both epidemiological and experimental studies (42).

ACKNOWLEDGEMENTS

This research was supported by the National Cancer Institute of Canada and the Medical Research Council of Canada. We wish to thank Cindy O'Brien for clerical assistance.

REFERENCES

1. Bartsch, H., Divorkin, C., Miller, E.C. and Miller, J.A. (1972): Biochim Biophys Acta 304: 42-55
2. Bartsch, H. and Hecker, E. (1971): Biochim. Biophys. Acta 237: 567-578.
3. Bartsch, H., Traut, M. and Hecker, E. (1971) Biochim. Biophys. Acta: 237: 556-566.
4. Beland, F.A., Allaben, W.T. and Evans, F.E. (1980): Cancer Res. 40: 834-840
5. Bennett, S., Marshall, W. and O'Brien, P.J. (1982): In: Prostaglandins and Cancer, edited by T.J. Powles, R.S. Bockman, K.V. Honn and P. Ramwell, pp. 143-148. A.R. Liss, Inc.
6. Bernheim, F., Bernheim, M.L. and Wilbur, K.M. (1948): J. Biol. Chem. 174: 257-264.
7. Boyd, J.A., Harvan, D.J. and Eling, T.E. (1983): J. Biol. Chem. 258: 8246-8254.
8. Brookes, P. and Lowley, P.D. (1964): Nature 202: 781-784
9. Clayson, D.B. and Garner, R.C. (1976): In: Chemical Carcinogenesis, ACS Monograph 173, Edited by C.E. Searle.
10. Cohen, A.J. and Grasso, P. (1981): Fd. and Cosmetics Toxicol. 19: 585-595.
11. DeBaun, J.R., Miller, E.C. and Miller, J.A. (1970): Cancer Res. 30: 577-595.
12. Degen, G.H., Eling, T.E. and McLachlan, J.A. (1982): Cancer Res. 42: 919-923.
13. Dix, T.A. and Marnett, L.J. (1983): Science 221: 77-79.
14. Floyd, R.A., Soong, L.M. and Culver, P.L. (1976): Cancer Res. 36: 1510-1519.
15. Floyd, R.A., Soong, L.M., Walker, R.N. and Stuart, M. (1976): Cancer Res. 36: 2761-2767.
16. Frederick, C.B., Mays, J.B., Ziegler, D.M., Guengerich, F.P. and Kadlubar, F.F. (1982): Cancer Res. 42: 2671-2677.
17. Fuchs, R. and Daune, M. (1972): Biochemistry 11: 2659-2664.
18. Gulumian, M., Sardianos, F., Kilroe-Smith, T. and Ockese, G. (1983): Chemico.-Biol. Interacns. 44: 111-118.

19. Haley, T.J. (1975): Clin. Toxicol. 8: 13-29.
20. Hochstein, P. and Ernster, L. (1963): Biochem. Biophys. Res. Commun. 12: 388-394
21. Irving, C.C. (1979): In: Carcinogenesis: Identification and Mechanism of Action, edited by A.C. Griffin and C.R. Shaw, pp.211-227. Raven Press, New York.
22. Irving, C.C., Janss, D.H. and Russell, L.T. (1971): Cancer Res. 31: 387-391.
23. Jain, S.K. and Hochstein, P. (1978): Biochim. Biophys. Acta 586: 128-137.
24. Kadlubar, F.F., Frederick, C.B., Weis, C.C. and Zenser, T.V. (1982): Biochem. Biophys. Res. Commun. 108: 253-258.
25. King, C.M. and Allaben, W.T. (1980): In: Enzymatic Basis of Detoxification, Vol. II, Edited by W.B. Jakoby, pp. 187-197, Academic Press, New York.
26. King, C.M. and Olive, C.W. (1975): Cancer Res. 35: 906-912.
27. Kriek, E. (1972): Cancer Res. 32: 2042-2048.
28. Krieg, T., Goerz, G, Lissner, R., Bolsen, K. and Ullrich, V. (1978): Biochem. Pharmacol. 27: 575-577
29. Kriek, E., Miller, J.A., Juhl, U. and Miller, E.C. (1967): Biochemistry 6: 177-182.
30. Kriek, E. and Reitserna, J. (1971): Chemico.-Biol. Interacns. 3: 397-403.
31. Lotlikar, P.D., Scribner, J.D., Miller, J.A. and Miller, E.C. (1966): Life Sci. 5: 1263-1267.
32. Lower, G.M. and Bryan, G.T. (1976): J. Toxicol. Environ. Health 1: 421-432.
33. Lowry, O.H., Rosebrough, N.J., Farr, A.L. and Randall, R.J. (1951): J. Biol. Chem. 193: 265-275.
34. Lucas, F.V., Neufeld, H.A., Utterbach, J.G., Martin, A.P. and Stotz, E. (1955): J. Biol. Chem. 214: 775-782.
35. Malejka-Giganti, D., McIver, R.C., and Rydell, R.E. (1980): J. Natl. Cancer Inst. 64: 1471-1477.
36. Malejka-Giganti, D., Ritter, C.L. and Ryzewski, C.N. (1983): Env. Health Persp. 49: 175-183.
37. Meerman, J.H.N., Beland, F.A., Ketterer, B., Srai, S.K.S., Bouins, A.P. and Mulder, G.J. (1982): Chemico.-Biol. Interacns. 39: 149-168.
38. Metzler, M. and MacLachlan, J.A. (1978): Biochem. Biophys. Res. Commun. 85: 874-884.
39. Miller, E.C. and Miller, J.A. (1981): Cancer 47: 2327-2345.
40. Morgenstern, R., DePierre, J.W., Lind, C., Guthenberg, C., Mannervik, B. and Ernster, L (1981): Biochem. Biophys. Res. Commun. 99: 682-690.
41. Morrison, M. and Allen, P.Z. (1967): Science 152: 1626-1628.
42. Mossman, B., Light, W. and Wei, E. (1983): Ann. Rev. Pharmacol. Toxicol. 23: 595-615.
43. O'Brien, P.J. (1982): In: Lipid Peroxides in Biology and Medicine, edited by K. Yagi,pp. 317-338, Academic Press, New York.
44. O'Brien, P.J. (in press): In: Free Radicals in Biology, edited by W. Pryor, Academic Press, New York. Vol. VI.
45. Osborne, J.C., Metzler, M. and Neumann, H.G. (1980): Cancer Lett. 8: 221-226.
46. Ramstock, E.R., Hoekstra, W.G. and Ganther, H.E. (1980): Toxicol. Appl. Pharmacol. 54: 251-156.

47. Razzouk, C., Mercier, M. and Roberfroid, M.B. (1980): Cancer Res. 40: 3540-3546.
48. Reigh, D.L., Stuart, M. and Floyd, R.A. (1978): Experientia 34: 107-115.
49. Sakai, S., Reinhold, C.E., Wirth, P.J. and Thorgeirsson, S.S. (1978): Cancer Res. 38: 2058-2067.
50. Sarma, I., Ghoshal, A. and Farber, E. (personal communication).
51. Scribner, J.D. and Naimy, N.K. (1973): Cancer Res. 33: 1159-1168.
52. Slater, T.S. (1982) : Free Radicals, Lipid Peroxidation and Cancer Ed. D.C. Mc Brien and Slater p. 243-274, Academic Press, N.Y.
53. Steward, J.E. and Floyd, R.A. (1980): Cancer Biochem. Biophys 5: 47-53.
54. Stohs, S.J., Hassan, M.Q. and Murray, W.J. (1983): Biochem. Biophys. Res. Commun. 111: 855-861.
55. Strum, J.M. (1978): Tissue Cell 10: 505-514.
56. Tsuruta, Y., Josephy, P.D., Rahimtula, A.D. and O'Brien, P.J. (submitted for publication).
57. Wagai, N. and Hosoya, T. (1982): J. Biochem. 91: 1931-1942.
58. Warren, J.R., Simon, V.F. and Reddy, J.K. (1980): Cancer Res. 40: 36-45.
59. Wattenberg, L.W. (1979): Adv. in Cancer Res. 28: 197-208.
60. Wattenberg, L.W. and Leong, J.L. (1971): In: Handbook of Experimental Pharmacology, edited by B.B. Brodie and J.R. Gillette, 27: pp. 422-430, Springer-Verlag, Berlin.
61. Wendel, A. (1982): Biochem. Pharmacol. 32: 665-672.
62. Wong, P.K., Hampton, M.J. and Floyd, R.F. (1982): In: Prostaglandins and Cancer, Edited by T.J. Powles, R.S Bockman, K.V. Honn and P. Ramwell, pp. 167-179, A.R. Liss, Inc., New York
63. Yamasaki, H., Pulkrabek, P., Grunberger, D. and Weinstein, I.B. (1977): Cancer Res. 37: 3756-3760.

Icosanoids and Cancer, edited by H. Thaler-Dao, et al. Raven Press, New York © 1984.

Metabolism of Carcinogens by Prostaglandin H Synthase

T. E. Eling, G. A. Reed, R. S. Krauss, R. P. Mason, and J. A. Boyd

National Institute of Environmental Health Sciences, Laboratory of Molecular Biophysics, Prostaglandin Group, Research Triangle Park, North Carolina 27709

The ubiquitous enzyme prostaglandin H synthase (PHS) catalyzes the conversion of arachidonic acid (AA) to the endoperoxide PGH_2. PGH_2 is a pivotal compound from which prostaglandins, thromboxane and prostacyclin arise. A unique aspect of PHS is that a single protein possesses two enzymatic activities. The fatty acid cyclooxygenase activity of PHS catalyzes the formation of the hydroperoxy-endoperoxide PGG_2, while the hydroperoxidase activity reduces the hydroperoxide moiety of PGG_2 to the alcohol, yielding PGH_2 (Fig. 1).

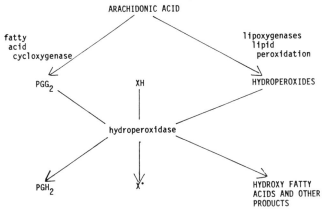

Fig. 1.   Scheme for the metabolism of chemicals by PHS hydroperoxidase.

A wide variety of chemicals (XH) are oxidized during this reduction of PGG_2 to PGH_2. This has been termed co-oxidation. In addition to PGG_2, other lipid hydroperoxides formed by lipoxygenases or lipid peroxidation, and hydrogen peroxide can support the oxidation of various chemicals. Non-steroidal anti-inflammatory drugs (i.e., indomethacin) only inhibit the fatty acid cyclooxygenase activity and not the peroxidase activity of PHS. Thus indomethacin inhibits AA-dependent PHS-catalyzed oxidation of chemicals by inhibiting the formation of PGG_2. Indomethacin does not inhibit the reaction initiated by other sources of hydroperoxide (For review see Ref. 10).

Metabolism of chemical carcinogens, particularly oxidation, is of importance in determining the carcinogenic activity of the chemical. It is generally accepted that many chemicals are not themselves carcinogenic but are metabolized or activated to electrophilic metabolite(s) which are the ultimate carcinogens (13,14). Considerable evidence testifies to the importance of mixed-function oxidases in chemical metabolism. However, PHS could serve as an alternate system for carcinogen metabolism, particularly in extra-hepatic tissues which are low in mixed-function oxidase activity and, in many cases, rich in PHS activity. To investigate this possibility, we have examined the metabolism of two classes of carcinogens by PHS.

Polycyclic aromatic hydrocarbons (PAH)

Extensive studies show that the ultimate carcinogenic metabolite of the polycyclic aromatic hydrocarbon benzo(a)pyrene (BP) is the anti-diol epoxide (anti-BPDE) formed by oxidation of trans-7,8-dihydroxy-7,8-dihydro-benzo(a)pyrene (BP-7,8-diol) (17,5). Ram seminal vesicle microsomal fractions and the microsomal fractions (11,19) from a variety of pulmonary tissues including human lung (20), catalyze the PHS dependent conversion of (±)-BP-7,8-diol to (±)-anti-BPDE. In contrast, the mixed function oxidase system converted (±)-BP-7,8-diol to a mixture of syn- and anti-BPDE (Fig. 2) (21,3). BP-7,8-diol became covalently bound to poly G added to incubations containing AA, BP-7,8-diol, and PHS (15). Furthermore, PHS converted BP-7,8-diol to a mutagen(s) as measured in a modified Ames test (4,12). Studies with C3H 10T$\frac{1}{2}$ fibroblasts and BP-7,8-diol demonstrated that stimulation of PHS activity leads to increased

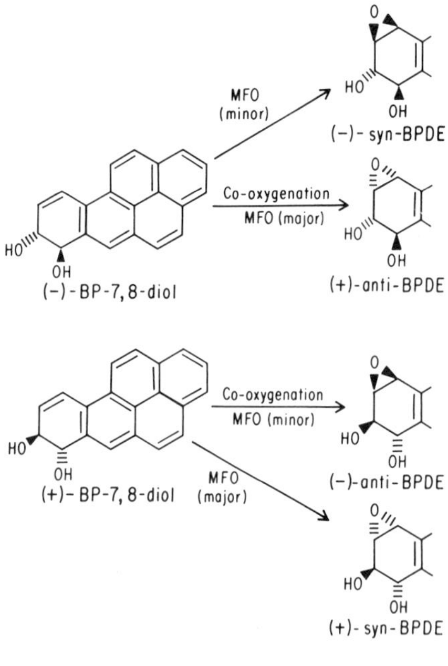

Fig. 2. Metabolism of (±) BP-7,8-diol by PHS and Mixed Function Oxidases.

epoxidation of the diol and increased cell transformation (2). These in vitro studies suggested a role for PHS in the initiation of tumors by PAH. However, further studies are clearly necessary to elucidate the importance of PHS in the initiation of neoplasia by PAH in vivo.

Aromatic Amines

Aromatic amines, in general, are excellent substrates for PHS hydroperoxidase. We have previously shown that a number of N-methyl substituted non-carcinogenic aromatic amines are extensively N-demethylated by PHS via a free radical mechanism (18). Primary aromatic amines are also good substrates for PHS hydroperoxidase. We have investigated the peroxidatic metabolism of benzidine, a human bladder carcinogen, and 2-aminofluorene (2-AF), a liver and bladder carcinogen. The formation of mutagens catalyzed by PHS was examined using a modified Ames bacterial tester system in which ram seminal vesicle microsomes, a source of PHS, were substituted for rat liver supernatant. Both benzidine and 2-AF were metabolized by PHS to mutagenic metabolites (16). 2-AF was metabolized to a more potent mutagen than benzidine.

PHS and horseradish peroxidase metabolize benzidine and its non-carcinogenic congener 3,5,3',5'-tetramethylbenzidine in a series of one electron oxidations to the radical cation and diimine (6,7,8) (Fig. 3).

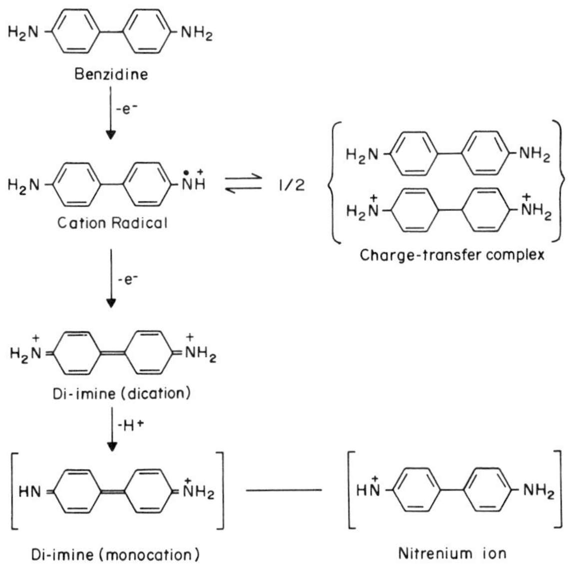

Fig. 3. Metabolism of benzidine by PHS.

The cation radical is in equilibrium with a blue colored charge transfer complex of benzidine and the benzidine diimine. The radical cation was detected directly by electron spin resonance spectroscopy, while the blue charge transfer complex was detected by optical spectroscopy. The major organic extractable metabolite of benzidine produced by oxidation with either horseradish peroxidase or PHS was the benzidine azo dimer. Furthermore, peroxidase-dependent benzidine metabolites reacted with phenolic compounds to yield benzidine/phenol adducts. Although the mechanism for the coupling is unknown, it appears to be a reaction between the diimine and phenol. The electrophlic and mutagenic metabolite of benzidine which reacts with tissue protein or DNA (9) may be either the radical cation or diimine. Note that the monoprotonated diimine is a resonance hybrid of the benzidine nitrenium ion.

We have also studied the metabolism of the liver and bladder carcinogen 2-aminofluorene (2-AF) by PHS and characterized the metabolites formed (1). The metabolites were isolated by HPLC and characterized by UV-visible spectrophotometry and mass spectrometry as 2-nitrofluorene and 2,2'-azobisfluorene (Table 1). In addition to the formation of organic extractable metabolites, AA-dependent co-oxidation of 2-AF resulted in products which were water soluble and covalently bound to the microsomal protein. The metabolism was dependent on AA, inhibited by the addition of indomethacin and also supported by H_2O_2 or 15-hydroperoxy-AA. The addition of glutathione depressed the overall metabolism of 2-AF by PHS and significantly increased the percentage of water soluble metabolite(s). These data suggest that 2-AF was metabolized by PHS to an electrophilic intermediate. The electrophiles could be N-hydroxy-2-AF and/or 2-nitrosoflourene, since both of these oxygenated metabolites are rapidly converted to 2-nitrofluorene by PHS. However, we were unable to detect either of these metabolites. Other data (1) suggest that 2-AF was oxidized to a free radical intermediate. The addition of butylated hydroxyanisole (BHA) significantly depressed the formation of 2-nitrofluorene, azofluorene, water soluble products and covalently

TABLE 1   ARACHIDONIC ACID - DEPENDENT CO-OXIDATION OF 2-AF BY PHS[a]

Incubation	2-Nitro-fluorene	Azo-fluorene	Water Soluble	Covalently Bound
Complete system[b]	5.0 ± 1.8	7.3 ± 1.1	3.0 ± 0.2	7.9 ± 0.6
-Arachidonic acid	0.9 ± 0.2	2.2 ± 0.3	0.2 ± 0.0	0.5 ± 0.0
+Indomethacin[c]	1.2 ± 0.6	2.4 ± 0.5	0.2 ± 0.1	0.9 ± 0.1
+Gluthathione[d]	1.1 ± 0.4	1.9 ± 0.8	4.1 ± 0.3	3.4 ± 0.3
-Arachidonic acid +NADPH[e]	0.8 ± 0.1	1.3 ± 0.6	0.3 ± 0.6	0.6 ± 0.1
+BHA[f]	3.0 ± 0.9	2.6 ± .3	1.3 ± .4	3.2 ± .5

[a]All values are nmol/incubation (mean ± standard deviation), n=4.
[b]The complete systems contains: 0.025 M potassium phosphate buffer, pH 7.8, 0.8 mg ram seminal vesicle microsomal protein, 50 μM (^{3}H)-2-AF, 100 μM arachidonic acid, and water to make 2 ml.
[c]Indomethacin = 100 μM.
[d]Gluthathione =500μM.   [e]NADPH = 1 mM.   [f]BHA = 100 μM.

bound metabolites. Furthermore, a pink colored product was formed which has been identified as an adduct between 2-AF and BHA. A free radical or nitrenium ion could be the electrophilic and mutagenic metabolite that binds to protein (see below). Further studies are clearly required to understand the metabolism of 2-AF by PHS and possible role of the metabolism in tumor development (Fig. 4).

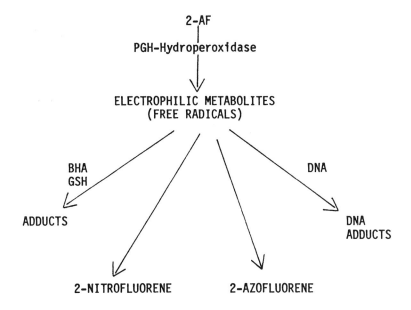

Fig. 4: Metabolism of 2-AF by PHS.

Formation of mutagens

Ample evidence exists for the formation of electrophilic metabolites from aromatic amines and polycyclic aromatic hydrocarbons by PHS. PHS, used in place of the mixed-function oxidase of rat liver microsomes, will metabolize these compounds to mutagens as measured in strains of <u>Salmonella typhimurium</u>. As seen in Table 2, PHS selectively activated dihydrodiol metabolites of PAH which contain an isolated bay-region double bond, to mutagens (4,12). The parent hydrocarbons and other diol metabolites were not activated. Thus, the proximate carcinogenic metabolites of PAH were activated by PHS to their ultimate carcinogenic forms.

Aromatic amines were also oxidized by PHS to derivatives mutagenic to <u>S. typhimurium</u>. 2-Aminofluorene, benzidine and β-naphthylamine were activated to mutagens by PHS, whereas 2-acetylaminofluorene and α-napthylamine were not (Table 2) (16). These results suggest that PHS is capable of activating a wide range of chemicals and may serve as an additional activating system to the mixed-function oxidases for use in the study and screening of chemicals as potential mutagens.

TABLE 2   CHEMICALS TESTED FOR MUTAGENICITY USING PHS AS THE ACTIVATING ENZYME

Chemical	Relative Mutagenicity	Bacterial Strain
Polycyclic Aromatic Hydrocarbons:		
Benzo[a]pyrene	–	TA98, TA100
Benzo[a]pyrene-7,8-diol	++++	TA98, TA100
Benzo[a]pyrene-4,5-diol	–	TA98
Benzo[a]pyrene-9,10-diol	–	TA98
Benzo[a]pyrene,7,8-dihydro-	+++++	TA98
Benzo[a]pyrene,9,10-dihydro-	–	TA98
Benzo[a]anthracene	–	TA100
Benzo[a]anthracene-3,4-diol	+++	TA100
Benzo[a]anthracene-1,2-diol	–	TA100
Benzo[a]anthracene-8,9-diol	–	TA100
Benzo[a]anthracene-10,11-diol	–	TA100
Chrysene	–	TA100
Chrysene trans-1,2-diol	+++	TA100
Chrysene trans-3,4-diol	–	TA100
Chrysene trans-5,6-diol	–	TA100
Chrysene cis-5,6-diol	–	TA100
Aromatic Amines		
2-Aminofluorene	+++	TA98
2-Acetylaminofluorene	+	TA98
Benzidine	++	TA98
2,4,-Diaminoanisole	+	TA1538
2,5,-Diaminoanisole	++	TA1538
α-Naphthylamine	–	TA1538
β-Naphthylamine	++	TA1538
Aniline	–	TA98
2-Aminoanthracene	–	TA98

SUMMARY

   Co-oxidation of chemicals during prostaglandin biosynthesis are hydroperoxide-dependent oxidations catalyzed by the hydroperoxidase component of PHS. Electrophilic derivatives of polycyclic aromatic hydrocarbons and aromatic amines were generated which bind to protein and DNA and, in certain cases, were mutagenic. Mechanisms of oxidations by PHS appear to be distinct from those of cytochrome P-450. Consequently, PHS may provide a complementary enzyme for the metabolic activation of toxins, mutagens, and carcinogens.
   Most of the research on co-oxidation has employed in vitro studies designed to determine whether PHS can catalyze the formation of toxic and/or carcinogenic derivatives of xenobiotics. Such studies have shown that it can. The focus of future investigations will shift to determine if this pathway of metabolism can play a role in chemically-induced toxicity in vivo.

REFERENCES

1. Boyd, J. A., Harvan, D.J., and Eling, T.E. (1983) J. Biol. Chem., 258, 8246-8254.

2. Boyd, J. A., Barrett, J. C., and Eling, T. E. (1982) Cancer Res., 42, 2628-2632.

3. Deutsch, J., Vatsis, K. P., Coon, M. J., Leutz, J. C., and Gelboin, H.V. (1979) Mol. Pharmacol., 16, 1011-1081.

4. Guthrie, J., Robertson, I. G. C., Zeiger, E., Boyd, J. A., and Eling, T. E. (1982) Cancer Res., 42, 1620-1623.

5. Huberman, E., Sach, L., Yang, S. K. and Gelboin, H.V. (1976) Proc. Natl. Acad. Sci. USA 73, 607-611.

6. Josephy, P. D., Mason, R. P., and Eling, T. E. (1982) Cancer Res., 42, 2567-2570.

7. Josephy, P. D., Eling, T. E., and Mason, R. P. (1982) J. Biol. Chem., 257, 3669-3675.

8. Josephy, P. D., Eling, T. E., and Mason, R. P. (1983) J. Biol. Chem., 258, 5561-5569.

9. Kadlubar, F., Fredrick, C., Weis, C. and Zenser, T. (1982) Biochem. Biophys. Res. Commun. 108, 253-258.

10. Marnett, L. J., and Eling, T. (1983) in: Hodgson, E., Bend, J.R. and Philpot, R. M. (Eds.), Review of Biochemical Toxicology, 5, 135-173 Elsevier Press.

11. Marnett, L. J., Johnson, J. T., and Bienkowski, M. J. (1979) FEBS Lett., 106, 13-16.

12. Marnett, L. J., Reed, G. A., and Dennison, D. J. (1978) Biochem. Biophys. Res. Comm., 82, 210-216.

13. Miller, E.C. and Miller, J.A. (1966) Pharmacol. Rev., 18, 805-827.

14. Miller, J.C. (1970) Cancer Res. 30,559-576.

15. Panthananickal, A., and Marnett, L. J. (1981) Chem.-Biol. Interactions, 33, 239-252.

16. Robertson, I. G. C., Sivarajah, K., Eling, T. E., and Zeiger, E. (1983) Cancer Res., 43, 476-490.

17. Sims, P. and Grover, P. L. (1974) Adv. Cancer Res. 20, 165-274.

18. Sivarajah, K., Lasker, J. M., Eling, T. E., and Abou-Donia, M. B. (1982) Mol. Pharmacol., 21, 133-141.

19. Sivarajah, K., Mukhtar, H., and Eling, T. E. (1979) FEBS Lett., 106, 17-20.

20. Sivarajah, K., Lasker, J. M., and Eling, T. E. (1981) Cancer Res., 41, 1834-1839.

21. Thakker, D. R., Yagi, H., Akagi, H., Koreeda, M., Lu, A.Y.H., Levin, W. Wood, A. W., Conney, A. H., and Jerina, D.M. (1977) Chem.-Biol. Interactions, 16, 281-300.

Icosanoids and Cancer, edited by H. Thaler-Dao, et al. Raven Press, New York © 1984.

Molecular Mechanism of Chemically-Induced Transitional Cell Carcinoma: Cooxidation by Prostaglandin H Synthase

*Terry V. Zenser, *Michael B. Mattammal, **Samuel M. Cohen, *Mark O. Palmier, *Ronald W. Wise, and *Bernard B. Davis

*Geriatric Research, Education and Clinical Center, VA Medical Center, and Departments of Medicine and Biochemistry, St. Louis University School of Medicine, St. Louis, Missouri 63125; and **Department of Pathology and Laboratory Medicine and the Eppley Institute for Research in Cancer, University of Nebraska Medical Center, Omaha, Nebraska 68105

Cancer of the renal urinary tract has long been associated with exposure to chemical agents. The high incidence of urinary bladder cancer among workers in dye and chemical industries has been attributed to their exposure to aromatic amines (3,10). Renal pelvic cancer has been associated with abuse of analgesics (1). Exposure to synthetic hormonal substances such as diethylstilbesterol (6) and to 5-nitrofurans such as N-[4-(5-nitro-2-furyl)-2-thiazolyl]formamide (FANFT), 2-amino-4-(5-nitro-2-furyl)-thiazole (ANFT), and 3-hydroxymethyl-1-[(3-(5-nitro-2-furyl)-allydidene)amino]-hydantoin (HMN) cause renal urinary tract cancers (for review, see 4). Interest in the nitroaromatic compounds has increased because they are components of diesel exhaust (5). In addition, 5-nitrofurans are probably one of the largest groups of nitroaryl chemicals commercially produced for use as human and veterinary medicinals and food additives (2).

FANFT is a potent urinary bladder carcinogen in rat, mouse, dog and hamster (4). When rats are fed a 0.2% FANFT diet, approximately 90% of the rats develop transitional cell carcinomas of the urinary bladder. ANFT, the deformylated metabolite of FANFT, is a weak bladder carcinogen in the rat. However, the mutagenicity of urine from FANFT-fed animals is correlated with the levels of ANFT rather than FANFT, suggesting that deformylation of FANFT to ANFT is an important step in FANFT carcinogenesis (4). Deformylation has been demonstrated in many tissues from several species (12).

In vivo effects of carcinogens are influenced by enzymatic activation and detoxification pathways. The balance between these opposing metabolic effects is an important determinant of the carcinogenic potential of a compound in its target tissue. In this regard, the present report will assess prostaglandin H synthase, mixed-function oxidase and nitroreductase metabolism of FANFT and ANFT. In view of the metabolism of these compounds by prostaglandin H synthase, a long-term FANFT feeding study assessing the effect of aspirin on bladder tumor formation was performed.

Metabolic Activation of FANFT and ANFT by Prostaglandin H Synthase
and Identification of a Prostaglandin H Synthase Metabolite of ANFT

Prostaglandin H synthase (PHS) catalyzed activation of both FANFT
and ANFT was assessed by measuring covalent binding to protein and DNA
(Table 1) (15). Control indicates that no binding was observed with
only ram seminal vesicle microsomes alone. However, following
addition of arachidonic acid, significant binding to protein was
observed with both FANFT and ANFT. The rate of ANFT binding was
approximately 5 times that of FANFT. In each case, binding was
inhibited by indomethacin. Arachidonic acid initiated binding to DNA
with ANFT but not FANFT. Similar results were observed with rabbit
renal medullary and dog bladder transitional epithelial microsomes.
The reduced rate of PHS catalyzed activation of FANFT relative to ANFT
along with the lack of detectable binding of FANFT to DNA is
consistent with previous studies suggesting that formation of ANFT may
be an intermediate step in FANFT-induced bladder cancer.

TABLE 1.   Prostaglandin H Synthase Catalyzed Binding of FANFT and ANFT
                       to Protein and DNA

	Protein Bound	DNA Bound
	pmol/mg protein/min	
FANFT		
Control	N.D.[a]	N.D.
Arachidonic Acid (0.06 mM)	410 + 30	N.D.
+ Indomethacin (0.1 mM)	26 + 8	
ANFT		
Control	N.D.	N.D.
Arachidonic Acid (0.06 mM)	2100 + 100	100 + 10
+ Indomethacin (0.1 mM)	200 + 30	N.D.

[a]N.D. = not detected, less than 2 pmol/mg protein

In separate experiments, aspirin, glutathione and vitamin E were
shown to inhibit arachidonic acid initiated binding of ANFT to protein
(7). In contrast, NADPH, a cofactor for mixed-function oxidase and
nitroreductase, did not initiate metabolism; and SKF-525A, a
mixed-function oxidase inhibitor, did not prevent binding. The
15-hydroperoxy analogue of arachidonic acid (15-HPETE) initiated
binding which was inhibited by propylthiouracil but not by aspirin or
indomethacin. Aspirin and indomethacin are inhibitors of the fatty
acid cyclooxygenase but not prostaglandin hydroperoxidase component of
PHS. These results are consistent with the hydroperoxidase activity of
PHS metabolizing ANFT. Mixed-function oxidase metabolism of FANFT and
ANFT could not be detected.
    GC/mass spectral analysis was used to tentatively identify a PHS
metabolite of ANFT (Figure 1) (15). This metabolite was found to have
oxygen in the 4-position of the furyl ring. Preliminary results
indicate that an additional product of ANFT metabolism is a lactone.

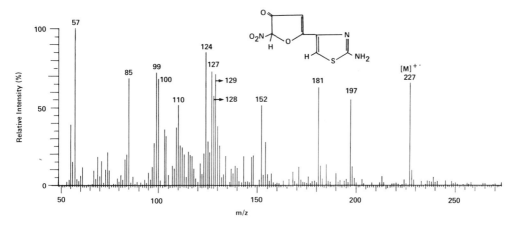

FIG. 1. The 70 electron volt electron impact spectrum of a PHS-catalyzed metabolite of ANFT.

The Role of Tissue Peroxidases in 5-Nitrofuran Activation

The mechanism of peroxidase catalyzed activation of ANFT and the aromatic amine bladder carcinogen benzidine has been assessed using electron paramagnetic resonance (Figure 2). PHS and horseradish peroxidase catalyze the oxidation of benzidine to the same free radical species (14). No radical was observed if either benzidine, H_2O_2 or enzyme was omitted. The similarity of the fine structure of this radical to a computer-simulated model of the free radical cation of benzidine suggests the formation of that species during the activation of benzidine (panel C). Further tests indicated neither superoxide nor hydroxyl radicals were involved in the cooxidation of benzidine by PHS. Production of the benzidine radical by PHS was inhibited by ANFT, acetaminophen, cyanide and ascorbate. ANFT was not metabolized by horseradish peroxidase (13). As a result, ANFT had no effect on either radical production or metabolism of benzidine by horseradish peroxidase. These results indicate that different peroxidases may exhibit specificity with respect to the carcinogens they activate. Other 5-nitrofurans which have a lower oxidation potential than ANFT, such as formic acid 2-[4-(5-nitro-2-furyl)-2-thiazolyl]-hydrazide (FNT), may be more susceptible to metabolism by additional peroxidases. The lack of ANFT metabolism by peroxidases other than PHS will make interpretation of ANFT in vivo metabolic studies less complicated. PHS did not appear to generate a radical during ANFT activation. The lack of a detectable radical during ANFT activation may be due to technical problems caused by the lower rate of ANFT metabolism compared to benzidine.

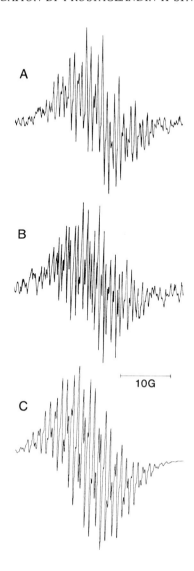

FIG. 2. Electron paramagnetic resonance signal of a free radical
species generated from the oxidation of benzidine by horseradish
peroxidase (A) and prostaglandin hydroperoxidase (B) using H_2O_2 as
cosubstrate. Scan C is a computer simulation of a benzidine cation
free radical.

Comparison of the Rates of ANFT Metabolic Activation
by PHS and Nitroreductase

Both ANFT and FANFT are metabolized by NADPH cytochrome c reductase
(8,16). Reduction results in the binding of carcinogen to

macromolecules. The product of ANFT reduction is an open chain nitrile, 1-(2-amino-4-thiazolyl)-3-cyano-1-propanone. Therefore, ANFT can be metabolized by both PHS and nitroreductase, with metabolites and characteristics of metabolism being distinct for each pathway. The relative rates of rabbit renal inner medullary microsomal metabolism of ANFT by these separate pathways was assessed (Table 2). Aerobic PHS catalyzed metabolism was defined as arachidonic acid initiated and aspirin inhibited. Nitroreductase catalyzed metabolism was defined as being initiated by NADPH and inhibited by oxygen. The rate of binding to both protein and DNA by PHS was approximately twice that of nitroreductase. Therefore, renal metabolism of ANFT by both enzymatic activation pathways can be demonstrated with more PHS than nitroreductase activity measurable under these experimental circumstances. Because specific in vivo modifications of the prostaglandin pathway are known, feeding studies were designed to assess the involvement of this pathway in FANFT-induced bladder carcinogenesis.

TABLE 2. Comparison of the Rates of ANFT Cooxidation by Prostaglandin H Synthase and Reduction by Nitroreductase with Microsomes Prepared from Rabbit Renal Inner Medulla

	Protein bound	DNA bound
	nmol/mg protein/min	
Prostaglandin H Synthase	900 ± 80	8.5 ± 0.7
Nitroreductase	420 ± 40	4.8 ± 0.4

Effect of the Prostaglandin H Synthase Inhibitor Aspirin on FANFT-Induced Bladder Tumor Formation

To assess the effect of PHS on FANFT-induced bladder carcinogenesis, a long-term feeding study was conducted (Table 3). Rats in group 1 were fed a control diet for two days and then 0.2% FANFT for 12 weeks (9). In group 2, rats were fed 0.5% aspirin two days before FANFT. These rats then received a diet of both aspirin and FANFT for 12 weeks. Group 3 received only 0.5% aspirin and group 4 was control. After 12 weeks, FANFT was removed from the diet of all rats, with group 2 rats receiving aspirin for an additional week. After 69 weeks, all animals were sacrificed. Rat bladder PGE_2

TABLE 3. Effect of Aspirin on the Incidence of Bladder Carcinoma Induced by 12 Weeks of Feeding FANFT

Group	Number of Rats	Carcinoma
1. F → C	21	18 (86%)
2. F + A → C	27	10 (37%)[a]
3. A	23	0
4. C	25	0

F = 0.2% FANFT; A = 0.5% aspirin; C = control diet.
[a]Group 1 versus Group 2, $p < 0.001$.

content during the 13 weeks of aspirin treatment was significantly
less than controls. Rats receiving only FANFT for the first 12 week
had an 86% incidence of bladder tumor formation (Table 3). However,
this was reduced to 37% by co-administration of aspirin. No tumors
were observed in the aspirin only or control group. These results are
consistent with PHS being involved in the initiation of FANFT induced
bladder carcinogenesis.

SUMMARY

Metabolic activation of the bladder carcinogens FANFT and ANFT
by PHS and nitroreductase has been demonstrated. The long-term FANFT
feeding study suggests that PHS may be involved in FANFT-induced
bladder carcinogenesis. Figure 3 depicts a model illustrating the

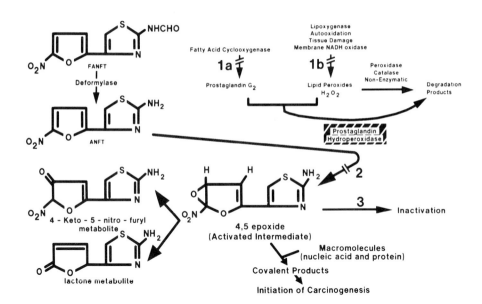

FIG. 3. A working model describing the genesis of FANFT-induced
bladder carcinogenesis and identification of possible sites of
intervention. The model is based on the hypothesis that prostaglandin
H synthase is involved in the initiation of FANFT-induced bladder
cancer.

involvement of PHS in FANFT-induced bladder cancer. The deformylation
of FANFT to ANFT is an important step in FANFT carcinogenesis. ANFT
is then activated by prostaglandin hydroperoxidase to the final
products which have tentatively been identified as a 4-keto and

lactone derivative of ANFT. This suggests the possibility of a
4,5-epoxide intermediate which binds DNA and initiates the
carcinogenic process. Our results show that aspirin can attenuate
this process by inhibiting peroxide generation at site 1a but would
not inhibit at site 1b. However, peroxidase substrates acting at site
2, such as propylthiouracil (11), would inhibit metabolism initiated
by peroxides from either pathway 1a or 1b. Glutathione can inactivate
the reactive intermediate by forming a conjugate (site 3). Although
other hemeprotein peroxidases are present in the mammalian tissues,
the hydroperoxidase component of PHS appears to be the only enzyme
thus far shown to activate ANFT. PHS activation of the aromatic amine
benzidine results in the formation of the benzidine cation radical. A
similar mechanism for PHS activation of ANFT may exist but could not
be demonstrated in the present studies. In addition to insertion of
oxygen into the furan ring, alternative modes of PHS metabolism of
ANFT at the amino group and at the nitrogen of the thiazole ring are
being investigated.

ACKNOWLEDGEMENTS

This research was supported by the Veterans Administration and
the U.S. Public Health Service Grant CA-28015 from the National Cancer
Institute through the National Bladder Cancer Project. The authors
wish to thank Miss Sharon Smith for skillful assistance in the
preparation of the chapter.

REFERENCES

1. Bengtsson, U., Johansson, S., and Angerwall, L. (1978): Kidney
   Int., 13:107-113.
2. Bryan, G.T. (1978): In: Nitrofurans: Chemistry, Metabolism,
   Mutagenesis, and Carcinogenesis, edited by G.T. Bryan, pp. 1-11.
   Raven Press, New York.
3. Case, R.A.M., Hosker, M.E., McDonald, D.B., and Pearson, J.T.
   (1954): Br. J. Ind. Med., 11:75-104.
4. Cohen, S.M. (1978): In: Nitrofurans: Chemistry, Metabolism,
   Mutagenesis, and Carcinogenesis, edited by G.T. Bryan, pp.
   171-232. Raven Press, New York.
5. Gorse, R.A., Riley, T.L., Ferris, F.C., Pero, A.M., and Skewes,
   L.M. (1983): Environ. Sci. Technol., 17: 198-202.
6. Kirkman, H., and Bacon, R. (1950): Cancer Res., 10:122-123.
7. Mattammal, M.B., Zenser, T.V., and Davis, B.B. (1981): Cancer
   Res., 41: 4961-4966.
8. Mattammal, M.B., Zenser, T.V., and Davis, B.B. (1982):
   Carcinogenesis, 3: 1339-1344.
9. Murasaki, G., Zenser, T.V., Davis, B.B., and Cohen, S.M. (in
   press): Carcinogenesis.
10. Rehn, L. (1895): Arch. Klin. Chir., 50:588.
11. Taurog, A. (1976): Endocrinology, 98: 1031-1046.
12. Wang, C.Y., and Bryan, G.T. (1974): Chem. Biol. Interact., 33:
    423-428.
13. Wise, R.W., Zenser, T.V., and Davis, B.B. (1983): Cancer Res.,
    43:1518-1522.
14. Wise, R.W., Zenser, T.V., and Davis, B.B. (1983): Carcinogenesis,
    4:285-289.

15. Zenser, T.V., Palmier, M.O., Mattammal, M.B., Bolla, R.I., and
    Davis, B.B. (in press, 1983): J. Physiol. Exp. Ther.
16. Zenser, T.V., Mattammal, M.B., Palmier, M.O., and Davis, B.B.
    (1981): J. Pharmacol. Exp. Ther., 219: 735-740.

Icosanoids and Cancer, edited by H. Thaler-Dao, et al. Raven Press, New York © 1984.

Arachidonate Cascade and Skin Tumor Promotion

Susan M. Fischer

The University of Texas System Cancer Center, Science Park-Research Division, Smithville, Texas 78957

Experimental chemical carcinogenesis studies in animals are valuable in identifying those biological events or agents that play either an essential or modulatory role in the development of neoplasias. Mouse skin has provided one of the best model systems for studying the multistage nature of carcinogenesis (2,24,26). Initiation is the result of a single application of a carcinogen, most commonly 7,12-dimethylbenz[a]anthracene, at a dose that causes no tumors by itself. The second stage, promotion, results from the repetitive treatment with a tumor promoter such as 12-O-tetradecanoylphorbol-13-acetate (TPA). This second stage can be further subdivided into additional stages in which the sequential use of incomplete or partial promoters such as the ionophore A23187 and mezerein can replace the use of a complete promoter such as TPA (25,26). These stages of promotion have been identified primarily through the use of agents that were found to inhibit specific biochemical events as well as inhibiting tumor development (21,25). Of all the biochemical and morphological responses of the epidermis to TPA, the most important and relevant appear to be the induction of ornithine decarboxylase, the induction of dark cells, hyperplasia and the development of an inflammatory state (23,26).

Our studies into the role of prostaglandins (PG) and the other metabolites of arachidonic acid were prompted in part by the observation that TPA induces cytotoxicity, inflammation, and vascular permeability changes (17,19). The critical nature of inflammation to tumor promotion was suggested by several studies (1,20) that demonstrated that the anti-inflammatory steroids dexamethasone and fluocinolone acetonide are able to completely suppress tumor promotion in mouse skin. These agents have also been shown to inhibit the production of arachidonic acid metabolites by inhibiting phospholipase A_2 (16). This may be the underlying mechanism by which these agents act as strong inhibitors of TPA-induced inflammation and epidermal DNA synthesis (1,20). Additionally, there are numerous reports on a variety of systems including mouse epidermis that TPA induces PG production (3,29,30), as well as work from other laboratories on the role of PGs in hyperplasia and tumor promotion (11,19).

79

TUMOR PROMOTION STUDIES

The above mentioned studies suggested that tumor promotion might be modified through the application of either exogenous PG's or inhibitors of various parts of the arachidonate cascade. Our initial approach to this question, made several years ago, was to determine the effect of the PGs when applied topically alone or with TPA on initiated mouse skin. The conclusions drawn from this series of experiments, summarized in Table 1, are that the effects of the different PGs on tumor production depend on both the particular agent used and the time of application with respect to TPA. None of the PGs tested had promoting activity when used alone on initiated mice (6).

Table 1. Effects of Topical Application of Several Prostaglandins and Precursors on TPA Tumor Promotion

Prostaglandin	Dose (μg)	Effect[a]
PGE_1	>1	↓
PGE_2	10	↑ ↓[b]
$PGF_{2\alpha}$	1-10	↑
arachidonic acid	>10	↓
linoleic acid	10-500	—

[a]Effect is evaluated as enhancement (↑), inhibition (↓), or no effect (-) on the mean number of papillomas per mouse. Data from ref. 6.

[b]Inhibition occurs when PGE_2 is applied within 45 min of TPA application; application 90 min before TPA results in a slight enhancement.

Although this approach indicated that PGs could be used to modify tumor yield, it is complicated by the fact that TPA induces PG synthesis on its own. The effect of the exogenously added PGs on endogenous PG biosynthesis in this system is unknown. For this reason, our next series of studies involved the use of inhibitors of various parts of the arachidonate cascade. Based on the fact PGs play a role in inflammation and that the steroidal anti-inflammatory agents are inhibitors of phospholipase A_2 (16) as well as being potent inhibitors of tumor promotion, it was originally thought that the nonsteroidal antiinflammatory agents, such as the cyclooxygenase inhibitors indomethacin or flurbiprofen, should also inhibit promotion. Additionally it was known that indomethacin suppresses TPA - induced ornithine decarboxylase activity and that this suppression can be overcome by PGE_2 (29). However, in the SENCAR mouse skin, we found that indomethacin can enhance TPA tumor promotion at applications of 25 to 100 µg while inhibiting at higher doses (7). This enhancing effect of indomethacin is even more striking in the multistage promotion protocol in which applications of TPA (first stage) are followed by repetitive applications of the weak promoter mezerein (second stage). When indomethacin is applied with TPA in the first stage, the tumor number is doubled that of TPA alone (data not shown).

Other tumor experiments were done using inhibitors that are effective in blocking both the cyclooxygenase and lipoxygenase pathways. A summary of this series of experiments may be found in Table 2. These studies indicated that cyclooxygenase inhibitors (at low doses) enhance promotion whereas inhibitors of both lipoxygenase and cyclooxygenase or phospholipase A_2 inhibit tumor promotion (9).

Table 2. Effects of Inhibitors of Arachidonate Metabolism on TPA Tumor Promotion

Inhibitor	Dose µg	% TPA Group
indomethacin	10	138
	25	210
	50	167
	100	108
	200	90
flurbiprofen	10	130
ETYA	100	45
phenidone	100	45
dibromoacetophenone	100	33
	250	25
	500	15

Each group consisted of 30 mice initiated with either 10 or 100 nmol (2.56 µg) dimethylbenz[a]anthracene (DMBA) and promoted with TPA twice weekly starting one week after initiation. Unless otherwise indicated, the inhibitors were applied concomitantly with TPA. The data is expressed as a percentage of the number of papillomas in the experimental group as compared to the TPA alone control group. Data from ref. 9.

Since these results indicated that the lipoxygenase pathway may be more important than the cyclooxygenase pathway, it was of interest to determine whether indomethacin could cause an elevation of the hydroperoxy fatty acids (HPETEs) in TPA-treated epidermal cells. HPETE production was determined in primary cultures of adult mouse epidermis, grown in the presence of [^{14}C]arachidonic acid, washed and then exposed to 1 μg/ml TPA with or without 35.8 μg/ml (10^{-4}M) indomethacin for appropriate time periods. Thin-layer chromatography was performed using the "A-9" solvent system of ethyl acetate, isooctane, acetic acid and water and HPETE references provided by L.J. Marnett. After the standards were visualized by iodine vapors, the appropriate corresponding sample zones were scraped for scintillation counting. The results show that the HPETEs are elevated about 45% over control with TPA alone while TPA + indomethacin gives an increase over control of 88%. These results indicated that indomethacin may shunt arachidonic acid into the lipoxygenase pathway, which further suggests that the HPETEs are initmately involved in tumor promotion.

AN IN VITRO MODEL

Since cell culture systems have the advantage over many in vivo systems of being easier to manipulate and control, it was felt that an in vitro model for particular events associated with tumor promotion would be of value in determining at least some of the mechanisms involved in promotion (4, 22). In this study, primary epidermal cell cultures were used to determine (a) the effect of inhibitors of arachidonate metabolism on TPA-induced DNA synthesis and (b) the effect of these inhibitors on PGE$_2$ and HPETE synthesis. These results were then correlated with in vivo DNA synthesis studies and tumor promotion experiments employing the same inhibitors.

Primary cultures of SENCAR newborn mouse epidermis were used for these experiments; the culture methods have been previously described (8). For the DNA synthesis studies, the cultures were treated with the appropriate drugs 24 hrs after plating and then pulse-labelled for 1 hr with [^{3}H] thymidine 5 days later, during the previously established optimum response time to TPA. PGE$_2$ and HPETE were measured using cultures prelabelled with [^{14}C] arachidonic acid for 12 hr (time of maximum incorporation into phospholipids) subsequently treated with the drugs for 4 hrs. The acidified media was extracted with ethyl acetate and the extracts subjected to thin layer chromatography in the "A-9" solvent system (14). The data for the in vitro DNA synthesis studies are shown in Table 3. Both the cyclooxygenase inhibitors indomethacin and flurbiprofen enhanced the rate of TPA-induced DNA synthesis; this enhancement correlates well with the increased number of tumors seen in the corresponding tumor experiments. Furthermore, the use of the inhibitors of both cyclooxygenase and lipoxygenase, ETYA and phenidone, resulted in a dose-response inhibition of TPA-induced DNA synthesis, as did the phospholipase A$_2$ inhibitor dibromoacetophenone. This also correlates well with the inhibition of tumor promotion by these same inhibitors.

Table 3. The Effects of Arachidonate Inhibitors on TPA-Induced DNA
Synthesis in Cultured Mouse Epidermal Cells

A. Cyclooxygenase Inhibitors

1. Flurbiprofen (Fl)	Dose μg/ml	Sp. Act. ± S.E.M.
Control	–	124.9 ± –
TPA	0.1	1329.1 ± 55.72
TPA + Fl	1.0	1464.0 ± 31.63
TPA + Fl	10	1701.5 ± 53.35
TPA + Fl	25	2056.4 ± 141.21

2. Indomethacin		
Control	–	362.3 ± 5.93
TPA	0.1	1265.9 ± 28.97
TPA + Indo	358	20.7 ± 8.23
TPA + Indo	35.8	1651.0 ± 3.56
TPA + Indo	3.6	1467.0 ± 226.77
TPA + Indo	.36	1642.6 ± 55.67

B. Cyclooxygenase-Lipoxygenase Inhibitors

1. ETYA	Dose μg/ml	Sp. Act. ± S.E.M.
Control	–	147.2 ± 2.25
TPA	0.1	2106.9 ± 92.05
TPA + ETYA	1	766.7 ± 47.94
TPA + ETYA	10	999.1 ± 21.63
TPA + ETYA	25	403.0 ± 67.76

2. Phenidone (Ph)		
Control	–	492.2 ± 42.63
TPA	0.1	3185.1 ± 563.93
TPA + Ph	1	2638.8 ± 304.50
TPA + Ph	10	1808.4 ± 236.07
TPA + Ph	25	960.6 ± 46.39

C. Phospholipase A_2 Inhibitor

1. Dibromoacetophenone (diBr)	Dose μg/ml	Sp. Act. ± S.E.M.
Control	–	223.0 ± 66.00
TPA	0.1	854.5 ± 103.60
TPA + diBr	1	466.6 ± 121.85
TPA + diBr	10	199.2 ± 20.55
TPA + diBr	25	TOXIC

Table 4

SUMMARY OF EFFECTS OF ARACHIDONATE INHIBITORS ON MOUSE EPIDERMIS

IN VITRO AND IN VIVO

INHIBITORS	IN VITRO			IN VIVO	
	DNA SYNTHESIS	PGE$_2$	HPETE	DNA SYNTHESIS	TUMOR PROMOTION
A. CYCLOOXYGENASE					
1. FLURBIPROFEN	↑	N.D.	N.D.	N.D.	↑
2. INDOMETHACIN	↑	↓	↑	↑	↑
B. CYCLO- AND LIPOXYGENASE					
1. ETYA	↓	↓	N.D.	↓	↓
2. PHENIDONE	↓	↓	↓	↓	↓
C. PHOSPHOLIPASE A$_2$					
1. STEROIDS	↓	N.D.	N.D.	↓	↓
2. DIBROMOACETOPHENONE	↓	N.D.	N.D.	↓	↓

N.D. = not determined
These experiments are described in the text.

In vivo DNA synthesis experiments were carried out on adult
mice treated in essentially the same manner as was done for the
tumor experiments. TPA induces DNA synthesis maximally at 24 hrs;
the effects of the inhibitors were therefore measured at this time
by 30 min. labelling with i.p. injected [^{3}H] thymidine. The results
of this study (data not shown) were essentially the same as for the
in vitro DNA synthesis studies.
    It was desireable to determine whether these inhibitors were
in fact inhibiting or enhancing either the cyclooxygenase or lipoxygenase pathways. As previously described, this was done by thin
layer chromatography on [14-C] arachidonate prelabelled cells. The
results of this study (data not shown) indicate that in this culture
system indomethacin is a cyclooxygenase but not lipoxygenase inhibitor, while ETYA and phenidone appear to inhibit both pathways.
Table 4 provides a graphic summary of the correlation between the
in vitro and in vivo systems.
    This in vitro system appears, therefore to be a good model for
particular events associated with in vivo tumor promoter treatment,
which is advantageous since cultures are easier to manipulate and
provide a 'sink' for the excretion of arachidonate metabolites.
Additionally, this information strengthens the hypothesis that
the lipoxygenase pathway is important if not essential in the
tumor promotion process.
    The question of which lipoxygenase products are synthesized
and responsible for the observed phenomens is currently under study.
Additionally, preliminary radioimmunoassay experiments done in col-
laboration with Ann Welton of Hoffmann-LaRoche utilizing these
epidermal cultures have shown that TPA induces the production of
leukotrienes of the C, D and E type.

ACTIVATED OXYGEN AND FREE RADICALS

    The role of activated oxygen species in tumor promotion has
been investigated recently through a variety of different approaches.
Work by Slaga et al. (27) showed that such free radical generating
compounds as benzoyl peroxide, lauroyl peroxide and chloroperbenzoic
acid have complete tumor promoting ability. Benzoyl peroxide was
also found to be positive (27) in an in vitro assay developed (30)
as a screen for tumor promoters. This assay utilizes wild-type
Chinese hamster V-79 cell (6-thioguanine sensitive) reduction in
the number of colonies formed by 6-thioguanine resistant cells
through metabolic cooperation. Since it was suggested that the
mechanism by which benzoyl peroxide promotes may involve membrane
changes caused by free radicals, it was of interest to determine
whether the HPETEs might also inhibit metabolic cooperation. As
previously reported by our laboratory (10) the HPETEs (a mixture
supplied by L. Marnett) do significantly inhibit cooperation although
to a lesser extent than TPA. It remains to be demonstrated whether
they have tumor promoting activity in whole animal experiments.

The involvement of free radicals in promotion has also been suggested by the TPA stimulation of superoxide anions in human polymorphonuclear leukocytes (PMNs) as measured by the rate of cytochrome c reduction (13). Using this system, it was demonstrated by Goldstein et al. (12) that such inhibitors of promotion as protease inhibitors, retinoids and anti-inflammatory steroids inhibit promoter induced free radicals. Another means of measuring the effect of TPA on human PMN utilization of oxygen is by measuring the photoemission or chemiluminescence that is accompanied by the generation and energy dissipation of superoxide anion and singlet oxygen (18). Several mechanisms by which TPA treatment of PMNs can result in the generation of excited oxygen species are presented in Figure 1. The degranulation reaction of PMN's is part of their normal response to a variety of foreign materials (13) and may result in extracellular singlet oxygen production (18). The normal oxidative metabolism and electron transport machinery also provides sources of active oxygen; TPA has been shown to enhance such oxidation metabolism (13). Thirdly, peroxidation reactions of lipids, including the intermediates in PG synthesis and the HPETEs are also contributors (18). It has been shown that the TPA - induced chemiluminescence is dose-responsive and that the activities of a series of phorbol esters corresponds with their relative activities as tumor promoters (18).

Figure 1. Possible Mechanisms for the Generation of Chemiluminesence by TPA in Human PMNs. Chemiluminescence occurs as a result of the emission of light when electronically excited states return to ground state. Scheme derived from ref. 18.

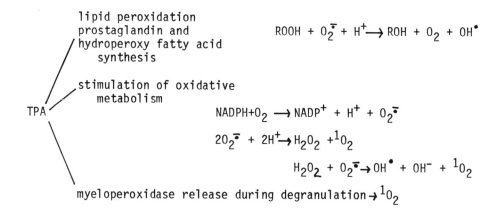

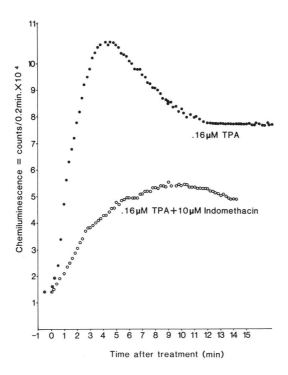

Figure 2. Chemiluminescence was measured after the addition of either .16 μM TPA (●) or .16 μM TPA + 10 μM indomethacin (o) to vials of 12 x 10^6 human PMN's.

We have recently been using human PMNs to determine whether some of the inhibitors of arachidonic acid metabolism would inhibit TPA - induced chemiluminescence. The measurements are made on samples of 12 x 10^6 freshly isolated PMNs in 3ml's of 0.1% glucose in Dulbecco's phosphate buffered saline using an ambient temperature scintillation counter in the out-of-coincidence mode (18). Figure 2 shows a typical chemiluminescence response to TPA treatment; there is an immediate peak (at about 5 min) followed by a more lengthly return to control levels (more than 30 min). The cells are totally refractory to subsequent TPA treatments. Since the arachidonate cascade can theoretically contribute to the pool of reactive oxygen species it was of interest to determine whether arachidonate inhibitors would have a significant inhibitory effect. As indicated in Table 5, all the inhibitors studied so far have considerably reduced the chemiluminescence response of TPA, which

suggests that at least part of the reactive oxygen generated is
from the arachidonate cascade. Additional work is needed to verify
this hypothesis, although it is interesting to note that the addition
of arachidonic acid resulted in a chemiluminescence response kinet-
ically similar to TPA.

Two other antipromoters, retinoic acid and a trimethylmethoxy-
phenyl analog also inhibit TPA-induced chemiluminescence. Retinoic
acid alone, but not the analog produces a quick but short-lived
burst of chemiluminescence which is believed to be indicative of
oxidative activation (18). The retinoic acid chemiluminescence is
interesting, however, in light of the recent report that it is a
tumor promoter when used by itself on the skin of initiated mice (15).

Table 5. Inhibitory Effect on TPA-induced Chemiluminescence in
          Human PMNs by Various Agents

Agent	Dose (μM)	% Inhibition of TPA Response
TPA	.16	100
acetone	-	0
retinoic acid	100	65
	10	49
retinoate analog	100	76
(RO-10-9359)	10	73
	1	57
	.1	12
indomethacin	100	68
	10	52
phenidone	100	84
	10	66
	1	47
flurbiprofen	100	64
	10	66
dexamethasone	100	42
	10	35

Measurements of this kind in mouse epidermal cells would clarify
further the relationship to tumor promotion. At the present time
this has not been possible, probably due to the fact PMNs possess
an enhanced metabolic capacity to reactive oxygen and a compart-
mentalized superoxide dismutase (5). It is of interest to note that
superoxide dismutase, which is thought to protect cells from the
toxic effects of free radicals, is inhibited in mouse epidermis by

TPA (28). Since reactive oxygen species or their products have been implicated in gene activation, it seems reasonable to continue to pursue the hypothesis that at least one of the mechanisms by which TPA can alter proliferation/differentiation is through changes in gene regulation that result from reactive oxygen generated in part by the arachidonate cascade.

SUMMARY

Tumor promotion studies using the phorbol ester TPA in SENCAR mice have shown that (1) exogenous application of various prostaglandins can modify the tumor yield, the direction being dependent on the particular prostaglandin used, and (2) the lipoxygenase pathway of arachidonic acid metabolism is important if not essential to promotion. An in vitro epidermal model system has been established such that there is good correlation in the response to inhibitors between in vitro DNA synthesis, PGE_2 and HPETE production and in vivo DNA synthesis and tumor promotion. Preliminary studies on the TPA - induced generation of reactive oxygen species in human PMNs have indicated that the inhibitors indomethacin, flurbiprofen, phenidone and dexamethasone can diminish this response considerably. This suggests that the arachidonate cascade may be a source of the free radicals that are thought to play a role in tumor promotion.

REFERENCES

1. Bellman, S. and Troll, W. (1972): Cancer Res., 32:450-454.
2. Berenblum, I. and Shubik, P. (1974): Br. J. Cancer I. 373-391.
3. Bresnick, E., Neunier, P., and Lamden, M. (1979): Cancer Letters 7:121-125.
4. Colburn, N.H., Vorder Bruegge, W.F., Bates, J.R., Gray, R.H., Rossen, J.D., Kelsey, W.H., and Shimada, T. (1978): Cancer Res. 28:624-634.
5. DeChatelet, L.R., McCall, C.E., McPhail, L.C., and Johnston, R.B. (1974): J. Clin. Invest. 53:1197.
6. Fischer, S.M., Gleason, G.L., Hardin, L.G., Bohrman, J.S., and Slaga, T.J. (1980): Carcinogenesis 1:245-248.
7. Fischer, S.M., Gleason, G.L., Mills, G.D., and Slaga, T.J. (1980): Cancer Letters 10:343-350.
8. Fischer, S.M., Viaje, A., Harris, K.L., Miller, D.R., Bohrman, J.S., and Slaga, T.J. (1980): In Vitro 16:180-188.
9. Fischer, S.M., Mills, G.D., and Slaga, T.J. (1982): Carcinogenesis 3:1243-1245.
10. Fischer, S.M., Mills, G.D., and Slaga, T.J. (1983): In: Adv. Prostaglandin, Thromboxane and Leukotriene Research, Vol. 12, edited by B. Sammuelsson, R. Paoletti, and P. Ramwell. Raven Press, New York, pp. 309-312.

11. Furstenberger, G. and Marks, F. (1983): In: Symp. on Cocarcino-genesis and Biological Effects of Tumor Promoters, edited by E. Hecker, F. Marks, N. Fusenig, and T.J. Slaga. Raven Press, New York, pp. 325-330.

12. Goldstein, B.D., Witz, G., Amoruso, M. and Troll, W. (1979): Biochem. Biophys. Res. Commun. 88:854-860.

13. Goldstein, B.D., Witz, G., Amoruso, M., Stone, D.S., and Troll, W. (1981): Cancer Letters 11:157.

14. Hamberg, M. and Samuelsson, B. (1966): Prostaglandins in human seminal plasma. J. Biol. Chem. 241:257.

15. Hennings, H., Wenk, M.L., and Donahue, R. (1982): Cancer Letters 16:1-5.

16. Hong, S.L., and L. Levine (1976): Proc. Natl. Acad. Sci. 73:1730.

17. Janoff, A., Klassen, A., and Troll, W. (1970): Cancer Res. 30:2568.

18. Kensler, T.W., and Trush, M.A. (1981): Cancer Res. 41:216-222.

19. Marks, F., Berry, D.L., Bertsch, S., Furstenberger, G. and Richter, H. (1980): In: Cocarcinogenesis and Biological Effects of Tumor Promoters, edited by E. Hecker, F. Marks, N. Fusenig and T.J. Slaga, pp. 331-346. Raven Press, New York.

20. Scribner, J.D., and Slaga, T.J. (1973): Cancer Res., 33:542-546.

21. Slaga, T.J., Fischer, S.M., Viaje, A., Berry, D.L., Bracken, W.M., LeClerc, S., and Miller, D.R.: (1978): In: Carcinogenesis, Vol. 2: Mechanisms of Tumor Promotion and Cocarcinogenesis, edited by T.J. Slaga, Sivak, A., and Boutwell, R.K. Raven Press, New York, pp. 173-195.

22. Slaga, T.J., Viaje, A., Bracken, W.M., Buty, S.G., Miller, D.R., Fischer, S.M., Richter, C.K., and Dumont, J.N. (1978): Cancer Res. 38:2246-2252.

23. Slaga, T.J., Fischer, S.M., Weeks, C.E., and Klein-Szanto, A.J.P.: (1980) In: Biochemistry of Normal and Abnormal Epidermal Differentiation. Univ. Tokyo Press, Tokyo, pp. 193-218.

24. Slaga, T.J., Fischer, S.M., Nelson, K., and Gleason, G.L. (1980): Proc. Natl. Acad. Sci. USA 77:3659-3663.

25. Slaga, T.J. and Klein-Szanto, A.J.P., Fischer, S.M., Weeks, C.E., Nelson, K., and Major, S.: (1980): Proc. Natl. Acad. Sci. USA 77:2251-2254.

26. Slaga, T.J., Fischer, S.M., Weeks, C.E., and Klein-Szanto, A.J.P. (1981): In: Rev. Biochem. Tox., (Eds. E. Hodgson, J.R. Bend, R.M. Philpot) Elsevier/North Holland, New York, pp. 231-282.

27. Slaga, T.J., Triplett, L.L., Yotti, L.P. and Trosko, J.E. (1981): Science 213:1023-1025.

28. Solanki, V., Rana, R.S., and Slaga, T.J. (1981): Carcino-genesis, 2:1141-1146.

29. Verma, A.K., Ashendel, C.L., and Boutwell, R.K. (1980): Cancer Res. 40:308-315.

30. Yotti, L.P., Chang, C.C., and Trosko, J.E. (1979): Science 206:1089-1091.

Icosanoids and Cancer, edited by H. Thaler-Dao,
et al. Raven Press, New York © 1984.

Involvement of Prostaglandins in the Process of Skin Tumor Promotion

G. Fürstenberger, M. Gross, and F. Marks

*Institute of Biochemistry, German Cancer Research Center, D-6900 Heidelberg,
Federal Republic of Germany*

In skin arachidonic acid metabolites such as prostaglandins, leukotrienes and hydroxylated arachidonic acid derivatives are involved in
inflammatory processes (4,15,28), wound repair (1,3) and in proliferative
diseases such as psoriasis (16,22). E-type prostaglandins have been
shown to play a key role as mediators of hyperplastic transformation of
epidermis which is at least in mouse skin the general response to chemical or mechanical irritation and injury (for review see 12,24). Among
agents which induce those responses, certain phorbol esters such as 12-
0-tetradecanoylphorbol-13-acetate (TPA) are of special interest since
they have been found to promote the development of tumors in mouse skin
initiated by a single treatment with a subthreshold dose of a carcinogen,
most commonly 7,12-dimethylbenz(a)anthracen (DMBA) (for review see 17).
Moreover, studies using inhibitors of the different pathways of arachidonic acid metabolites as inhibitors of tumor promotion by phorbol esters
indicate a crucial role of arachidonic acid metabolites in the process
of tumor promotion ((7,8,12,26,29).

Investigations into the role of arachidonic acid metabolites in the
process of tumor promotion are impaired by the multiplicity of biological effects evoked by phorbol ester tumor promoters i.e. causation of
inflammatory reactions, of epidermal hyperproliferation and of tumor formation and by the fact that tumor promotion is a long term process. A
more detailed analysis can now be achieved since we and others have shown
that the process of tumor promotion consists of at least two separate
steps (11,27) confirming an experimental protocol originally reported by
Boutwell (5). In the following presentation, the role of prostaglandins
in both stages of the process of tumor promotion will be discussed.

II. TWO-STAGE TUMOR PROMOTION IN MOUSE SKIN

The tumor promoting potency of TPA-type phorbol esters can be almost
completely abolished when conjugated double bonds are introduced into the
long chain fatty acid or when the tetradecanoic acid residue is replaced
by retinoic acid (11,13). The ability of the phorbol esters to act as an
irritant skin mitogen is not impaired by these manipulations. Indeed,

both TPA and 12-0-retinoylphorbol-13-acetate (RPA) induce irritation and hyperplasia to a similar degree and along the same prostaglandin E-dependent pathway (10,11,23; see below). In the two-stage approach to skin tumorigenesis, RPA acts as an "incomplete" promoter in that the sequential treatment of initiated mouse skin with a few TPA applications (which by themselves are insufficient for promotion) followed by twice weekly RPA applications yields tumor responses comparable to those obtained by prolonged TPA treatment (11,13). Under these conditions, TPA treatment can even be restricted to only one application thus achieving for the first time the possibility of studying those TPA effects which are critical and obligatory for promotion and which are completely camouflaged by pleiotypic side effects in the course of chronic TPA treatment.

TABLE 1. Characteristics of the first and second stages of skin tumor promotion

First stage	Second stage
Single treatment with TPA or wounding	Repetitive treatments with RPA or other agents which induce chronic epidermal hyperplasia
Irrversible	Reversible
Transient epidermal hyperplasia is necessary	Sustained epidermal hyperplasia is necessary

Properties of the first and second stages of tumor promotion as revealed by the TPA-RPA regimen are summarized in Table 1. A unique and unexpected feature of the first TPA-dependent stage of promotion is its irreversibility: no significant decrease of the tumor response is observed when the time interval between stage 1 and stage 2 is increased up to 3 months (ref. 14 and unpublished results), whereas the symptoms of irritation and hyperplastic transformation cease within 2 weeks (2). Two lines of evidence support an obligatory role of epidermal hyperproliferation and hyperplasia in the first stage of promotion (Table 1). First, hydroxyurea applied 18 hours after a single TPA treatment leads to an almost complete inhibition of both epidermal DNA synthesis and first stage promotion being not due to cytotoxic effects of the drug (21). Second, transmaternally initiated neonatal mouse skin has been found to be resistant to the first stage-promoting effect of TPA as long as it does not respond to TPA by hyperplastic growth (25). Obviously, the sensitivity of neonatal mouse skin to the stimulation of both hyperplasiogenic and tumor promoting activities shows a similar time course of ontogenetic development (25). Both experiments indicate that the induction of epidermal hyperproliferation is a necessary condition of the first stage of promotion. In addition to TPA, skin wounding exerts a moderate effect as first stage promoter when followed by repetitive RPA treatments (13). This is in accordance with previous results showing a complete promoting activity of repeated skin wounding (2,6,18).

To perform the second stage of promotion, RPA has to be applied twice weekly over a period of at least 10 weeks. RPA can be replaced by a limited number of other irritant skin mitogens such as the unsaturated phorbol esters of the Ti_8-type (13). As for the first stage, hyperplastic transformation of epidermis seems also to be a necessary condition for the second stage of promotion (Table 1). Extending the time interval between RPA applications up to 4 weeks results in a dramatic decrease of tumor development indicating that the effects of the second stage promoter are reversible in nature and that generation of a sustained epidermal hyperplasia is a necessary and perhaps a sufficient condition of the second stage of tumor promotion (ref. 14 and unpublished results). The previously reported reversibility of tumor promotion (5) is thus most probably related to the second stage.

III. INVOLVEMENT OF PROSTAGLANDINS IN THE PROCESS OF TUMOR PROMOTION

Two lines of evidence support a role of prostaglandins in tumor promotion. First, in NMRI (12) and CD-1 (29) mouse skin, the cyclooxygenase inhibitor indomethacin inhibits the tumor promoting effect of TPA in a dose-dependent manner when applied one hour prior to or simultaneously with repetitive TPA treatments. This inhibition can be reversed by simultaneous treatment with $PGF_{2\alpha}$, indicating that products of the cyclooxygenase pathway are involved (12). Second, epidermal hyperplasia has proved to be an integral part of both stages of promotion (see above).

1. Role of prostaglandins in epidermal hyperproliferation and hyperplasia as an integral part of tumor promotion

TPA-induced epidermal hyperplasia is mediated by an accumulation of prostaglandin E in epidermis (10,23). TPA induces two early waves of prostaglandin E synthesis 10 minutes and 90 minutes after treatment probably corresponding to the stimulation of different cell populations. Inhibition of the first wave by indomethacin leads to an inhibition of epidermal hyperproliferation, whereas prevention of the second wave of PGE synthesis does not result in such an effect (10,23). PGE_2 but not $PGF_{2\alpha}$ is able to release the indomethacin inhibition of TPA-induced cell proliferation (29 and Fig. 1). However, both PGE_2 and $PGF_{2\alpha}$ show a comitogenic effect, when applied simultaneously with TPA, indicating that TPA gives rise to both PGE_2- and $PGF_{2\alpha}$-responsive cells in the course of the stimulation of epidermal cell proliferation (Fig. 1). Apparently, both E- and F-type prostaglandins are involved in the hyperproliferative response induced by TPA, with prostaglandin E being particularly involved in the trigger process. TPA induces indeed two waves of epidermal prostaglandin F synthesis, peaking at about 2.5 hours and between 3.5 hours and 4 hours after treatment (Fig. 2).

The incomplete tumor promoter RPA induces epidermal hyperproliferation and hyperplasia to a comparable extent and along the same prostaglandin E-dependent pathway as TPA (11). With respect to the stimulation of prostaglandin F synthesis there is, however, a significant difference between both phorbol esters (Fig. 2) in that RPA is not capable of inducing the second wave of PGF synthesis peaking between 3.5 and 4 hours.

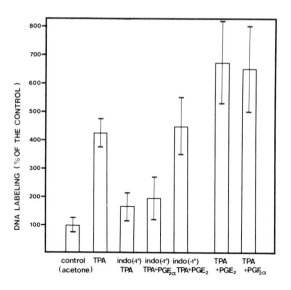

FIG. 1. Effects of prostaglandins E2 and F2α on epidermal DNA
        synthesis induced by simultaneous treatment with TPA
        with or without indomethacin pretreatment.

Mice were treated with either 0.1 ml acetone or 1.1 μmol indomethacin in 0.1 ml acetone one hour prior to application of
either 0.1 ml acetone, 10 nmol TPA, 10 nmol TPA + 60 nmol PGE2
or 10 nmol TPA + 60 nmol PGF2α, dissolved in 0.1 ml acetone,
and killed 18 hours after TPA treatment. Labeled thymidine was
injected one hour prior to sacrifice. The isolation of DNA and
measurement of radioactivity are described in ref. 9. Each experimental point represents the mean ± S.D. for 10 mice (55 ± 15
cpm/μg DNA = 100%).

2. Role of prostaglandins in the first stage
of promotion

Since prostaglandin E-mediated induction of epidermal hyperproliferation and hyperplasia is a necessary event in the first stage of tumor
promotion, it is conceivable that indomethacin may act as an inhibitor
for this stage. This is shown in Table 2. When applied one hour prior to
TPA, indomethacin causes an inhibitory effect on both the induction of
epidermal hyperplasia (9) and the first stage of promotion (Table 2)
induced by TPA. However, PGE2 which has been shown to release the indomethacin inhibition of the hyperproliferative response upon simultaneous
application with TPA does not reverse the inhibition of the first stage
of promotion, and PGF2α overcomes neither the inhibition of hyperplastic
growth (9) nor that of promotion (Table 2).
Whereas for an inhibition of epidermal hyperplasia indomethacin has to
be applied prior to TPA treatment, the maximal inhibitory effect on the
first stage of promotion is observed when the cyclooxygenase inhibitor
is applied 3 hours <u>after</u> TPA (Fig. 3). Indomethacin treatment 6 to 9

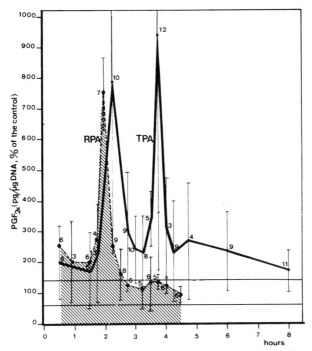

FIG. 2. Levels of prostaglandin in mouse epidermis in vivo
         after topical application of TPA or RPA

Mice were treated with 0.1 ml acetone, 10 nmol TPA or 10 nmol
RPA, dissolved in 0.1 ml acetone, and killed at the times indicated. The prostaglandins were extracted from frozen epidermis,
isolated by thin-layer chromatography and determined by radio-
immunassay (10). Each experimental point represents the mean
± S.D. for 3-12 mice. The number of animals (experiments) is
given beside each point. The horizontal lines represent the
average ± S.D. of the control values as obtained with 45 mice
$(4.3 \pm 1.7$ PGF/μg DNA = 100%).

hours after TPA yields only a marginal inhibitory effect on tumor promotion. Indomethacin applied 3 hours after TPA inhibits first of all the
second wave of prostaglandin F synthesis induced by TPA (Fig. 2). Accordingly, $PGF_{2\alpha}$ is able to overcome the inhibition of the first stage of
promotion when applied simultaneously with indomethacin, i.e. 3 hours after TPA treatment (Fig. 3). These results indicate that the second wave
of prostaglandin F synthesis observed 3 to 4 hours after TPA treatment
is critically involved in the first stage of tumor promotion. Such an
assumption would be consistent with the fact that the incomplete tumor
promoter RPA does not evoke an accumulation of prostaglandin F at this
time point (Fig. 2). Investigations are now underway to characterize the
role of $PGF_{2\alpha}$ in the first stage of promotion in more detail.

3. Role of prostaglandins in the second stage of promotion

As already mentioned, prostaglandin-mediated epidermal hyperplasia is
a necessary and perhaps a sufficient condition of the second stage of pro-

TABLE 2. Effects of indomethacin and prostaglandins E_2 and $F_{2\alpha}$ on the first stage promoting activity of TPA

| Treatment | | Tumor formation[a] | | | |
| First (no. of appl.; dose/animal) | Second (no. of appl.; dose/animal) | After 15 weeks | | After 18 weeks | |
		Rate[b]	Yield[c]	Rate[b]	Yield[c]
acetone (2x;100µl) 60 min later TPA (2x;10nmol)	RPA (34x;10nmol)	69	4.8	69	5.3
indomethacin (2x;550nmol) 60 min later TPA (2x;10nmol)	RPA (34x;10nmol)	31	1.9	31	2.5
indomethacin (2x;550nmol) 60 min later TPA (2x; 10nmol) + PGE_2 (2x; 28 nmol)	RPA (34x;10nmol)	19	1.7	33	2.6
indomethacin (2x;550nmol) 60 min later TPA (2x; 10nmol) + $PGF_{2\alpha}$ (2x; 28 nmol)	RPA (34x;10nmol)	38	1.6	38	2.3

[a] For each group 16 female NMRI mice (7 weeks old) were initiated by topical application of 100 nmol DMBA (dissolved in 0.1 ml acetone) onto the shaved back skin. Treatment with indomethacin, prostaglandins E_2 and $F_{2\alpha}$ and TPA was started one week later. The compounds were dissolved in 0.1 ml acetone and applied twice weekly. One week later, treatment with RPA was started. All tumor promotion experiments have been performed at last twice, yielding similar results.

[b] number of tumor bearers/survivors (94% or more survivors in all groups)

[c] number of papillomas/survivor

motion. Accordingly, indomethacin inhibits the second stage promoting activity induced by repetitive RPA treatments (Table 3). Considering the fact that the induction of epidermal hyperplasia depends on PGE_2, it was surprising to find that only $PGF_{2\alpha}$ but not PGE_2 when applied simultaneously with RPA is able to release the indomethacin inhibition of the second stage of promotion (Table 3). One possible interpretation of this result would be that PGE_2 is only necessary to trigger the tissue from a more quiescent into the hyperproliferative state and that the maintenance of epidermal hyperplasia is then mediated by $PGF_{2\alpha}$. Contrary to the situation during the first stage of promotion where $PGF_{2\alpha}$ has to be applied several hours after TPA, indomethacin inhibition of the second stage can be reversed when $PGF_{2\alpha}$ is administered simultaneously with RPA. Although this result may be taken as an indication that $PGF_{2\alpha}$ has different effects on both stages of promotion, a detailed kinetic analysis of these effects is not possible since the situation may change profoundly due to repetitive phorbol ester treatments during the second stage.

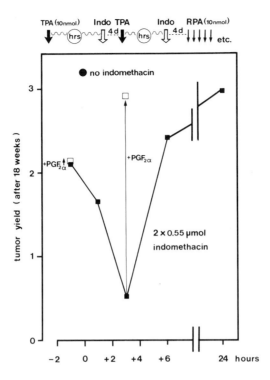

FIG. 3. Effect on first-stage promotion activity of varying the
time interval between indomethacin or indomethacin and
PFG$_{2\alpha}$ treatment and TPA application

For each group 16 female NMRI mice (7 weeks old) were initiated by
topical application of 100 nmol DMBA (dissolved in 0.1 ml acetone)
onto the shaved back skin. One week later, first stage treatment
was performed as schematically depicted. Mice were treated with TPA
(10 nmol), indomethacin (0.55 µmol) and PGF$_{2\alpha}$ (60 nmol), dissolved
in 0.1 ml acetone, followed by repetitive treatments with RPA
(10 nmol/0.1 ml acetone). The tumor response is measured as tumor
yield, i.e. papillomas/survivors after 18 weeks of promotion. The
negative sign refers to indomethacin or indomethacin and PGF$_{2\alpha}$
application before, the positive sign after TPA treatment.

IV. CONCLUSIONS

Our results indicate that prostaglandins are associated with the stimulation by phorbol esters of epidermal cell proliferation in mouse skin
in vivo in that E-prostaglandins appear to be involved in triggering the
tissue from the quiescent into the hyperproliferative state and F-prosta-
glandins in maintaining epidermal hyperproliferation and hyperplasia
(see also ref. 12). Both prostaglandins do not stimulate cell proliferation in normal mouse epidermis indicating that prostaglandins act with
the exogenous stimulus itself or with endogenous growth factors induced
by the exogenous stimulus in a synergistic manner. The nature of this
synergism remains to be elucidated. In various cell lines, PGF$_{2\alpha}$ was

TABLE 3. <u>Effects of indomethacin and prostaglandins E_2 and $F_{2\alpha}$ on the</u>
<u>second stage of promotion</u>

First (no.of appl.; dose/animal)	Treatment Second (no.of appl.; dose/animal)	Tumor formation[a]			
		After 15 weeks		After 18 weeks	
		Rate[b]	Yield[c]	Rate[b]	Yield[c]
TPA (2x; 20 nmol)	RPA (34x; 10 nmol)	50	2.6	66	3.1
TPA (2x; 20 nmol)	indomethacin (34x; 550 nmol) 60 min later RPA (34x; 10 nmol)	27	1.1	33	1.2
TPA (2x; 20 nmol)	indomethacin (34x; 550 nmol) 60 min later RPA+PGE$_2$ (34x; 10 nmol+ 28 nmol)	27	1.3	27	1.2
TPA (2x; 20 nmol)	indomethacin (34x; 550 nmol) 60 min later RPA+PGF$_{2\alpha}$ (34x; 10 nmol + 28 nmmol)	60	2.0	66	2.6

[a] For each group 16 female NMRI mice (7 weeks old) were initiated by topical application of 100 nmol DMBA (dissolved in 0.1 ml acetone) onto the shaved back skin. Treatments with TPA were started one week later. Twice-weekly treatments with RPA, indomethacin and prostaglandins E_2 and $F_{2\alpha}$ were started another week later. The compounds were dissolved in 0.1 ml acetone. All tumor promotion experiments have been performed at least twice, yielding similar results.

[b] number of tumor bearers/survivors (94% or more survivors in all groups)

[c] number of papillomas/survivor

found to stimulate the initiation of DNA synthesis either by itself as in quiescent 3T6 and Swiss 3T3 cells (20) or with growth factors such as EGF in a synergistic manner (19,20).

Moreover, $PGF_{2\alpha}$, appearing as one distinct wave of prostaglandin F synthesis 3 to 4 hours after TPA application seems to be critically involved in the first stage of promotion. The distinct prostaglandin peaks observed after TPA treatment could indicate that different epidermal cell populations are subsequently triggered to proliferate and that the activation of one of the prostaglandin F responsive cell populations may provide a critical step in the first stage of promotion. In this respect, it is remarkable that the second stage promoter RPA does not give rise to the accumulation of prostaglandin F 3 to 4 hours after application as obtained after TPA treatment. The precise role of $PGF_{2\alpha}$ in the first stage of promotion is subject to ongoing investigations in our laboratory.

REFERENCES

1. Anggard, E., and Jonsson, C.E. (1972): In: Prostaglandins in Cellular Biology, edited by P.W. Ramwell, and B.B. Pharris, Vol. 1, pp. 269-291. Plenum Press, New York.
2. Argyris, T.S. (1982): J. Cutaneous Pathol., 9: 1-18.
3. Bertsch, S., and Marks, F. (1982): Cell Tissue Kinet., 15: 81-87.
4. Bonta, J.L., and Parnham, M.J. (1978): Biochem. Pharmacol., 27: 1611-1623.
5. Boutwell, R.K. (1964): Progr. Exp. Tumor Res., 4: 207-250.
6. Clark-Lewis, J., and Murray, A.W. (1978): Cancer Res., 38: 494-497.
7. Fischer, S.M., and Slaga, T.J. (1982): In: Prostaglandins and Related Lipids, edited by T.J. Powles, R.S. Bockmann, K.V. Honn, and P.W. Ramwell, Vol. 2, pp. 255-264. Alan R. Liss, New York.
8. Fischer, S.M., Mills, G.D., and Slaga, T.J. (1982): Carcinogenesis, 3: 1243-1245.
9. Fürstenberger, G., and Marks, F. (1978): Biochem. Biophys. Res. Commun., 84: 1103-1108.
10. Fürstenberger, G., and Marks, F. (1980): Biochem. Biophys. Res. Commun., 92: 749-756.
11. Fürstenberger, G., Berry, D.L., Sorg, B., and Marks, F. (1981): Proc. Natl. Acad. Sci. USA, 78: 7722-7726.
12. Fürstenberger, G., Gross, M., and Marks, F. (1982): In: Prostaglandins and Related Lipids, edited by T.J. Powles, R.S. Bockmann, K.V. Honn, and P.W. Ramwell, Vol. 2, pp. 239-254. Alan R. Liss, New York.
13. Fürstenberger, G., and Marks, F. (1983): J. Invest. Dermatol., 81: 157s-161s.
14. Fürstenberger, G., Sorg, B., and Marks, F. (1983): Science 220: 89-91.
15. Goetzl, E.J., Wood, J.M., and Gorman, R.R. (1977): J. Clin. Invest., 59: 179-183.
16. Hammarström, S., Hamberg, M., Samuelsson, B., Duell, M., Stawiski, M., and Vorhees, J.J. (1975): Proc. Natl. Acad. Sci. USA, 72: 5130-5134.
17. Hecker, E., Fusenig, N.E., Kunz, W., Marks, F., and Thielmann, H.W. eds. (1982): Cocarcinogenesis and biological effects of tumor promoters. Carcinogenesis, a Comprehensive Survey, Vol. 7. Raven Press, New York.
18. Hennings, H., and Boutwell, R.K. (1970): Cancer Res., 30: 312-320.
19. Jimenez de Asua, L., Richmond, K.M.V. and Otto, M.A. (1981): Proc. Natl. Acad. Sci. USA, 78: 1004-1008.
20. Jimenez de Asua, L., Otto, A.M., Ulrich, M.O., Martin-Perez, J., and Thomas, G. (1982): In: Prostaglandins and Related Lipids, edited by T.J. Powles, R.S. Bockmann, K.V. Honn, and P.W. Ramwell, Vol. 2, pp. 309-331.
21. Kinzel, V., Fürstenberger, G., Richards, J., Goerttler, K., Loehrke, H., and Marks, F. (1983): In: Proceedings of the Symposium "Role of Cocarcinogens and Promoters in Human and Experimental Carcinogenesis", IARC Monographs, in press. International Agency For Research on Cancer, Lyon.
22. Marcelo, C.L., and Vorhees, J.J. (1980): Pharmac. Ther., 9: 297-310.
23. Marks, F., Fürstenberger, G., and Kownatzki, E. (1981): Cancer Res., 41: 696-702.

24. Marks, F., Bertsch, S., Fürstenberger, G., and Richter, H. (1983): In: Psoriasis: Cell Proliferation, edited by N.A. Wright and R.S. Lamplejohn, pp. 173-188. Churchill Livingstone, Edinburgh.
25. Marks, F., and Fürstenberger, G. (1983): In: Proceedings of the Symposium "Role of Cocarcinogens and Promoters in Human and Experimental Carcinogenesis", IARC Monographs, in press. International Agency For Research on Cancer, Lyon.
26. Nakadate, T., Yamamoto, S., Iseki, H., Sonoda, S., Takemura, S., Ura, A., Hosoda, Y., and Kato, R. (1982): Gann, 73: 841-843.
27. Slaga, T.J., Fischer, S.M., Nelson, K., and Gleason, G.L. (1980): Proc.Natl.Acad.Sci. USA, 77: 3659-3663.
28. Samuelsson, B. (1983): Science, 220: 568-575.
29. Verma, A.K., Ashendel, C.L., and Boutwell, R.K. (1980): Cancer Res., 40: 308-315.

Icosanoids and Cancer, edited by H. Thaler-Dao, et al. Raven Press, New York © 1984.

Involvement of Lipoxygenase Products of Arachidonic Acid in Tumor-Promoting Activity of TPA

Ryuichi Kato, Teruo Nakadate, and Satoshi Yamamoto

Department of Pharmacology, School of Medicine, Keio University, Tokyo 160, Japan

The application of 12-O-tetradecanoylphorbol-13-acetate (TPA[1]) to mouse skin or certain cells in culture causes a number of biochemical alterations and of changes in cellular functions, and skin tumor promotion (2,3). Inductions of epidermal ornithine decarboxylase (ODC) and DNA synthesis are the typical and prominent biochemical alterations elicited by TPA and have been thought to be representative biochemical parameters of phorbol diesters with strong tumor promoting activity (21,11).

Considerable evidence suggests the involvement of prostaglandins in TPA-induced responses in various types of cells (14,16,28). In epidermis and epidermal cells, it was suggested that TPA releases arachidonic acid and prostaglandins (9) by phospholipase A_2 stimulation (4). Verma et al. (27) reported that pretreatment with prostaglandin synthesis inhibitor such as indomethacin markedly inhibits the induction of epidermal ODC by TPA. The application of prostaglandin E_2 (PGE$_2$) to skin counteracts the inhibitory effect of indomethacin upon ODC induction. They suggested that PGE$_2$ may play a crucial role in ODC induction by TPA (27). Since there has been reported the presence of lipoxygenase activity in mouse epidermis (10), part of the released arachidonic acid would be oxidized through lipoxygenase pathway to hydroperoxy and hydroxy derivatives of arachidonic acid as well as through cyclooxygenase pathway to prostaglandins. These findings

---

[1] Abbreviations used are: TPA, 12-O-tetradecanoylphorbol-13-acetate; DMBA, 7,12-dimethylbenz[a]anthracene; NDGA, nordihydroguaiaretic acid; BPB, p-bromophenacyl bromide; PGE$_2$, prostaglandin E$_2$; FA, fluocinolone acetonide; BHA, butylated hydroxyanisole

urged us to investigate the possible involvement of lipoxygenase products in the mechanism of TPA actions such as ODC induction, enhancement of DNA synthesis and tumor promotion in mouse epidermis.

MATERIALS AND METHODS

Chemicals

7,12-Dimethylbenz[a]anthracene (DMBA), TPA, mepacrine, arachidonic acid, indomethacin, fluocinolone acetonide (FA), nordihydroguaiaretic acid (NDGA), esculetin and α-tocopherol were purchased from Sigma Chemicals Co., St. Louis, MO, USA, quercetin, morin, phenidone and (+)catechin were from Tokyo Chemical Industry Co., Tokyo, Japan, p-bromophenacyl bromide (BPB) and butylated hydroxyanisole (BHA) were from Wako Pure Chemical Industries Ltd., Osaka, Japan. Prostaglandin E_2 (PGE_2) was supplied from Ono Pharmaceutical Co. Ltd., Osaka, Japan. DL-[1-^{14}C]Ornithine (51.3mCi/mmol), [methyl-^{3}H]thymidine (78.9Ci/mmol) and [1-^{14}C]arachidonic acid (52.9mCi/mmol) were obtained from New England Nuclear, Boston, MA, USA.

Animals and Treatments

Female CD-1 mice (Charles River, Atsugi, Japan), 7-8 week of age were used. Mice were housed in an air-conditioned room (22-23°C) under indoor illumination from 6 a.m. to 6 p.m. Food and water were available ad libtum. The dorsal hair of each mouse was shaved with clippers at least 2 days before use, and only those mice in a resting phase of the hair cycle were used. All chemicals were dissolved in reagent grade acetone, acetone:ethanol (4:1, v/v) or acetone:water (12.5:1, v/v), and applied to the shaved area in a volume of 0.2 ml using a micropipette. Mice were topically treated with vehicle, mepacrine, BPB, NDGA, phenidone, quercetin, BHA, esculetin, α-tocopherol, (+)catechin or fluocinolone acetonide prior to the application of TPA. The same amounts of the inhibitors except BPB were applied again to the mice concurrently with TPA. Topical application of indomethacin was performed concurrently and 2 h prior to TPA treatment. PGE_2 were applied twice concurrently with indomethacin or mepacrine. Arachidonic acid was applied once concurrently with TPA.

Assay of ODC Activity

Five hours after the TPA administration, the mice were killed by cervical dislocation. Epidermis was separated by a brief heat treatment (21) and ODC activities of the soluble epidermal supernatants were determined by measuring the release of $^{14}CO_2$ from [1-^{14}C]ornithine, as described previously (18). The results are expressed as nmol CO_2/60 min/mg protein.

[³H]Thymidine Incorporation into Epidermal DNA

Mice were killed 18 h after topical application of TPA and 30 μCi of [³H]thymidine was injected intraperitoneally 1 h before sacrifice. Animal sacrifice was performed during 10 a.m.- 11 a.m. of a day in order to avoid circadian variation in epidermal DNA synthetic activity. Epidermis from each mouse was isolated by a brief heat treatment (21), and homogenized in 2.0 ml of 0.4 M perchloric acid at 4 °C. The homogenate was filtered through gauze to remove connective tissue and centrifuged at 4 °C for 15 min at 3,000 rpm. The pellet was washed twice (2 x 2.0 ml) with ice-cold 0.4 M perchloric acid and twice with 100% ethanol (2.0 ml). DNA in the pellet was hydrolyzed in 0.5 M perchloric acid by heating at 95 °C for 10 min. After centrifugation at room temperature for 15 min at 3,000 rpm, aliquots of hydrolysates were taken for determination of radioactivity and DNA content. DNA content was determined by Burton's method (5).

Tumor Promotion Experiment

A group of 24 mice was initiated by applying 200 nmol of DMBA to the dorsal skin. Promotion with 20 nmol of TPA applied twice weekly was begun 10 days after initiation. BPB (10 μmol) was applied topically 30-40 min before each TPA treatment. NDGA (30 μmol), quercetin (30 μmol), morin (30 μmol), esculetin (30 μmol), α-tocopherol (30 μmol) and (+)catechin (30 μmol) were applied topically 30-40 min before each TPA treatment and concurrently with TPA. These treatments were continued for 18 weeks.

Epidermal Lipoxygenase Activity

The skin of a non-treated mouse was placed on an ice-cold plate and epidermis was removed free from dermis and fat by scraping with a razor blade. The epidermal sheets were homogenized in 100 mM Tris-HCl buffer containing 1 mM EDTA, pH 7.2, in a Polytron PT-10 homogenizer for 10 to 15 sec at 4 °C, and centrifuged for 10 min at 12,000 x g. The supernatant was re-centrifuged for 60 min at 105,000 x g and the obtained supernatant was used for lipoxygenase assay. An aliquot (500 μl) of supernatant (1.1 mg protein) supplemented with calcium ion (final 2 mM) was preincubated in the presence or absence of NDGA, phenidone, quercetin, BHA, esculetin or indomethacin for 5 min at 37°C. The reaction was started by the addition of [¹⁴C]arachidonic acid (final 3.6 μM) and the incubation was carried out for 10 min at 37°C. The reaction was terminated by the addition of 2.0 ml of a solvent containing 15 parts ethyl acetate, 2 parts methanol and 1 part 0.4 M citric acid. The mixture was vortexed vigorously, centrifuged, and the organic phase was transferred into another tube and was dried under N_2 gass. The dried residue was dissolved by a small amount of

chloroform and methanol (1:1, v/v) and spotted on silica gel
LK6D (Whatman) plates. The plates were developed in the
solvent system : benzene/ether/ethanol/acetic acid
(50:40:2:0.2, by vol.). After the development was
performed, the plates were dried and fractions of silica gel
(0.5 cm each) were scraped by a razor blade and transferred
into vials. Methanol (0.5 ml) was added to each vial in
order to extract [14C]arachidonic acid and its labeled
metabolites. The radioactivity was measured in a liquid
scintillation counter (Beckman LS 3800).

RESULTS

A single application of TPA (20 nmol) resulted in a
substantial and transient increase in mouse epidermal ODC
activity with peak activity at about 5 h after TPA treatment
(12,18,19,21). ODC induction by TPA was inhibited by the
treatment of mouse skin with mepacrine (TABLE 1, Exp.2)
which has been shown to be a phospholipase A_2 inhibitor.
BPB, another phospholipase A_2 inhibitor, also inhibited the
epidermal ODC induction by TPA(TABLE 1, Exp.1). The
inhibition of ODC induction by mepacrine could not be
reversed by treatment of mice with 140 nmol of PGE_2 (TABLE
1, Exp.2). The above dose of PGE_2 restored the ODC
induction suppressed by indomethacin (1.12 μmol) (TABLE 2,
Exp.3 and 4). Further increase in the doses of PGE_2 also

TABLE 1. Inhibition of TPA-caused ODC induction by BPB and
mepacrine, and effects of PGE_2 and arachidonic acid on the
inhibition of TPA-caused ODC induction by mepacrine

Treatment	ODC activity[a] (nmol CO_2/60min/mg protein)
Experiment 1	
Vehicle	0.05 ± 0.03
TPA (20 nmol)	1.17 ± 0.30
TPA + BPB (10 μmol)	0.19 ± 0.10[c]
Experiment 2	
Vehicle	0.09 ± 0.08
TPA (20 nmol)	1.04 ± 0.15
TPA + mepacrine (20 μmol)	0.08 ± 0.02[b]
TPA + mepacrine + PGE_2 (140 nmol)	0.13 ± 0.02[d]
Experiment 3	
Vehicle	0.02 ± 0.02
TPA (20 nmol)	1.08 ± 0.21
TPA + mepacrine (20 μmol)	0.28 ± 0.05[b]
TPA + mepacrine + arachidonic acid (1 μmol)	0.58 ± 0.05[e]

[a] Mean ± S.E. of individual determinations from 4-5 mice.
[b] $P < 0.01$ vs TPA. [c] $P < 0.05$ vs TPA. [d] not significantly
different from TPA plus mepacrine. [e] $P < 0.01$ vs TPA plus
mepacrine.

TABLE 2. Inhibition of TPA-caused ODC induction by NDGA, phenidone, quercetin, BHA and esculetin, and effects of NDGA and phenidone on the restorative action of PGE_2 on TPA-caused ODC induction inhibited by indomethacin

Treatment	ODC activity[a] (nmol CO_2/60min/mg protein)
Experiment 1	
Vehicle	0.05 ± 0.01
TPA (20 nmol)	1.58 ± 0.14
TPA + NDGA (30 μmol)	0.45 ± 0.07[b]
Experiment 2	
Vehicle	0.10 ± 0.01
TPA (20 nmol)	1.15 ± 0.15
TPA + phenidone (30 μmol)	0.33 ± 0.04[b]
Experiment 3	
Vehicle	0.03 ± 0.03
TPA (20 nmol)	1.03 ± 0.07
TPA + indomethacin (1.12 μmol)	0.34 ± 0.06[b]
TPA + indomethacin + PGE_2 (140 nmol)	0.69 ± 0.05[d]
TPA + indomethacin + PGE_2 + NDGA (30 μmol)	0.32 ± 0.06[g]
Experiment 4	
Vehicle	0.06 ± 0.02
TPA (20 nmol)	1.46 ± 0.18
TPA + indomethacin (1.12 μmol)	0.46 ± 0.06[b]
TPA + indomethacin + PGE_2 (140 nmol)	1.14 ± 0.19[e,f]
TPA + indomethacin + PGE_2 + phenidone (30 μmol)	0.41 ± 0.07[g]
Experiment 5	
Vehicle	0.20 ± 0.04
TPA (20 nmol)	2.64 ± 0.54
TPA + quercetin (10 μmol)	0.83 ± 0.14[b]
TPA + quercetin (30 μmol)	0.75 ± 0.25[b]
Experiment 6	
Vehicle	0.11 ± 0.02
TPA (20 nmol)	1.36 ± 0.27
TPA + BHA (10 μmol)	0.80 ± 0.07[c]
TPA + BHA (30 μmol)	0.51 ± 0.13[b]
Experiment 7	
Vehicle	0.15 ± 0.05
TPA (20 nmol)	2.66 ± 0.48
TPA + esculetin (10 μmol)	1.76 ± 0.43
TPA + esculetin (30 μmol)	1.42 ± 0.12[c]

[a] Mean ± S.E. of individual determinations from 5 mice. [b] $P < 0.01$ vs TPA. [c] $P < 0.05$ vs TPA. [d] $P < 0.01$ vs TPA plus indomethacin. [e] $P < 0.05$ vs TPA plus indomethacin. [f] not significantly different from TPA. [g] $P < 0.01$ vs TPA plus indomethacin plus PGE_2; not significantly different from TPA plus indomethacin.

failed to counteract the inhibitory effect of mepacrine (18). On the contrary, topical application of arachidonic acid (1 µmol) significantly restored the TPA-caused ODC induction which was suppressed by mepacrine (20 µmol) (TABLE 1, Exp.3). Arachidonic acid also partially restored the TPA-caused ODC induction which was inhibited by BPB (18).

NDGA (30 µmol) and phenidone (30 µmol), well-known lipoxygenase inhibitors, inhibited the induction of ODC by TPA (TABLE 2, Exp.1 and 2). The treatment of mice skin with quercetin (10-30 µmol) also inhibited TPA-caused induction of ODC (TABLE 2, Exp.5). In addition, BHA (10-30 µmol) (13) and esculetin (30 µmol) significantly but less potently inhibited the induction of ODC by TPA (TABLE 2, Exp.6 and 7). Actually, quercetin potently inhibited epidermal lipoxygenase activity in this strain of mouse (FIG. 3). BHA and esculetin also inhibited epidermal lipoxygenase activity (FIG. 3). As shown in TABLE 2, Exp.3, in the presence of indomethacin NDGA (30 µmol) inhibits the PGE_2-induced restoration of TPA-caused ODC induction. As in the case of NDGA, phenidone (30 µmol) also inhibits the restorative effect of PGE_2 (TABLE 2, Exp.4).

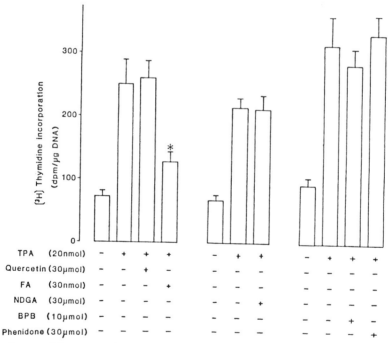

FIG. 1. Effects of quercetin, FA, NDGA, BPB, and phenidone on TPA-induced [^{3}H]thymidine incorporation into epidermal DNA. Details are given in "MATERIALS AND METHODS". Each value is the mean of individual determinations from 5 mice. Vertical bars indicate S.E. * P < 0.05 vs TPA.

A single application of TPA (20 nmol) to mouse skin stimulated the incorporation of [^{3}H]thymidine into epidermal DNA with the first peak at about 18 h after TPA treatment. As shown in FIG. 1, treatment of mouse skin with either BPB (10 μmol), NDGA (30 μmol), phenidone (30 μmol) or quercetin (30 μmol) failed to affect the TPA-induced [^{3}H]thymidine incorporation into epidermal DNA. In the same condition, treatment of mouse skin with FA (30 μmol), an anti-inflammatory agent, reduced TPA-induced [^{3}H]thymidine incorporation into DNA (Fig. 1) as previously reported by Schwarz et al. (23).

Effect of BPB, NDGA, quercetin, morin, esculetin, α-tocopherol and (+)catechin on the incidence of TPA-induced skin papilloma formation was examined (TABLE 3). Treatment of initiated mice with 20 nmol of TPA alone resulted in about 20 - 25 papillomas per mouse 18 weeks after the start of promotion. Application of 10 μmol of BPB 30 - 40 min before each TPA treatment resulted in 94% inhibition in the number of papillomas per mouse compared to mice receiving only TPA. Pretreatment of mouse skin with 30 μmol of NDGA, quercetin and morin 30 - 40 min prior to each promotion also markedly reduced the production of papillomas. In addition, pretreatment with 30 μmol of esculetin, α-tocopherol and (+)catechin slightly reduced the production of papillomas.

To demonstrate the inhibitory effect of NDGA, phenidone, quercetin, esculetin and BHA on epidermal lipoxygenase

TABLE 3. Inhibitory effects of BPB, NDGA, quercetin, morin, esculetin, α-tocopherol and (+)catechin on the TPA-caused tumor promotion and ODC induction

Treatment	% Inhibition of tumor promotion[1]	% Inhibition of ODC induction[2]
BPB	94%	83%
NDGA	82%	57%
Quercetin	71%	74%
Morin	86%	57%[3]
Esculetin	34%	34%[4]
α-Tocopherol	37%	27%[4]
(+)Catechin	27%	36%[4]

1) % Inhibition of the number of papillomas per mouse at 18th week.
2) % Inhibition of epidermal ODC induction by single TPA treatment. The used dose of inhibitors was 10 μmol except morin.
3) The dose of morin was 3 μmol.
4) not significantly different from TPA.

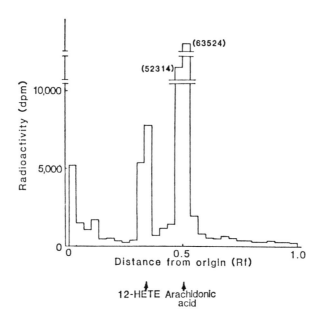

FIG. 2. Thin-layer chromatogram of products formed from
[14C]arachidonic acid during 10 min incubation at 37°C with
cytosol fraction obtained from homogenate of mouse
epidermis.

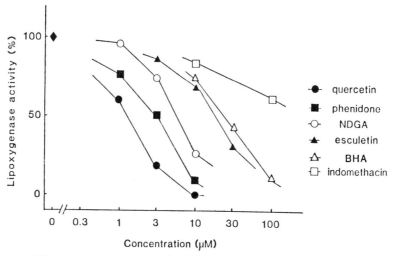

FIG. 3. Effects of NDGA, phenidone, quercetin, esculetin,
BHA and indomethacin on the epidermal lipoxygenase activity.
The results are expressed as the percent formation of
[14C]12-hydroxyeicosatetraenoic acid from [14C]arachidonic
acid.

activity, we used cytosol fraction of mouse epidermis. We
observed that the cytosol fraction of mouse epidermis
effectively converted arachidonic acid to lipoxygenase
products i.e. 12-hydroxyeicosatetraenoic acid (12-HETE,
major product) and 15-hydroxyeicosatetraenoic acid (15-HETE,
minor product), by the analyses of thin-layer chromatography
and high-performance liquid chromatography (12). FIG. 2
showes a typical thin-layer chromatogram. The conversion of
arachidonic acid to 12-hydroxyeicosatetraenoic acid was
potently inhibited by NDGA, phenidone and quercetin. The
inhibition by esculetin and BHA was less potent (FIG. 3).
Indomethacin, a selective cyclooxygenase inhibitor, failed
to inhibit it. The 50 percent inhibition of lipoxygenase
was observed by NDGA at 5.4 μM, phenidone at 3.2 μM,
quercetin at 1.3 μM, esculetin at 18 μM, BHA at 24 μM and
indomethacin at more than 100 μM (FIG. 3).

DISCUSSION

Verma et al. (27) suggested that a cyclooxygenase product
such as PGE_2 may play a crucial role in the mechanism of ODC
induction by TPA. In the present study, we confirmed the
above findings and further postulated a hypothesis that some
lipoxygenase product(s) as well as cyclooxygenase product(s)
such as PGE_2 are involved in the mechanism of ODC induction
and tumor promotion caused by TPA (12,17-19).

When ODC induction by TPA was inhibited by mepacrine, a
phospholipase A_2 inhibitor, PGE_2 failed to overcome the
inhibitory effect of mepacrine. This finding indicates the
idea that PGE_2 is an essential factor but not one sufficient
to induce ODC activity by TPA (18). The inhibitory effect
of mepacrine, however, was partially overcome by arachidonic
acid. Similar restorative effect of arachidonic acid was
observed when the TPA-caused ODC induction was suppressed by
BPB, another phospholipase A_2 inhibitor (18). The results
indicate that not only cyclooxygenase product(s) but also
lipoxygenase product(s) of arachidonic acid are involved in
the mechanism of ODC induction by TPA (18). Moreover,
present data clearly show that TPA-caused ODC induction was
inhibited by treatment of mice with, well known lipoxygenase
inhibitors, NDGA, phenidone and quercetin which potently
inhibited mouse epidermal lipoxygenase activity (12,18,19).
The TPA-caused ODC induction was less potently inhibited by
esculetin and BHA which were shown to be less potent
lipoxygenase inhibitors compared to NDGA, phenidone and
quercetin in mouse epidermis. The potency of the inhibitory
action of the drugs on the TPA-caused ODC induction is
apparently correlated with the potency of their lipoxygenase
inhibition. These findings also support above contention
that lipoxygenase products are involved in the mechanism of
ODC induction.

As often pointed out, the above lipoxygenase inhibitors may also inhibit cyclooxygenase as well as lipoxygenase (1,22). However, we observed that quercetin (3-30 μM) and NDGA (10-30 μM) failed to inhibit epidermal cyclooxygenase (data not shown), whereas lipoxygenase activity was completely inhibited by quercetin and NDGA at 3-30 μM and 10-30 μM, respectively. Thus, the inhibitory effect of NDGA and quercetin are clearly selective to lipoxygenase in CD-1 mice epidermis. However, it is very difficult to estimate the local drug concentrations after the topical applications of these drugs. Thus, there still remains a slight possibility that the inhibition of TPA-caused ODC induction by lipoxygenase inhibitors is due to the inhibition of cyclooxygenase by these drugs. We carried out, therefore, the further experiments. As described above, PGE_2 counteracted the inhibition of TPA-caused ODC induction by indomethacin. This restoring effect of PGE_2 was inhibited by NDGA and phenidone. Since indomethacin, at the concentration we used, exerts its maximal effect by inhibiting epidermal cyclooxygenase (27), it is highly possible that the inhibitory effects of NDGA and phenidone on the restorative action of PGE_2 is mediated through the inhibition of lipoxygenase (19).

It has been reported that teleocidin, which is structurally different from the phorbol esters, shares many biochemical and biological effects in various cell systems with TPA, including ODC induction and tumor promotion in mouse epidermis (7,8,25). It was also reported that TPA and teleocidin bind to common membrane located receptors (24,26). We observed that teleocidin-caused ODC induction was inhibited by BPB, NDGA and indomethacin (Nakadate et al., manuscript in preparation). PGE_2 counteracted the indomethacin-caused inhibition of ODC induction, but failed to counteract the BPB-caused inhibition. However, arachidonic acid partially but significantly restored the teleocidin-caused ODC induction which was inhibited by BPB. In addition, NDGA inhibited the restoring effect of PGE_2 on the teleocidin-caused ODC induction which was inhibited by indomethacin. These results further support our hypothesis that lipoxygenase product(s) are involved in the mechanism of actions of tumor promoter such as TPA and teleocidin (Nakadate et al., manuscript in preparation).

Our present results clearly show that treatment of mice with NDGA or BPB markedly inhibits the skin tumor promotion induced by TPA in CD-1 strain mice (17). Quercetin (12) and morin also markedly inhibited the skin tumor promotion caused by TPA. The TPA-induced skin tumor promotion was slightly suppressed by esculetin. In addition, α-tocopherol and (+)catechin were less potent in the inhibition of skin tumor promotion in accordance with ODC induction (TABLE 3). α-Tocopherol and (+)catechin failed to inhibit epidermal lipoxygenase activity (umpublished data). These results suggest that phospholipase A_2 stimulation and lipoxygenase product(s) are also involved in the mechanism of tumor promotion induced by TPA (12,17). Recently, Fischer et al. also suggested that lipoxygenase products are essential for tumor promotion (6).

The DNA synthesis in mouse epidermis is enhanced by a single topical application of TPA and the stimulation of DNA synthesis is thought to be one of the representative biochemical parameters of phorbol esters with strong tumor promoting activity (11). In the present study, BPB, NDGA, phenidone and quercetin failed to affect the TPA-induced [^{3}H]thymidine incorporation into DNA. In the same conditions, FA, which is a potent inhibitor of tumor promotion (23), but not an inhibitor of ODC induction (15), inhibited the TPA-induced DNA synthesis in agreement with the data of Schwarz et al. (23). These results suggest that inhibition of TPA-induced DNA synthesis is not always in parallel with the inhibition of the TPA-caused ODC induction and tumor promotion (12). O'Brien et al. (20) have also reported that the induction of ODC and the stimulation of DNA synthesis following TPA treatment are regulated independently.

CONCLUSION

1. TPA-caused ODC induction was inhibited by phospholipase A_2 inhibitors, mepacrine and BPB, and lipoxygenase inhibitors, NDGA, phenidone, quercetin and morin. PGE_2 counteracted the indomethacin-caused inhibition of ODC induction by TPA, but failed to counteract the mepacrine-caused inhibition. However, arachidonic acid partially but significantly restored the TPA-caused ODC induction which was inhibited by mepacrine. In addition, NDGA and phenidone inhibited the restoring effect of PGE_2 on the TPA-caused ODC induction which was inhibited by indomethacin.
2. TPA-caused tumor promotion on mouse skin was inhibited by BPB, NDGA, quercetin and morin.
3. Mouse epidermis have high activity in lipoxygenase and the formation of 12-hydroxyeicosatetraenoic acid was clearly inhibited by putative inhibiters.
4. These results indicated a possible involvement of lipoxygenase product(s) in the mechanism of TPA-caused epidermal ODC induction and tumor promotion.

ACKNOWLEDGEMENT

We are grateful to Miss Eriko Aizu and Miss Miki Ishii for technical assistance. A part of this work was supported by Grants-in-Aid for Cancer Research and for Encouragement of Young Scientists, from the Ministry of Education, Science and Culture of Japan.

REFERENCES

1. Blackwell, G.J., and Flower, R.J. (1978): <u>Prostaglandins</u>, 16: 417-425.
2. Blumberg, P.M. (1981): <u>CRC Crit. Rev. Toxicol.</u>, 9: 199-234.
3. Boutwell, R.K. (1978): In: <u>Carcinogenesis, a Comprehensive Survey, Vol. 2</u>, edited by T.J. Slaga, A.Sirak, and R.K. Boutwell, pp. 49-58. Raven Press, New York.
4. Bresnick, E., Bailey, G., Bouney, R.J., and Wightman, P. (1981): <u>Carcinogenesis</u>, 2: 1119-1122.
5. Burton, K.A. (1956): <u>Biochem. J.</u>, 62: 315-322.
6. Fischer, S.M., Mills, G.D., and Slaga, T.J. (1982): <u>Carcinogenesis</u>, 3: 1243-1245.
7. Fujiki, H., Mori, M., Nakayasu, M., Terada, M., and Sugimura, T. (1979): <u>Biochem, Biophys. Res. Commun.</u>, 90: 976-983.
8. Fujiki, H., Mori, M., Nakayasu, M., Terada, M., Sugimura, T., and Moore, R.E. (1981): <u>Proc. Natl. Acad. Sci. USA</u>, 78: 3872-3876.
9. Fürstenbergar, G., Richter, H., Fusenig, N.E., and Marks, F. (1981): <u>Cancer Lett.</u>, 11: 191-198.
10. Hammarström, S., Lindgren, J.A., Marcelo, C., Duell, E.A., Anderson, T.F., and Voorhees, J.J. (1979): <u>J. Invest. Dermatol.</u>, 73: 180-183.
11. Hennings, H., and Boutwell, R.K. (1970): <u>Cancer Res.</u>, 30: 312-320.
12. Kato, R., Nakadate, T., Yamamoto, S., and Sugimura, T. (1983): <u>Carcinogenesis</u>, 4: (in press).
13. Kozumbo, W.J., Seed, J.L., and Kensler, T.W. (1983): <u>Cancer Res.</u>, 43: 2555-2559.
14. Levine, L., and Ohuchi, K. (1978): <u>Cancer Res.</u>, 38: 4142-4146.
15. Lichti, U., Slaga, T.J., Ben, T., Patterson, E., Hennings, H., and Yuspa, S.H. (1977): <u>Proc. Natl. Acad. Sci. USA</u>, 74: 3908-3912.
16. Mufson, R.A., DeFeo, D., and Weinstein, I.B. (1979): <u>Mol. Pharmacol.</u>, 16: 569-578.
17. Nakadate, T., Yamamoto, S., Iseki, H., Sonoda, S., Takemura, S., Ura, A., Hosoda, Y., and Kato, R. (1982): <u>Gann</u>, 73: 841-843.
18. Nakadate, T., Yamamoto, S., Ishii, M., and Kato, R. (1982): <u>Cancer Res.</u>, 42: 2841-2845.
19. Nakadate, T., Yamamoto, S., Ishii, M., and Kato, R. (1982): <u>Carcinogenesis</u>, 3: 1411-1414.
20. O'Brien, T.G., Lewis, M.A., and Diamond, L. (1979): <u>Cancer Res.</u>, 39: 4477-4480.
21. O'Brien, T.G., Simsiman, R.C., and Boutwell, R.K. (1975): <u>Cancer Res.</u>, 35: 1662-1670.
22. Panganamala, R.V., Miller, J.S., Gwebu, E.T., Sharma, H.M., and Cornwell, D.G. (1977): <u>Prostaglandins</u>, 14: 261-271.

23. Schwarz, J.A., Viaje, A., Slaga, T.J., Yuspa, S.H., Hennings, H., and Lichti, U. (1977): Chem.-Biol. Interact., 17: 331-347.
24. Solanki, V., and Slaga, T.J. (1981): Proc. Natl. Acad. Sci. USA, 78: 2549-2553.
25. Sugimura, T. (1982): Gann, 73: 499-507.
26. Umezawa, K., Weinstein, I.B., Horowitz, A., Fujiki, H., Matsushima, T., and Sugimura, T. (1981): Nature, 290: 411-413.
27. Verma, A.K., Ashendel, C.L., and Boutwell, R.K. (1980): Cancer Res., 40: 308-315.
28. Yamasaki, H., Mufson, R.A., and Weinstein, I.B. (1979): Biochem. Biophys. Res. Commun., 80: 1081-1025.

Icosanoids and Cancer, edited by H. Thaler-Dao, et al. Raven Press, New York © 1984.

Arachidonic Acid Metabolism by Cells in Culture: Effects of Tumor Promoters

L. Levine, S. M. Goldstein, G. T. Snoek, and A. Rigas

Department of Biochemistry, Brandeis University, Waltham, Massachusetts 02254

One of the pleiotropic biochemical responses to tumor-promoting phorbol ester treatment in mouse skin and cultured cells is increased prostaglandin synthesis (7). Some phorbol esters are known to be potent tumor promoters in the two-stage model of carcinogenesis. This model was originally demonstrated in skin (4), but it also has been shown to be operative in liver (1,26,27), bladder (12), mammary gland (2), stomach (9), and cultured cells (23).

Although prostaglandin production has been associated with tumor formation, a causal relationship has never been demonstrated (18). The most compelling evidence that prostaglandin production is involved in the process of tumor formation has come from inhibition of tumor formation in vivo. Several inhibitors of prostaglandin synthesis are capable of inhibiting tumor promotion by a particularly potent tumor promoter, 12-0-tetradecanoyl phorbol-13-acetate (TPA), and this inhibition can be overcome by addition of specific prostaglandins (20,21). The possible relationship between prostaglandin synthesis and tumor formation has increased interest in mechanisms involved in regulation of prostaglandin synthesis and especially in mechanisms leading to stimulation of arachidonic acid metabolism by tumor promoters.

Arachidonic acid, the precursor of prostaglandins, is metabolized by a complex series of reactions. Inhibitors that act at different steps of the overall reaction have been described. For example, non-steroidal anti-inflammatory drugs, such as aspirin and indomethacin, inhibit the enzyme cyclooxygenase and block prostaglandin, prostacyclin and thromboxane synthesis (32). Anti-oxidants, such as butylated hydroxyanisole, inhibit both cyclooxygenase and lipoxygenase activities and block production of prostaglandins, prostacyclins, thromboxanes, hydroxyeicosatetraenoic acids (HETEs) and 6-sulfidopeptide-containing hydroxyeicosatetraenoic acids, the leukotrienes (LTs). The anti-inflammatory steroids, such as dexamethasone, inhibit expression of acylhydrolase activity (11,15), possibly by inducing the synthesis of a polypeptide inhibitor (8,13); and, as a result, besides inhibiting deacylation of cellular phospholipids, they also inhibit formation of both cyclooxygenase and lipoxygenase products. Most of the above inhibitors of arachidonic acid metabolism have been shown to block tumor production in vivo (17).

Retinoids, synthetic and natural derivatives of Vitamin A, also block
the formation of tumors, in vivo (30). Retinoids can block TPA-
stimulated prostaglandin production by some, but not all, cells (17,19,
25). For example, all trans retinoic acid (RA) inhibits 6-keto-PGF$_{1\alpha}$
production in bovine aorta smooth muscle cells (SMC) stimulated by TPA
(10 ng/ml) (Fig. 1) (10). Inhibition is seen with doses of RA as low as

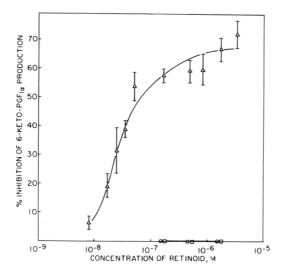

FIG. 1. Inhibition of 6-keto-PGF$_{1\alpha}$ production in SMC stimulated by TPA and treated with either RA ($\triangle$), retinol ($\square$), or
retinyl acetate ($\bigcirc$). Inhibition was determined by comparison
of RIAs of individual TPA-retinoid treated dishes (n=4) to
mean of dishes treated with TPA alone (0% inhibition) minus
mean of dishes without TPA (no stimulation). Values of inhibition for individual dishes were averaged and are expressed
as mean ± s.e.m. Significance was determined by comparison of
means by t test. Curve was fitted by a non-linear computer
plotting program (from 10).

16.6 μM. The dose response curve is steep, and shows saturation behavior, with maximal inhibition of 70%. Half maximal inhibition is caused
by RA at 27 nM. Retinol and retinyl acetate in doses as high as 1.7 μM
and 1.5 μM respectively do not inhibit significantly. Inhibition by RA
at 1.7 μM is not due to cytotoxicity as assessed by trypan blue exclusion. RA inhibition is not immediate; no difference between cells
stimulated by TPA and those treated with TPA and RA can be seen for the
first 90 minutes (10). Preincubation of cells with RA (1.7 μM) prior
to TPA stimulation increases the inhibition caused by RA, and the additional inhibition is proportional to the length of time of preincubation
with RA. The effect of a 3-hour preincubation of SMC with RA prior to
TPA stimulation is shown in Fig. 2. There is a lag before the stimulating effects of RA are seen, and this lag can be decreased by exposure
of cells to RA prior to TPA stimulation.

RA at 1.7 μM has no effect on binding of PDBU to SMC (10). Nor is

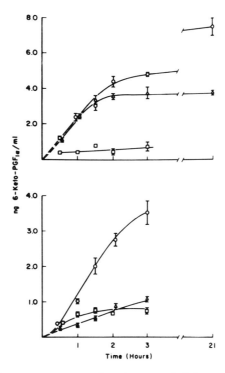

FIG. 2. (Top) Time course of release of 6-keto-PGF$_{1\alpha}$ into media after TPA stimulation. Points = mean ± s.e.m. of (○) cells treated with TPA (n=4), (△) cells treated with TPA and RA (n=4), and (□) minimal essential medium, no serum supplement (MEM) control cells (n=3). (Bottom) Effect of a 3-hour preincubation of RA on 6-keto-PGF$_{1\alpha}$ production. (○) cells preincubated with MEM prior to TPA. (△) cells preincubated with RA prior to TPA + RA, (□) control cells preincubated in MEM (from 10).

RA inhibition specific for SMC treated with TPA. RA at 1.7 µM inhibits 6-keto-PGF$_{1\alpha}$ production stimulated by serotonin, melittin, A-23187, and 10% fetal calf serum (10). RA seems to inhibit only stimulated cells and has no statistically significant effect on baseline levels in unstimulated cells. The stimulated 6-keto-PGF$_{1\alpha}$ production by exogenous arachidonic acid (5 µg/ml) also is not inhibited by RA. However, SMC are capable of yet further stimulation by TPA in the presence of exogenous arachidonic acid (AA), and RA (at 3.3 µM) does inhibit this additional 6-keto-PGF$_{1\alpha}$ production. When SMC, labeled with [^{14}C]AA, are treated with RA (1.7 µM) for 2 hours prior to TPA stimulation and then analyzed for release of radioactivity, the cpm/ml of media are similar between the two groups: 24,070 (TPA) vs. 21,570 (TPA + RA). However, duplicate assays of 6-keto-PGF$_{1\alpha}$ in each pool by RIA show a large inhibition: 6.0 ng/ml (TPA) vs. 2.0 ng/ml (TPA + RA). Analyses of these culture fluids by HPLC show that AA accounts for most of the released radioactivity, and the two radioactive fractions differ by only 4%, as does the total radioactivity eluting from the HPLC column. However, the 6-keto-PGF$_{1\alpha}$ radioactive fraction in the chromatogram from TPA + RA SMC media is only 47% as large as that for TPA stimulated cells.

Tumor promoters stimulate PGI_2 production by rat liver cells (29) (the C-9 cell line) in culture in a dose-dependent manner (Fig. 3). Indomethacin (0.34×10^{-6} M) and aspirin (6.0×10^{-5} M) inhibit the TPA-stimulated production of 6-keto-$PGF_{1\alpha}$. The C-9 liver cells synthesize PGE_2 and $PGF_{2\alpha}$ as well as PGI_2, but only 4% and 3% as much, respectively. Stimulation of arachidonic acid metabolism by TPA, increases the synthesis of PGE_2 and $PGF_{2\alpha}$ to the same extent as that of 6-keto-$PGF_{1\alpha}$. Increased levels of 6-keto-$PGF_{1\alpha}$ after TPA treatment are found also when measured after resolution by reversed phase high performance liquid chromatography. Stimulation of 6-keto-$PGF_{1\alpha}$ production in the C-9 cells after addition of 30 nM TPA takes 4 hours for completion (Fig. 4).

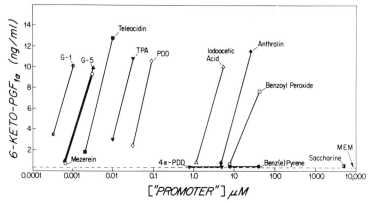

FIG. 3. Dose-response of 6-keto-$PGF_{1\alpha}$ production by C-9 liver cells after stimulation with gnidimacrin (G-1), gnilatimacrin (G-5), mezerein, teleocidin, TPA, PDD, iodoacetic acid, anthralin, and benzoyl peroxide. Benz(e)pyrene, saccharine and 4-α-PDD did not stimulate at the levels tested.

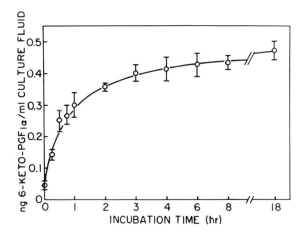

FIG. 4. Effect of time on stimulation of 6-keto-$PGF_{1\alpha}$ synthesis by TPA. Each point is the mean of at least 3 dishes; the bars indicate the standard deviation. The TPA concentration was 0.3×10^{-7} M.

Inhibition of protein synthesis by cycloheximide (by incubation of the cells with nM levels of cycloheximide for 4 hours) blocks the stimulation of 6-keto-$PGF_{1\alpha}$ synthesis by TPA (after the 4-hour treatment, the cycloheximide concentrations do not affect the cell viability as measured by trypan blue exclusion). The dose-dependent inhibition of TPA-stimulated 6-keto-$PGF_{1\alpha}$ production and protein synthesis are parallel. The identity of the protein whose synthesis is being inhibited by cyclo-heximide and is required for complete expression of TPA-stimulated 6-keto-$PGF_{1\alpha}$ production is unknown. The TPA-stimulated 6-keto-$PGF_{1\alpha}$ production is particularly sensitive to regulation by this short-lived protein, since stimulated 6-keto-$PGF_{1\alpha}$ production by combined epidermal growth factor (EGF) and vasopressin (ADH) treatment is not inhibited by a similar treatment with cycloheximide (Levine, unpublished). Several proteins must be considered as possible short-lived protein(s): 1. Acyl-hydrolase. In dog kidney cells, like in C-9 cells, arachidonic acid metabolism was stimulated by TPA and the TPA-stimulation was inhibited by cycloheximide. TPA stimulated acylhydrolase activity in the dog kidney cells and cycloheximide inhibited this as well. Thus, the essential short-lived protein could be an acylhydrolase. If so, mechanisms for liberation of arachidonic acid during TPA- and EGF-ADH stimulation are different (only TPA stimulation was inhibited by cycloheximide). 2. Growth factor. TPA could be inducing the synthesis of a growth factor which then stimulates prostaglandin production. Cultured cells can be stimulated to produce prostaglandins by EGF, platelet derived growth factor, sarcoma growth factor, interleukin 1 and interleukin 2 (17). 3. Regulation of acylhydrolase activity. Just as the anti-inflammatory steroids induce the synthesis and/or activation of a protein that inhibits phospholipase A_2 (8,13), TPA could be inducing the synthesis and/or activation of a protein that stimulates liberation of arachidonic acid. It could be the same protein as that induced by the anti-inflammatory steroid, but in a different conformation or in a different chemical state, e.g. a different state of phosphorylation. Some of this hypothetical polypeptide could exist preformed in a "neutral" or even an "inhibit" conformation and when stimulated by tumor promoters, it could be changed to the "not inhibit" conformation. This change of "neutral" or "inhibit" to "not inhibit" conformation could be mediated by a recently described TPA-induced Ca^{2+}, phospholipid dependent protein kinase (16). 4. Ca^{2+}, phospholipid dependent protein kinase. The short-lived protein could be this Ca^{2+}, phospholipid dependent protein kinase whose phosphorylated product regulates prostaglandin production. 5. TPA-receptor. This short-lived protein could also be the cell receptor for TPA, which as a result of binding to TPA is no longer available; e.g., it is internalized. More receptor must be synthesized before TPA-stimulation can continue.

The C-9 cells, treated with the Ca^{2+} ionophore, A-23187 (2 μM) for 1 hour, produce 20-50 times more 6-keto-$PGF_{1\alpha}$. The dependence on Ca^{2+} for TPA-stimulated prostaglandin synthesis in C-9 rat liver cells can be demonstrated with the use of reagents that inhibit Ca^{2+} function by different mechanisms. EGTA, which chelates Ca^{2+} ions, inhibits the TPA stimulation of 6-keto-$PGF_{1\alpha}$ in a dose-dependent manner (Fig. 5). The concentration of Ca^{2+} in the medium is 1.8 nM; 2 nM EGTA completely inhibits 6-keto-$PGF_{1\alpha}$ production in our experimental conditions. At 4 hours, 2 mM EGTA does not affect 6-keto-$PGF_{1\alpha}$ in the non-stimulated cells. Stimulation of 6-keto-$PGF_{1\alpha}$ synthesis by TPA is inhibited also

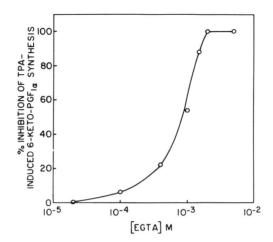

FIG. 5. Inhibition of TPA-stimulated 6-keto-PGF$_{1\alpha}$ synthesis
by increasing levels of EGTA ($\bigcirc$). Each <u>point</u> is the mean of
at least 3 dishes; analysis of each culture dish agreed within
20% (from 29).

by both nifedipine which blocks Ca^{2+} channels in the cell membrane and
TMB-8 which inhibits the translocation of the intracellular Ca^{2+} ions.
When both Ca^{2+} antagonists are added at low concentrations, they are
found to act synergistically. At the concentrations used, these Ca^{2+}
antagonists do not affect basal 6-keto-PGF$_{1\alpha}$ production, viability as
measured by trypan blue exclusion, or protein synthesis when measured
at 4 hours.

Anti-inflammatory steroids are effective inhibitors of tumor promotion <u>in vivo</u> (17). They also inhibit arachidonic acid metabolism <u>in
vivo</u> and in cell culture (8,11,13,15). Dexamethasone inhibits stimulation of 6-keto-PGF$_{1\alpha}$ synthesis by TPA in C-9 cells (Fig. 6), even at
nM levels (2.55 x 10^{-8} M dexamethasone inhibits the TPA-stimulated 6-
keto-PGF$_{1\alpha}$ synthesis 50%). Inhibition by dexamethasone does not occur
immediately: there is a lag of 45-60 minutes before inhibition is seen
and maximum inhibition is seen only after 6 hours.

It is generally accepted that metabolism of arachidonic acid via
cyclooxygenase and lipoxygenase pathways is limited by the availability
of free arachidonic acid (33). Arachidonic acid is esterified in phospholipids in most eukaryotic cells, so that liberation of arachidonic
acid by deacylation of the cellular lipids is a prerequisite for arachidonic acid metabolism. Several mechanisms for such deacylation have
been described (3,5,6,14,28), one of which is a phospholipase C attack
to form diacylglycerol followed by deacylation of the diacylglycerol by
a diacylglycerol lipase (3,14,28). Recently, an inhibitor of diacylglycerol lipase, which does not affect phospholipase C or phospholipase
A$_2$ activities, has been described (31). This inhibitor, RHC 80267 (1,6-
di-(0-(carbamoyl)-cyclohexanone oxime)hexane), should block arachidonic
acid metabolism in cells that utilize a diacylglycerol lipase for
liberation of free arachidonic acid. RHC 80267 inhibits 6-keto-PGF$_{1\alpha}$
production by the C-9 liver cells when stimulated by thrombin, vasopressin and synergistic stimulation by epidermal growth factor and

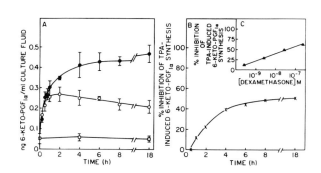

FIG. 6. Effect of time on the inhibition of TPA-stimulated 6-keto-PGF$_{1\alpha}$ synthesis by dexamethasone. A: ●, 0.3 x 10^{-7} M TPA. ○, 0.3 x 10^{-7} M TPA 2.6 x 10^{-8} M dexamethasone; □, 2.6 x 10^{-8} M dexamethasone. Each <u>point</u> is the mean of at least 3 culture dishes; <u>bars</u>, S.D. In the presence of MEM 6-keto-PGF$_{1\alpha}$ (0.034 ± 0.005 ng/ml) was produced. B: difference curve. X, TPA minus TPA-dexamethasone (A); C: percentage of inhibition (dose-response curve) of TPA-stimulated 6-keto-PGF$_{1\alpha}$ synthesis by dexamethasone, ▲. Each <u>point</u> is the mean of at least 5 dishes; analysis of each dish agreed to within 20% (from 29).

TABLE 1. <u>Effect of the diacylglycerol lipase inhibitor, RHC 80267</u>
<u>[1,6-di-(0-(carbamoyl)cyclohexanone oxime)hexane], on</u>
<u>arachidonic acid metabolism by rat liver (C-9) cells</u>

Treatment	6-keto-PGF$_{1\alpha}$ ng/ml
MEM	0.12 ± 0.021 (6)[a]
RHC (60 µM)	0.19 ± 0.015 (6)
Thrombin (0.1 unit/ml)	0.77 ± 0.026 (3)
RHC (60 µM) + thrombin (0.1 unit/ml)	0.40 ± 0.029 (3)
ADH (0.05 µM)	0.78 ± 0.041 (3)
RHC (60 µM) + ADH (0.05 µM)	0.32 ± 0.01 (3)
EGF (0.01 µg/ml) + ADH (0.05 µM)	14.83 ± 0.025 (4)
RHC (60 µM) + EGF (0.01 µg/ml) + ADH (0.05 µM)	4.39 ± 0.198 (4)
TPA (0.017 µM)	2.36 ± 0.56 (4)
RHC (60 µM) + TPA (0.017 µM)	2.28 ± 0.78 (4)

[a]Each value given is the mean ± SD for the number of dishes in parentheses.

vasopressin but not when stimulated by TPA (Table 1). It is possible that TPA's stimulation of AA metabolism proceeds through liberation of AA by a mechanism different than that of other agonists, but because TPA's stimulation depends on synthesis of a new protein, an explanation for the lack of inhibition by RHC 80267 may not be that simple. At the level of RHC 80267 used (60 μM), cyclooxygenase activity is not affected.

Oligomycin, antimycin and 2,4-dinitrophenol, inhibitors of cellular ATP accumulation, also stimulate arachidonic acid metabolism by C-9 cells, and their stimulation is synergistic with other agonists. The synergistic stimulations of arachidonic acid metabolism by TPA and oligomycin and TPA and antimycin are inhibited by RHC 80267 (120 μM) (Table 2). As with 60 μM RHC 80267, cyclooxygenase activity in C-9 cells is not affected by 120 μM RHC 80267.

The enzyme mechanisms leading to liberation of arachidonic acid by TPA in the C-9 liver cells appear to include hydrolysis of diacylglycerol by a diacylglycerol lipase (most likely, a Ca^{2+}-dependent phospholipase C attacks a phospholipid and produces the diacylglycerol). Mechanisms leading to stimulation of arachidonic metabolism by oligomycin, antimycin and 2,4-dinitrophenol are less clear. One possibility is that the diacylglycerol is phosphorylated to form phosphatidic acid and it is the relative rates of deacylation and phosphorylation of the diacylglycerol that regulates arachidonic acid metabolism in the C-9 cells. A scheme that illustrates such a mechanism is shown in Fig. 7.

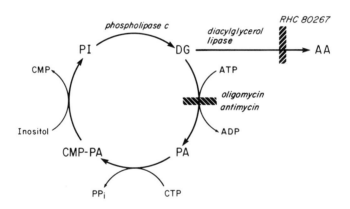

FIG. 7. Schematic pathways leading to liberation of arachidonic acid in rat liver cells (the C-9 cell line).

In this scheme, the phosphatidylinositol cycle is depicted (22), but, as yet, the metabolic pool of phospholipids in C-9 cells giving rise to arachidonic acid has not been identified. Another possibility is that more than one mechanism for liberation of arachidonic acid in the C-9 liver cells exists; the second being hydrolysis by a phospholipase A_2 or phospholipase A_1 followed by hydrolysis of the arachidonic acid by a lysophospholipase. Thus, the stimulation of arachidonic acid metabolism by inhibitors of cellular ATP accumulation would reflect inhibition of Acyl·COA synthetase activity and blocked reesterification of the liberated arachidonic acid. Inhibition of arachidonic acid metabolism by ATP in rat liver homogenates has been reported (24). Whereas the diacylglycerol lipase inhibitor blocks arachidonic acid metabolism by the C-9 liver cells, it does not inhibit prostaglandin production by all cells (Levine, unpublished).

TABLE 2. Effect of the diacylglycerol lipase inhibitor, RHC 80267 [1,6-di-(O-(carbamoyl)-cyclohexanone oxime)hexane], on arachidonic acid metabolism by rat liver cells (C-9) stimulated by TPA in the presence of oligomycin or antimycin

Treatment	6-keto-PGF$_{1\alpha}$ ng/ml[a]	PGE$_2$	PGF$_{2\alpha}$
MEM	0.24 ± 0.025 (4)	<0.05[b]	<0.05[b]
TPA	3.18 ± 0.327 (4)	0.078	0.056
Oligomycin (6.2 µM) + TPA (0.034 µM)	80.5 ±14.24 (4)	0.354	0.363
Oligomycin (6.2 µM) + TPA (0.034 µM) + RHC (120 µM)	4.45 ± 0.726 (4)	0.079	0.068
Antimycin (1.8 µM) + TPA (0.034 µM)	29.0 ± 1.73 (4)	0.178	0.191
Antimycin (1.8 µM) + TPA (0.034 µM) + RHC (120 µM)	5.8 ± 0.86 (4)	0.086	0.099

[a]Each value given is the mean ± SD for the number of dishes in parentheses.
[b]For PGE$_2$ and PGF$_{2\alpha}$ analyses, appropriate dishes were pooled, and RIAs performed in duplicate.

ACKNOWLEDGEMENTS

This work was supported by Grants GM-27256 and CA-17309 from the National Institutes of Health. L.L. is an American Cancer Society Professor of Biochemistry (Award PRP-21). G.T.S. was a Queen Wilhelmina Foundation Fellow from the Netherlands. S.G. was supported by NIH National Research Service Award AM06999-01.

We thank Dr. Charles A. Sutherland of the Revlon Health Care Group, Research & Development Division, Tuckahoe, New York, for the gift of the RHC-80267.

REFERENCES

1. Armuth, V., and Berenblum, I. (1972): Cancer Res., 32:2259-2262.
2. Armuth, V., and Berenblum, I. (1974): Cancer Res., 34:2704-2707.
3. Bell, R. L., Kennerly, D. A., Stanford, N., and Majerus, P. W. (1979): Proc. Natl. Acad. Sci. U.S.A., 76:3238-3241.
4. Berenblum, I. (1975): In: Cancer a Comprehensive Treatise, Vol. 1, edited by F. F. Becker, pp. 323-344. Plenum Press, New York.
5. Billah, M. M., Lapetina, E. G., and Cuatrecasas, P. (1981): J. Biol. Chem., 256:5399-5403.
6. Bills, T. K., Smith, J. B., and Silver, M. J. (1977): J. Clin. Invest., 60:1-6.
7. Diamond, L., O'Brien, T. G., and Baird, W. M. (1980): Adv. Cancer Res., 32:1-74.
8. Flower, R. J., and Blackwell, G. J. (1979): Nature (London), 278:456-459.
9. Goerttler, K., Loehrke, H., Schweizer, J., and Hesse, B. (1979): Cancer Res., 39:1293-1297.
10. Goldstein, S. M., Moskowitz, M. A., and Levine, L. (1983) (submitted for publication).
11. Gryglewski, R., Panczenko, B., Korbut, R., Grodzinska, L., and Ocetkiewicz, A. (1975): Prostaglandins, 10:343-355.
12. Hicks, R. M., Chowaniec, J., and Wakefield, J. (1978): In: Carcinogenesis, Vol. 2, edited by T. J. Slaga, A. Sivak, and R. K. Boutwell, pp. 475-489, Raven Press, New York.
13. Hirata, F., Schiffmann, E., Venkatasubramanian, K., Salomon, D., and Axelrod, J. (1980): Proc. Natl. Acad. Sci. U.S.A., 77:2533-2536.
14. Hong, S. L., and Deykin, D. (1979): J. Biol. Chem., 254:11463-11466.
15. Hong, S. L., and Levine, L. (1976): Proc. Natl. Acad. Sci. U.S.A., 73:1730-1734.
16. Kraft, A. S., and Anderson, W. B. (1983): Nature (London), 301:621-623.
17. Levine, L. (1982): In: Prostaglandins and Cancer, First International Conference, Prostaglandins and Related Lipids, Vol. 2, edited by T. J. Powles, R. S. Bockman, K. V. Honn, and P. Ramwell, pp. 189-204, Alan R. Liss, Inc., New York.
18. Levine, L. (1981): Adv. Cancer Res., 35:49-79.
19. Levine, L., and Ohuchi, K. (1978): Nature (London), 276:274-275.
20. Lupulescu, A. (1978): Nature (London), 272:634-636.
21. Marks, F., Berry, D. L., Bertsch, S., Furstenberger, G., and Richter, H. (1982): In: Carcinogenesis, Vol. 7, edited by E. Hecker, N. E. Fusenig, W. Kunz, F. Marks, and H. W. Thielmann, pp. 69-73. Raven Press, New York.

22. Mitchell, R. H. (1975): Biochim. Biophys. Acta, 415:81-147.
23. Mondal, S., Brankow, D. W., and Heidelberger, C. (1976): Cancer Res., 36:2254-2260.
24. Morita, I., and Murota, S.-I. (1980): Biochim. Biophys. Acta, 619: 428-431.
25. Mufson, R. A., DeFoe, D., and Weinstein, I. B. (1979): Molec. Pharmacol., 16:569-578.
26. Peraino, C., Fry, R. J. M., and Grube, D. D. (1978): In: Carcino-genesis, Vol. 2, edited by T. J. Slaga, A. Sivak, and R. K. Boutwell, pp.421-432, Raven Press, New York.
27. Pitot, H. C., and Sirica, A. E. (1980): Biochim. Biophys. Acta, 605: 191-215.
28. Rittenhouse-Simmons, S., and Deykin, D. (1981): In: Platelets in Biology and Pathology, Vol. 2, edited by J. L. Gordon, pp. 349-372. Elsevier/North Holland, Amsterdam, New York, and Oxford.
29. Snoek, G. T., and Levine, L. (1983): Cancer Res. (in press).
30. Sporn, M. B., Dunlop, N. M., Newton, D. L., and Smith, J. M. (1976): Fed. Proc., 35:1332-1338.
31. Sutherland, C. A., and Amin, D. (1982): J. Biol. Chem., 257:14006-14010.
32. Vane, J. R. (1971): Nature New Biol., 231:232-235.
33. Vogt, W., Suzuki, T., and Babilli, S. (1966): Mem. Soc. Endocrinol., 14:137-142.

Icosanoids and Cancer, edited by H. Thaler-Dao, et al. Raven Press, New York © 1984.

Icosanoids and Chromosome Damage

I. Emerit and P. Cerutti

Institut Biomédical des Cordeliers, Paris 6, France; and Départment of Carcinogenesis, Swiss Institute for Experimental Cancer Research, CH-1066 Epalinges/Lausanne, Switzerland

The role of chromosome mutation at the origin of cancer has been intensely investigated since the first observations of abnormal chromosomes in malignant cells in the end of the nineteenth century. Ionizing radiation, certain viruses and a great variety of chemical substances are clastogenic i.e. able to induce chromosome breakage, and at the same time carcinogenic, i.e. able to initiate the malignant process. The notion of a correlation between chromosome breakage and cancer is supported by the high risk of cancer in patients with the so-called congenital breakage syndromes (Bloom's syndrome, Fanconi's anemia and Ataxia telangiectasia) (18). The postulated effect of chromosome damaging agents on DNA is especially intriguing when viewed in conjunction with recent research suggesting that cellular oncogenes (c-onc genes) are activated as a result of the chromosomal rearrangements associated with certain cancers (17).

Nature has developed enzyme systems to repair DNA damage, but besides possible repair deficiencies, DNA damage may exceed the capacity of a normal repair system. This may be true in particular in conditions, in which chromosome damage is produced in a chronic self-sustained process. Free radicals and so-called clastogenic factors (CF) may play a role in this process.

CF were first described by radiobiologists as an indirect effect of ionizing radiation (19, 22, 34). They exist also in the plasma and in supernatants of blood cultures from patients with chronic inflammatory diseases such as progressive systemic sclerosis, lupus erythematosus, dermatomyositis, rheumatoid arthritis and Crohn's ileocolitis (for review see 7) as well as from patients with the cancer-prone genetic diseases Ataxia telangiectasia (35) and Bloom's syndrome (10,13). In the latter conditions the supernatant of fibroblast cultures was studied, too, and contained clastogenic activity. Recently we showed that CF play a role in the clastogenic action of the tumor promoter phorbol-12-myristate-13-acetate (PMA) (11, 12). This phorbolester has not only tumor promoting properties, but causes also important inflammatory changes in mouse skin. PMA is known to stimulate the oxidation of arachidonic acid (AA), and its inflammatory properties can be blocked by compounds which inhibit the conversion of AA to prostaglandins, thromboxanes and leukotrienes (36). In the following we will illustrate using PMA as an example that icosanoids may be involved in the clastogenic mechanisms of this tumor promoter and in the production of chromosome damage by the other CF mentioned.

PMA, A CLASTOGENIC AGENT

The mouse skin tumor promoter PMA does not form covalent adducts with DNA and its mutagenic potency in several systems is low or absent (38). Therefore until recently it appeared that PMA exerts its pleio - tropic effects via epigenetic mechanisms without causing DNA damage. However it is now evident that PMA is a potent clastogen for human lymphocytes (11, 12) and mouse epidermal cells (6), and that it induces aneuploidy in yeast (30) and single strand breaks in neutrophils (3). Reports on the effects of PMA on SCE frequencies were discordant, probably because of variable culture conditions (27). In our laboratory, we obtain a clastogenic effect (with rare exceptions) using PMA (CCR, Eden Prairie, MN) at a dose of 10-100ng/ml, dissolved in acetone at final concentrations not exceeding 0.1 %. The incidence of structural chromosome aberrations was 33.5 ± 8.2 for 100ng/ml and 26.4 ± 7.5 for ng/ml PMA. Even doses of 1ng/ml were still clastogenic (13.0 ± 5.3) compared to acetone treated (7.2 ± 8.6) and untreated controls (5.7 ± 2.7). The SCE-rates for the doses of 10 and 100ng/ml were 7.7 ± 3.4 and 8.0 ± 2.4 respectively relative to 5.2 ± 2.2 SCE per mitosis for untreated controls.

It is important to establish the cultures with a medium which possesses low radical scavenging potential (23) such as TC medium 199 from Flow laboratories and to supplement this medium rather with human AB serum than with fetal calf serum which, probably due to hemolysis, may show considerable variation in superoxide dismutase levels (1).

The chromosome aberrations induced by PMA are mainly of the chromatid type. Aberrations involving both chromatids represented only 18-19 % in 72 h cultures, Rings, dicentrics and structurally rearranged chromosomes were only present at 1.7 %. There were also cells with numerous chromatid breaks, minute fragments and reunion figures, scored as "fragmentations", which represented 1.6 % of the total cells with aberrations. Polyploid cells were frequent in 72 h cultures (18.5 ± 5.2), but were not found in 48 h cultures. Almost all were tetraploid and many showed premature chromosome condensation (S-phase, G_1 and G_2 phase PCC's).

The weak promoter 4-O-methyl PMA induced a statistically significant increase in aberrations only at a dose of 1000ng/ml and the non - promoter phorbol was completely inactive.

INDUCTION OF A CLASTOGENIC FACTOR

The supernatants of blood or lymphocyte culture from normal donors treated with 10 or 100 ng/ml PMA were collected after 72 h and purified by ultrafiltration (7). Under these conditions media components in the 1-10000 molecular weight range are isolated and concentrated 20 times. If small aliquots of these concentrated ultrafiltrates are added to test cultures set up with blood or lymphocytes from normal donors, the frequency of structural chromosome aberrations (mostly chromatid aberrations) is increased in these cultures compared to simultaneous controls receiving identically prepared ultrafiltrates from solvent instead of PMA treated cultures. Experiments using radioactive PMA allowed to determine the PMA concentrations of the ultrafiltrates. More than 99 % of the radioactivity was eliminated during the isolation procedure of CF and the residual PMA concentrations in the test cultures varied between 0.005 and 0.008ng /ml depending on the sizes of the aliquots added (12). PMA at this concentration is no longer clastogenic. It could thus be concluded that the clastogenic effect of the ultrafiltrates was not due to contamination by residual PMA, but produced by low molecular weight components released by the cells in response to PMA treatment.

No simple dose relationship was observed between the concentration of PMA and the potency of the clastogenic components which were induced. In contrast to PMA the non-promoter phorbol was not clastogenic and did not induce clastogenic activity in the supernatants of cell cultures.

CONTRIBUTION OF THE DIFFERENT BLOOD CELLS TO THE FORMATION OF CF

Conventional cytogenetic analysis is based on chromosome preparations derived from cultures of whole blood or "regular" lymphocytes which are contaminated with platelets, monocytes and polymorphonuclear leukocytes (PMN). Since specific receptors for phorbolesters are present not only on lymphocytes but also on the other blood cells with the exception of erythrocytes, it seemed probable that PMA acted in blood cultures not only on lymphocytes but also on the other blood cells present. According to date from the literature, the biological responses to PMA vary from one cell type to the other :

- PMN respond with a respiratory burst and produce superoxide and hydrogen peroxide. The PMA effect is analogous to the phagocytic process (5, 20, 24).
- Monocytes also display increased O_2^- production and stimulated cells manifest enhanced cytotoxic efficacy (24).
- Platelets aggregate upon PMA treatment and release serotonin and other pharmacologic mediators (45, 46).
- Lymphocytes are producing little or no O_2^- but respond in other ways. PMA is mitogenic, induces the formation of a mitogenic factor, (37) the production of T-cell growth factor (33) and increases phospholipid metabolism (44).

TABLE 1. <u>Effect of addition of monocytes and PMN to 2.5 x 10^6 "pure" lymphocytes for CF formation.</u>

Number of cells added	% cells with aberrations in CF-treated cultures	
x 10^4	Monocytes	PMN
0	8.3 $\pm$ 4.4	8.4 $\pm$ 4.4
5	19.8 $\pm$ 4.8	
10	23.5 $\pm$ 5.3	
15	29.0 $\pm$ 6.8	
25	26.4 $\pm$ 10.9	13.5 $\pm$ 6.6
50		14.0 $\pm$ 3.5
100		15.0 $\pm$ 3.5
250		17.7 $\pm$ 7.3
500		20.5 $\pm$ 6.0

The result of our study showed that ultrafiltrates from "pure"
lymphocytes (residual monocytes and PMN not exceeding 1-2 %, absence of
platelets and erythrocytes) were essentially inactive. Addition of monocytes, PMN and platelets regularly resulted in supernatants with clastogenic activity (16).

Cultures of purified monocytes and PMN were capable also of producing CF in the absence of lymphocytes. In 4 experiments, monocytes atta-
ched to plastic were washed with medium and then treated with PMA for
1 h. The ultrafiltrates from media conditioned by 1 to 1.8×10^6 monocytes yielded aberration rates in the test system of 18.5 % compared
to 6.0 % obtained with ultrafiltrates of similar numbers of monocytes
which had not been exposed to PMA. When the monocytes were first deta-
ched from the plates with ice-cold PBS and then exposed to PMA for 1 h,
the aberration rates induced by the medium ultrafiltrates were lower,
although significant clastogenicity was still observed relative to untreated controls (10.8 and 4.0 % respectively).

CF preparations from PMA-treated PMN consistently showed clastogenic activity that was detected already after 60min incubation of the
PMN with PMA and did not change up to 48 h. Increasing numbers of PMN
induced increasing frequencies of aberrations in the test culture system:
50, 100 and 500×10^4 PMN yielded aberration rates of 10.0, 15.0 and
18.8 % respectively.

The comparaison of results obtained with lymphocyte preparations
from heparinized blood which contain 5-10 platelets per lymphocyte and
preparations which are platelet-free from defibrinized blood suggest
that also platelets can contribute to the formation of CF (both types of
lymphocyte cultures were essentially free of monocytes and PMN). The CF-
preparations from platelet-containing cultures were considerably active
(13.0 ± 4.1 % mitosis with aberrations) relative to those from platelet-
free cultures (2.6 ± 1.6 %).

We may conclude from these data that the CF isolated from blood
cultures after 72 h cultivation in presence of PMA consists of accumulated clastogenic material produced by the different types of blood cells.
In this system the lymphocytes, as the only dividing cells in culture ,
are the indicators for the presence of clastogenic material, but their
contribution in the formation of CF seems to be minimal compared to the
other blood cells.

EFFECT OF PMA ON AA-METABOLISM OF HUMAN LYMPHOCYTES

PMA represents the prototype of a membrane active agent and interacts with membrane receptors in a hormone-like fashion. Receptor binding
and calcium-calmodulin mediated activation of phospholipase A_2 results
in the release of free AA which is converted to prostaglandins, thromboxanes, prostacyclines and leukotrienes via the cyclooxygenase and the
lipoxygenase pathways. PMA has been shown to stimulate the synthesis of
prostaglandins in mouse skin and dog kidney cells. Increased levels of
prostaglandins were found in the supernatants of PMA treated fibroblast
cultures (36). In bovine lymphocytes, rapid stimulation of phospholipid
metabolism was observed after exposure to tumor promoting phorbolesters
(44). For this reason, we studied a possible relationship between PMA
effects on AA-metabolism and formation of CF.

Regular human lymphocytes (i.e. Ficoll-hypaque preparations from heparinized blood which are contamined with a small number of platelets, monocytes and other leukocytes) were labelled in their membrane phospholipids with ^{3}H-AA and incubated in TC medium 199 plus 20 % heat-inactivated human AB serum for 48 hours in presence of PMA. The long incubation period was chosen in analogy to our cytogenetic studies. The culture media were then acidified to pH 3.5 and extracted with ethylacetate. The total radioactivity of the samples was counted and the content of the extracts determined by thinlayer chromatography. Authentic markers of AA-metabolites were used for product identification.

Approximately 30 % more ^{3}H-AA label was released by the PMA treated lymphocytes relative to untreated controls. Most of the additional radioactivity in the PMA treated samples was AA, while the content in prostaglandins , thromboxane A_2 and HETEs (HPETES) was comparable. However approximately four times more radioactivity accumulated at the start of the chromatogram relative to controls. This highly polar material remains unidentified.

TABLE 2. Release of ^{3}H-AA and metabolites from ^{3}H-AA labelled human lymphocytes exposed to PMA

	Extractable radioactivity	Start	PG	TX	H(P)ETE	AA
Control	20.0	1.3	0.7	2.1	2.2	10.1 %
PMA 10ng/ml	33.4	4.2	0.7	2.2	2.0	20.5 %
PMA 50ng/ml	30.2	5.1	0.3	1.6	2.4	19.1 %

ANTICLASTOGENIC EFFECT OF INHIBITORS OF AA METABOLISM

The mechanism of action of a variety of structurally different antipromoters may involve the inhibition of a step in the oxidative metabolism of AA. For example the anti-inflammatory steroid fluocinolone-acetonide exerts its antipromotional effect probably via inhibition of phospholipase A_2. Similarly non-steroidal anti-inflammatory agents which inhibit AA-cyclooxygenase and/or lipoxygenase appear to possess antipromotional properties (40,41). The data in table 3 show that these drugs inhibit also completely or partially PMA-induced chromosome damage.

TABLE 3. Anticlastogenic effect of inhibitors of the AA-cascade

Inhibitor	conc. μM	PMA (100 ng/ml)	PMA + inhibitor	
fluocinolone	22	26.5 $\pm$ 5.7	8.7 $\pm$ 3.1	oo
indomethacin	28	26.2 $\pm$ 9.5	9.0 $\pm$ 4.9	oo
flufenamic acid	36	25.2 $\pm$ 6.1	4.0 $\pm$ 2.8	oo
NDGA [a]	20	26.0 $\pm$ 4.0	7.0 $\pm$ 7.0	oo
BN 1048 [b]	36	29.6 $\pm$ 7.4	11.5 $\pm$ 4.4	oo
BN 1015	33	28.5 $\pm$ 9.1	9.4 $\pm$ 6.4	oo
ETYA [c]	52	26.6 $\pm$ 8.2	17.1 $\pm$ 4.2	oo
imidazole	150	24.6 $\pm$ 4.8	17.7 $\pm$ 7.7	ns

oo $p < 0.001$ ns = not significant. a nordihydroguaiaretic acid b BN 1048 and BN 1015 were kindly provided by Dr Braquet, Institut Beaufour, Paris .c 5, 8, 11, 14-eicosatetraynoic acid.

Fluocinolone, a known phospholipase inhibitor, indomethacin and flufenamic acid, which preferentially inhibit the cyclooxygenase pathway, as well as the lipoxygenase inhibitors NDGA, BN 1048, and BN 1015 were anticlastogenic. The AA analogue ETYA which inhibits both pathways was only moderately active at concentrations from 50 to 250 μM. Similarly imidazol, an inhibitor of thromboxane synthetase, was only a moderate anticlastogen in a mM dose range.

From these data it can be concluded that AA-metabolism is involved in the induction of aberrations by PMA, but since inhibitors of both pathways possessed substantial activity, it is not possible to relate a particular metabolic step to the clastogenic action (15).

Certain of these drugs were also studied for their influence on the clastogenic action of CF in the test culture system. Indomethacin, flufenamic acid and NDGA again reduced the chromosome aberration rate in the CF treated cultures. Also ETYA was clearly anticlastogenic at a dose of 52 μM, while imidazole was only moderately protective.

Since there is no simple procedure to remove these drugs quantitatively from the media, it could not be tested whether they also inhibited formation of CF.

ANTICLASTOGENIC EFFECT OF ANTIOXIDANTS

As already mentioned leukocytes respond to PMA with a respiratory burst. It was therefore of interest to determine whether scavenging of O_2^- by superoxide dismutase (SOD) would have a protector effect against PMA induced chromosome damage. Furthermore in previous work with CF from irradiated blood, patients with chronic inflammatory diseases and subjects with Bloom's syndrome, SOD was found to be anticlastogenic.

The data in table 4 show that the clastogenic action of PMA on human lymphocytes can also be fully suppressed by bovine CuZn SOD. The chromosome aberration rate induced by PMA (100ng/ml) was 36.7 % and only 5.3 % in presence of SOD ($p < 0.001$). Also the clastogenic effect of CF in the test culture system was suppressed, if SOD was added before addition of CF to the cultures (24.4 and 4.4 %mitoses with aberrations respectively). Since bovine erythrocyte SOD has a molecular weight of about 30,000, it is removed by our standard ultrafiltration procedure for the preparation of CF. Therefore we also compared the clastogenicity of CF preparations induced by PMA in the presence and absence of SOD. The potency of the CF was decreased from 17.3 ± 2.1 % to 5.0 ± 3.6 % mitoses with aberrations when SOD at 10 ug/ml was present together with PMA (10, 11, 15). Also the increased production of CF after addition of 2.5 millions of PMN to pure lymphocytes was prevented when SOD was present from the beginning of the cultivation period (8.4 ± 4.0 % abnormal mitoses in presence of SOD relative to 18.0 ± 2.0 without SOD) ; similarly the formation of CF by monocytes and PMN in absence of lymphocytes was prevented by the addition of 10 μg/ml SOD (16).

In conclusion, SOD inhibited the clastogenic activity of PMA, formation of CF and the activity of previously formed CF.

Since O_2^- is dismutated to molecular oxygen and H_2O_2 and since H_2O_2 is also produced during the respiratory burst, the influence of catalase on the breakage phenomenon was studied. No consistent results could be obtained with a dose of 50 μg/ml, which is a protective dose in radiation induced chromosome damage (28). In 4 of 12 experiments, the PMA induced aberration rate was decreased, but no significant effect was observed on the mean breakage rate derived from the entire data. On the other hand identical concentrations of catalase prevented the formation of CF by isolated PMN. Glutathione peroxidase in the range of 0.06 to 0.3 μU/ml decreased the PMA induced aberrations rate but had only a minor effect on CF formation by PMN.

Interaction of O_2^- with H_2O_2 may lead to $OH^{\cdot}$ radical formation in a metal catalyzed Haber-Weiss reaction. The protective effect of mannitol was an indication for the involvement of $OH^{\cdot}$ in the production of chromosome damage, while dimethylfuran, a scavenger of singlet oxygen was not protective (15).

Also antioxidants such as butylated hydroxytoluene (BHT) and butylated hydroxyanisole (BHA) were protective at concentrations of 1 μM.

TABLE 4. Anticlastogenic effect of antioxidants

Inhibitor conc.		PMA	PMA + antioxidant
		% cells with aberrations	
SOD	10 μg/ml	36.7	5.3 oo
Catalase	50 μg/ml	24.8	23.4 ns
GSH peroxid.	0.06 μU/ml	29.4	14.0 oo
Mannitol	100 mM	31.0	15.5 oo
Dimethylfuran	0.5 mM	31.0	28.0 ns
BHT	1 μM	28.2	12.1 oo
BHA	1 μM	28.2	11.4 oo

oo $p < 0,001$ ns = not significant

MEMBRANE-MEDIATED CHROMOSOME DAMAGE

From the observation that both active oxygen species and products of the AA-cascade represent intermediates in PMA induced clastogenicity, we have derived the model of "membrane-mediated chromosomal damage" (4, 15). It proposes that membrane-active agents induce chromosomal damage by eliciting an oxidative burst, stimulating the AA-cascade or creating conformational changes in membranes. The relative contribution of the two pathways depends on the cell type and the agent. The release of free AA which is converted to prostaglandins, prostacyclins, thromboxanes and leukotrienes via the cyclooxygenase and the lipoxygenase pathways, is the consequence of the interaction of PMA with membranes. Lipid hydroperoxides are formed with the participation of active oxygen and release active oxygen upon their transformation into more stable derivatives. Together with aldehydic breakdown products and free AA they represent probably the principal components of the clastogenic material called CF. This CF is not only the mediator between the events at the membranes and the genome of the stimulated cell, but communicates clastogenic activity also to other cells and is transferable into other culture systems.

According to preliminary chromatographic data, there is increase in free AA of about 30 % in supernatant of PMA treated lymphocytes. This increased availability of free AA may further contribute to the production of clastogenic material by other cells. For instance, monocytes synthesize icosanoids from T-lymphocyte derived AA (21) and the initiation of the AA-cascade of platelets is also dependent on the availability of free AA. Recent reports describe complexe interregulatory relationships between blood cells and the products obtained via the cyclooxygenase and the lipoxygenase pathways (25,39). It is likely that the components of CF preparations also react among each other and not only with cell membranes. Free radical reactions certainly play a role as indicated by the inhibitory effect of SOD and mannitol. It is interesting that CF preparations exposed during 30 min to 10 ug/ml SOD and subsequently filtered through membranes retaining the SOD are less clastogenic than the initial preparations (chromosome aberration rates 20.0 and 6.0 % respectively). The oxidation of membranes in response to PMA may further impair membrane integrity and result in additional stimulation of phospholipid degradation. In this case a self-sustaining autocatalytic process may establish itself.

As a consequence of its membrane-active properties PMA is an "indirect" DNA damaging agent, i.e. it interacts first with a non-DNA target which produces the ultimate clastogen. Maximal concentration of clastogen may be produced with a considerable delay following PMA addition and continue to the end of the incubation period. This could explain why the frequency of chromosome aberrations varies considerably as a function of exposure time (10) and also why 72 h cultures, in which about 50 % of mitoses are at their 2nd division, show a predominance of chromatid type aberrations. Another characteristic of membrane-mediated chromosome damage is the discrepancy between the potency of production of chromosome damage and the relative low capacity for the induction of SCE (15).

ANALOGOUS MECHANISMS WITH CLASTOGENIC FACTORS FROM OTHER SOURCES.

Low doses of ionizing radiation create oxidative damage to membranes with formation of lipid-peroxidation products such as lipid peroxide radicals ($ROO^\bullet$), lipid hydroperoxides (ROOH) and fragmentation products such as malonaldehyde (31). The latter have been shown to be mutagenic, carcinogenic and clastogenic (2).

O_2^- from endogenous sources could be at the origin of the CF occuring in the various diseases with spontaneous chromosome instability. The causes for the increased fluxes of O_2^- may be different from one disease to the other. The importance of activated oxygen species for bacterial killing by phagocytosing cells has been demonstrated as well as their possible role in tissue damage during inflammation as a consequence of the O_2^- release from inflammatory cells into the extracellular space poor in endogenous SOD (32). O_2^- production by inflammatory cells may lead to lipid peroxidation of membranes resulting in phospholipase activation (29) and the formation of icosanoids from released AA via the cyclooxygenase and the lipoxygenase pathways.

At present we dispose of results with CF preparations from patients with lupus erythematosus and from the classical animal model for this disease, New Zealand Black (NZB) mice. These mice are of further interest in the context of this study because of the high incidence of malignant lymphomas well-known for this strain. CF was prepared from serum of patients or mice according to published procedures (8, 9) and added to test cultures set up with blood from healthy blood donors. In analogy to our study with CF from the supernatants of PMA treated cells, we added various antioxidants and inhibitors of AA metabolism to these cultures before exposure of the cells to CF.

TABLE 5. Anticlastogenic effect of antioxidants and inhibitors of AA-metabolism.

	% mitoses with chromosome aberrations	
	CF from lupus patients	CF from NZB mice
CF	20.3 ± 4.7	18.0 ± 4.6
CF + antioxidants [a]		
SOD	7.0 ± 2.6	4.0 ± 2.0
Catalase	10.5 ± 3.4	10.7 ± 2.3
GSH peroxidase	10.0 ± 5.3	12.0^{b}
Mannitol	9.0 ± 3.6	4.7 ± 5.0
Dimethylfuran		6.0
BHT	10.0 ± 3.5	7.0
BHA	14.7 ± 6.1	2.0
CF + inhibitors of AA-metabolism [a]		
indomethacine	18.5 ± 5.3	12.7 ± 4.2
flufenamic acid	6.8 ± 2.5	9.0
ETYA	5.8 ± 5.9	9.3 ± 5.0
NDGA	10.3 ± 9.3	4.5 ± 4.4
BN 1015	14.0 ± 7.2	10.0
p-bromophenacylbromide	12.7 ± 4.2	
imidazole	21.0 ± 3.5	18.0

a The doses correspond to those given in PMA treated cells
b Only 2 exp. have been done in the columns without standard deviation.

Similar to the results obtained with PMA and with PMA induced CF inhibitors of cyclo-and lipoxygenase pathways proved to be anticlastogenic, while imidazole, an inhibitor of thromboxane synthetase was inactive. Indomethacin was not as protective against the CF from lupus patients and NZB mice as in PMA induced damage. Bromophenacylbromide, an inhibitor of phospholipase A_2 (26), was moderately anticlastogenic.

In agrement with our previous work (8, 9), SOD was highly protective. By scavenging O_2^- radicals it protects membranes and thus prevents phospholipase activation. It was suggested that the antiinflammatory properties of SOD may depend at least in part on the inhibition of phospholipase activation, since it inhibited prostaglandin formation (29). Other antioxidants were only moderately anticlastogenic.

CONCLUDING REMARKS

Chronic inflammation may be associated with cancer. This association is well documented for patients with Crohn's disease, who have a 20-fold risk of developing colon cancer compared to the general population (42). Also dermatomyositis is frequently associated with cancer. For progressive systemic sclerosis, the statistical analysis of large series could not confirm an increase in the incidence of cancer as suggested by numerous case reports. NZB mice, however, the classical animal model for the study of lupus erythematosus clearly show an increased tumor incidence, not only for lymphomas, but also for epitheliomas in older animals (35). The example of the tumor promoter PMA documents again the association between inflammatory reactions and the development of cancer. Furthermore antiinflammatory drugs may have antipromotional properties.

Chromosome damage is observed in chronic inflammatory states as well as after exposure to tumor promoters. It may be in part due to oxygen metabolites produced by inflammatory cells, since phagocytes that were activated to produce oxygen radicals induce an increase in sister chromatid exchanges in cultured CHO cells (43). Also generation of O_2^- in the growth medium of lymphocyte cultures results in an increase of chromosome damage and sister chromatid exchanges (14). However the action of short-lived free radicals with a limited range of diffusion cannot alone explain the cytogenetic damage. The present data support the notion that more long-lived clastogenic compounds are formed as a consequence of lipid peroxidation of membranes. Icosanoids seem to be constituents of these clastogenic factors and further identification of these DNA damaging metabolites may be of interest for the elucidation of the role of icosanoids at the origin of cancer.

REFERENCES

1. Baret, A., and Emerit, I. (1983): Mutation Res., in press.

2. Bird, R., Draper, H., and Basrur P. (1982): Mutation Res., 101: 237-246.

3. Birnboim, H. (1982): Science, 215: 1247-1249.

4. Cerutti, P., Emerit, I., and Amstad, P. (1983): In: Genes and Proteins in Oncogenesis, edited by H. Vogel and I. Weinstein. Academic Press, New York, in press.

5. DeChatelet, L.R., Shirley, P.S., and Johnston, Jr., R.B. (1976): Blood, 47: 545-554.

6. Dzarlieva, R. and Fusenig, N. (1982): Cancer Letters, 16: 7-17.

7. Emerit, I. (1982): In: Progress in Mutation Research, edited by A.T. Natarajan, G. Obe and H. Altmann. Elsevier Biomedical, Amsterdam, 4: 61-74.

8. Emerit, I., Michelson, A., Levy, A., Camus, J. and Emerit, J. (1980): Hum. Genet., 55: 341-344.

9. Emerit, I., Levy, A. and de Vaux Saint-Cyr, D. (1980): Cytogenet. Cell Genet., 26: 41-48.

10. Emerit, I. and Cerutti, P. (1981): Proc. nat. Acad. Sci. (Wash.), 78: 1868-1872.

11. Emerit, I. and Cerutti, P. (1981): Nature, 293: 144-146.

12. Emerit, I. and Cerutti, P. (1982): Proc. nat. Acad. Sci. (Wash.), 79: 7509-7513.

13. Emerit, I., Jalbert, P. and Cerutti, P. (1982): Hum. Genet, 61: 65-67.

14. Emerit, I., Keck, M., Levy, A., Feingold, J. and Michelson, A.M. (1982): Mutation Res., 103: 165-172.

15. Emerit, I., Levy, A. and Cerutti, P. (1983): Mutation Res., 110: 327-335.

16. Emerit, I. and Cerutti, P. (1983): Carcinogenesis, in press.

17. Erikson, J., Ar-Rushdi, A., Drwinga, H., Nowell, P. and Croce, C. (1983): Proc. nat. Acad. Sci. (Wash.), 80: 820-824.

18. German, J. (1969): Amer. J. hum. Genet., 21: 196-227.

19. Goh, K.O. and Sumner, H. (1968) : Radiat. Res., 35: 171-174.

20. Goldstein, B.D., Witz, G., Amoruso, M., Stone, D.S. and Troll, W. (1981): Cancer Letters, 11: 257-262.

21. Goldyne, M.E. and Stobo, J.D. (1982): Prostaglandins, 24: 623-631.

22. Hollowell, J.G. and Littlefield, L.G. (1968); Proc. Soc. exp. Biol. (N.Y.), 129: 240-243.

23. Keck, M. and Emerit, I. (1979): Hum. Genet., 50: 277-283.

24. Lehrer, R.I. and Cohen, L. (1981): J. clin. Invest., 68: 1314-1320.

25. Maclouf, J., Fruteau de Laclos, B. and Borgeat, P. (1982) : Proc. nat. Acad. Sci. (Wash.), 79: 6042-6046.

26. Mitchell, S., Poysen, M. and Wilson, N. (1977): Brit. J. Pharmacol., 59: 107-113.

27. Nagasawa, H. and Little, J. (1981): Carcinogenesis, 2: 601-607.

28. Nordenson, I., Beckman, G. and Beckman, L. (1976): Hereditas, 82: 125-126.

29. Parente, L. (1982): Prostaglandins, 23: 725-730.

30. Parry, J., Parry, E. and Barret, J. (1981) Nature (Lond.), 294: 263-265.

31. Petkau, A. (1980) Acta physiol. scand. Suppl. 492: 81-90.

32. Salin, M.L. and Mc Cord, J.M. (1975): J. clin. Invest., 24: 1319-1323.

33. Sando, J.J., Hilfiker, M.L., Salomon, D.S. and Farrar, J.J. (1981): Proc. nat. Acad. Sci. (Wash.), 78: 1189-1193.

34. Scott, D. (1968): Cell. Tiss. Kinet., 2: 295-298.

35. Shaham, M., Beeker, J. and Cohen M.M. (1980): Cytogenet. Cell Genet. 27: 155-161.

36. Slaga, T. (1978): In: Carcinogenesis, edited by T. Slaga, A. Sivak, and R. Boutwell. Raven Press, New-York, 2:

37. Sundar, S.K., Ablashi, D.V., Levine, P.H., Wallen, W.C. and Armstrong, J.R. (1981): Biomedicine, 35: 11-13.

38. Thompson, L.H., Baker, R.M., Carrano, A.V. and Brookman K.W. (1980): Cancer Res., 40: 3245-3251.

39. Vanderhoek, J.Y., Bryant, R.W. and Bailey, J.M. (1982): Biochem. Pharmacol., 31: 3463-3467.

40. Verma, A., Ashendel, C. and Boutwell, R. (1980): Cancer Res., 40: 308-315.

41. Viaje, A.T., Slaga, T., Wigler, M. and Weinstein, I. (1977): Cancer Res., 37: 1530-1536.

42. Weedon, D.D., Shorter, R.G., Ilstrup, D.M., Huizenga, K.A., Taylor, W.F. (1973): New Engl. J. Med., 289: 1099.

43. Weitberg, A.B., Weitzman, S.A., Destrempes, M., Latt, S.A. and Stossel, T.P. (1983): New Engl. J. Med.,

44. Wertz, P.W. and Mueller, G.C. (1978), Cancer Res. 38: 2900-2904.

45. White, J.G., Rao, G.H.R. and Estensen, R.D. (1974): Amer. J. Path., 75: 301-314.

46. Zucker, M.B., Troll, W. and Belman, S. (1974): J. Cell Biol., 60: 325-336.

Icosanoids and Cancer, edited by H. Thaler-Dao, et al. Raven Press, New York © 1984.

Prostaglandins and the Proliferation of Swiss Mouse 3T3 Cells: A Model System for Studying Growth Control

*Luis Jimenez de Asua, **Colin Macphee, **Alan H. Drummond, and *Angela M. Otto

*Friedrich Miescher-Institut, CH-4002 Basel, Switzerland; and **Department of Pharmacology, University of Glasgow, Glasgow, G12 8QQ Scotland

One of the most challenging problems in modern biology and medicine is to understand the molecular changes that induce normal cells to undergo malignant transformation. During the last decade it has become clear that the proliferation of normal cells and tissues, in vivo as well as in vitro is controlled by complex regulatory mechanisms (1,14,20). These mechanisms are in turn modulated by the intrinsic requirements of specific tissues, the spatial relationship among cells within an organ and by a delicate balance of interaction between different mitogens, non-mitogenic hormones, ions, nutrients and cellular inhibitors which are present in the extracellular millieu (20,25,43,47).

Most of these mitogens or inhibitors initially interact with specific receptors present on the cell surface and from there elicit a repertoire of intracellular signals. These signals, which interact with specific targets, determine whether a cell will remain quiescent, or will divide (21). Many of the rapidly proliferating cells isolated from malignant tumours, or cells transformed by chemicals or oncogenic viruses, have apparently lost their mechanisms for restricting cell division. Thus it appears that their rate of proliferation is no longer regulated by mitogens or inhibitors present in the extracellular environment (14,20,48, 56).

Prostaglandins are a group of closely related lipid molecules, which are synthesized from arachidonic acid and released by mammalian cells in response to physiological changes and pathological conditions (30, 44). Numerous studies have shown that in vivo as well as in vitro, prostaglandins can regulate the rate of proliferation and differentiation of certain mammalian cells (41). In a number of malignant tumours the synthesis and release of prostaglandins is markedly increased (2,30,33,42,49,54). When inhibitors of prostaglandin synthesis are added to induced, spontaneous or transplanted tumours in rodents, the growth of these tumours is inhibited (19,39,40,48,50). Similarly, the production and release of prostaglandins E_1, E_2 or $F_{2\alpha}$ is increased in several cell lines transformed by chemicals or oncogenic viruses, and the proliferation of these cell lines is reduced when prostaglandin synthesis is inhibited (15,17,18,34). These observations suggest a correlation of the increased prostaglandin production with changes in the rate of proliferation of transformed and malignant cells. Furthermore, the tumour promotor tetradecanoylphorbol acetate (TPA) as well as several growth factors, including some isolated from malignant cells, increase the synthesis of prostaglandins E_1, E_2 and/or $F_{2\alpha}$ in mammalian cell culture (32). It is not clear, however, whether the increase in the synthesis and release of prostaglandins is the cause or the effect of increased proliferation rates, or whether it merely accompanies this phenomenon (29).

Burk (3-5) and Todaro and his coworkers (10,11,36,53) have independently proposed that the lack of control by extracellular factors on the proliferation of malignant or transformed cells can be partially accounted for by the intracellular production and release of their own mitogenic factors. These factors, once released from the cells, can bind to their own receptors, and could thereby autostimulate cell proliferation. Thus the rate of proliferation becomes independent of the mitogens present in the extracellular fluid (4,36). Furthermore, these investigators have shown that these secreted factors consists of a number of different polypeptides, and it was suggested that some of them may even have similar properties to those that may be present in the bloodstream or in the interstitial fluid surrounding normal cells. This type of autonomous control has been called ectopic auto-stimulation of growth (4). One of the predictions of this model or hypothesis is that addition of these polypeptide factors secreted by malignant or transformed cells to their normal counterparts, the normal cells should at least partially mimic the expression of the phenotype of transformed cells. This phenotype includes changes in the morphological arrangement of the cells in the monolayer, increases in nutrient uptake and dramatic increases in the rate of initiation of DNA replication and cell division as well as other changes in gene expression.

Our objective here is to present some experimental evidence indicating that $PGF_{2\alpha}$, PGE_1 and PGE_2, when added to resting Swiss 3T3 cells, can affect their morphology, biochemical events and rate of DNA replication in a way which resembles both normal proliferation and some of the characteristics considered to be typical of transformed cells in culture (22-29,38). We shall discuss here five aspects of the interaction of $PGF_{2\alpha}$ with Swiss 3T3 cells and the control of cell proliferation: 1) Changes in arrangement of cells in the monolayer; 2) Interactions of PGE_1 and PGE_2 with $PGF_{2\alpha}$ and changes in the rate of proliferation; 3) Interaction of prostaglandins and epidermal growth factor; 4) Biochemical events stimulated by prostaglandins; 5) The relevance of mitogenic stimulation by prostaglandins and other mitogens in Swiss 3T3 cells to the origin of transformation.

MATERIALS AND METHODS

Cell Cultures

Swiss mouse 3T3 cells (52) were propagated in Vogt-Dulbecco's modified Eagle's medium (VDMEM) containing 100 µg/ml of streptomycin, 100 units/ml of penicillin and 10% v/v of fetal calf serum as previously described (24).

Assay for the initiation of DNA synthesis

Subconfluent cultures were trypsinized and plated in 35 mm petri dishes in 2 ml of VDMEM supplemented with 6% (v/v) fetal calf serum and low molecular weight nutrients as described before (24). For the determination of the labelling index (percentage of cells having initiated DNA synthesis by a given time) the cultures were labelled by adding 3 μCi/ml of [methyl-^{3}H] thymidine from 0 to 28 hours. Cultures were fixed and processed for autoradiography as previously described (24).

Morphological observations

Cells were plated in the same conditions as for the assay of initiation of DNA synthesis and were exposed to different compounds for 4 days. Thereafter, the medium was aspirated and the cells were washed twice with 0.9% NaCl at 24°C and a coverslip was placed on top of the monolayer. The cells were photographed using phase contrast optics at a magnification of 125x with XP1 400 Ilford Film.

Determination of phosphatidylinositol turnover

Swiss 3T3 cells were plated as for the assay of the initiation of DNA synthesis, except that the concentration of phosphate in the medium was reduced to 100 μM. Resting cultures were prelabelled with [^{32}P]PO$_4$ 2.5 hours prior to use, and the stimulation with mitogens and non-mitogenic hormones as well as the determination of phosphatidylinositol turnover were as described by Macphee et al. (35).

RESULTS AND DISCUSSION

1. Morphological changes in response to prostaglandin $F_{2\alpha}$, E_1 and insulin

Confluent resting Swiss mouse 3T3 cells have an appearance that resemble a well-organized mosaic, referred to as cobblestone appearance. The nuclei and cytoplasm show little optical density and the borders of the cells are obscure (Fig. la). Addition of insulin, PGE$_1$, or both insulin and PGE$_1$ together for 48 hrs or 96 hrs did not change the morphological appearance observed for the resting culture (Fig. lb,c,d).

When PGF$_{2\alpha}$ was added to the resting cells for 48 hrs, the cells appeared slightly elongated and they tended to have a parallel arrangements(Fig. le). In cultures in which PGF$_{2\alpha}$ was added with insulin or PGE$_1$, the cells lost more of their original arrangement, leaving empty spaces between cells which became more elongated (Fig. lf,g). These changes became more dramatic when the cells were treated with PGF$_{2\alpha}$, PGE$_1$ and insulin (Fig. lh) for a 48 hr period: The nuclei were optically denser, the cytoplasmic processes overlapped each other and the cells exhibited irregular patters of arrangement. Treatment for a period of 96 hrs showed that cells treated with PGF$_{2\alpha}$ or PGF$_{2\alpha}$ and insulin tend to reorganize to the original cobblestone appearance although the cell bodies had not yet returned to their original cobblestone form (Fig. li,j). In contrast, the cells treated by PGF$_{2\alpha}$ and PGE$_1$ continued exhibiting their disorganized morphology characteristic of transformed cells. In the presence of the PGF$_{2\alpha}$, PGE$_1$ and insulin together the cells continued dividing, giving rise to more crowded cultures with cells overlayering each other without discernible pattern, similar to that observed in cells transformed by viruses (Fig. lk,l). Yet, such stimulated cells failed to form colonies in agar (Jimenez de Asua and Poskocil, unpublished results). Furthermore, when cells

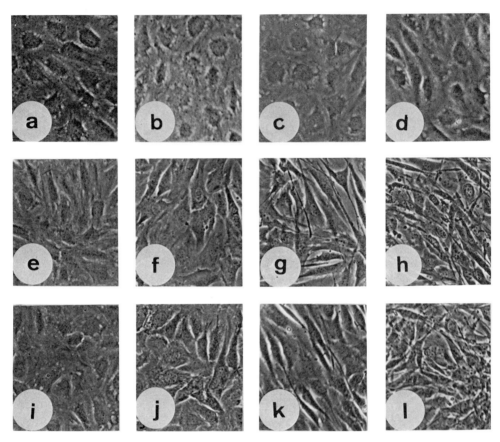

FIG. 1. Morphological changes of confluent resting Swiss 3T3 cells in
response to $PGF_{2\alpha}$, PGE_1 and insulin after 48 or 96 hours of stimulation.
In: A to H the changes were observed after 48 hours. Additions were
as follows: A) control; B) insulin; C) PGE_1; D) PGE_1 + insulin;
E) $PGF_{2\alpha}$; F) $PGF_{2\alpha}$ + insulin; G) $PGF_{2\alpha}$+ PGE_1; H) $PGF_{2\alpha}$ + PGE_1 + insulin.
In I to L the changes were observed after 96 hrs. Additions were as
follows: I) $PGF_{2\alpha}$; J) $PGF_{2\alpha}$ + insulin; K) $PGF_{2\alpha}$ + PGE_1 ;and L) $PGF_{2\alpha}$ +
PGE_1 + insulin. The concentrations were: for $PGF_{2\alpha}$ (100 ng/ml),insulin
(50 ng/ml) and PGE_1 (100 ng/ml).

which had been treated with $PGF_{2\alpha}$, PGE_1 and insulin together for 96 hr
were replated in medium with 6% fetal calf serum and low molecular
weight nutrients (as for assay of DNA synthesis), they grow to confluency and form a monolayer with morphology characteristic of quiescent
cells. This shows that normal cells do not retain their altered morphology upon removal of the prostaglandins, indicating that the resemblance
to transformed morphology is temporary and dependent on the combination
of mitogens and hormones present in the culture medium.

2. Prostaglandin E₁ and E₂ enhance the mitogenic effect of Prostaglandin F₂α, alone or with insulin

PGF$_{2\alpha}$ added alone at a saturating concentration of 300 ng/ml to resting Swiss 3T3 cells stimulated the initiation of DNA synthesis resulting in 20% labelled nuclei after 28 hr (Fig. 2). PGE$_1$, PGE$_2$, and PGD$_2$ which

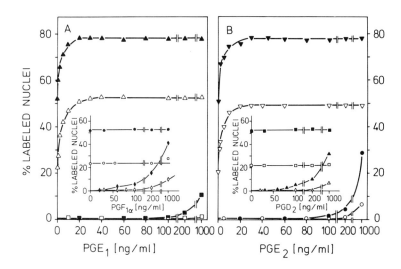

FIG. 2. Enhancement by PGE$_1$ (A) and PGE$_2$ (B) of the initiation of DNA synthesis stimulated by PGF$_{2\alpha}$ (300 ng/ml) alone or with insulin (60 ng/ml) (A) △ , PGF$_{2\alpha}$ + PGE$_1$; ▲ , PGF$_{2\alpha}$ + insulin + PGE$_1$; □ , PGE$_1$; ■ , PGE$_1$ + insulin. (Inset: ○, PGF$_{2\alpha}$ + PGF$_{1\alpha}$; ● , PGF$_{2\alpha}$ + insulin + PGF$_{1\alpha}$; ◇, PGF$_{1\alpha}$; ◆, PGF$_{1\alpha}$ + insulin. (B) ▽ , PGF$_{2\alpha}$ + PGE$_2$; ▼, PGF$_{2\alpha}$ + insulin + PGE$_2$; ○, PGE$_2$; ●, PGE$_2$ + insulin (inset) □, PGF$_{2\alpha}$ + PGD$_2$; ■ , PGF$_{2\alpha}$ + insulin + PGD$_2$; △, PGD$_2$; ▲,PDG$_2$ + insulin. Cultures were exposed to [methyl-^{3}H]thymidine for 0-28 hrs after additions and then processed for autoradiography. Reprinted from Otto et al. (38).

have closely related structures to PGF$_{2\alpha}$, only marginally stimulate DNA synthesis in these cells even at much higher concentrations (Fig. 2). Insulin, at a concentration that in these cells does not stimulate DNA synthesis, enhanced the effect of PGF$_{2\alpha}$ on the labelling index to 50%. The small stimulatory effect of the other prostaglandins was also enhanced by insulin, but the synergistic effect was always less than that observed with PGF$_{2\alpha}$ (Fig. 2). However, when PGE$_1$ or PGE$_2$ at 2 ng to 1 µg/ml was added to cells stimulated by PGF$_{2\alpha}$, it markedly enhanced the value of the labelling index up to 50%. The concentration of PGE$_1$ or PGE$_2$ giving maximal enhancement was 20 ng/ml. In the presence of insulin the labelling index was further enhanced, giving a value of about 80%. Addition of PGE$_1$ (100 ng/ml) or PGE$_2$ (100 ng/ml) together did not produce further enhancement than that observed by either

PGE_1 or PGE_2 separately (38). This effect on the stimulation of the initiation of DNA synthesis was also reflected in an increase in cell numbers 48 hrs after additions (38). Neither $PGF_{1\alpha}$ nor PGD_2 at a concentration up to 1 µg/ml had any effect on cells stimulated by $PGF_{2\alpha}$ alone or with insulin (Fig. 3 AB inserts). Other prostaglandins such as A_1, A_2, B_1 or I_2 (prostacyclin), which alone do not have any stimulatory effect, likewise did not have a synergistic effect with $PGF_{2\alpha}$ (38).

The mitogenic effect of $PGF_{2\alpha}$ on Swiss mouse 3T3 cells is expressed through two different phenomena: a) The length of the prereplicative phase of about 15 hrs and b) the final rate at which stimulated cells enter S phase (24-27). Analysis of the kinetics revealed that the synergistic interaction of PGE_1 or PGE_2 with $PGF_{2\alpha}$ led to a marked increase in the rate of initiation of DNA synthesis without changing the length of the prereplicative phase (38). Increase in the rate of entry into the S phase also observed when PGE_1 or PGE_2 was added at 9 or 15 hrs of the lag phase (38). Insulin did not change the pattern of interaction of the prostaglandins but it increased the value of the final rate (38).

3. Interaction of prostaglandins and epidermal growth factor

Confluent resting Swiss 3T3 cells can also be stimulated to proliferate by epidermal growth factor (EGF) (8,26,27, Table 1). Addition of EGF at 20 ng/ml, like $PGF_{2\alpha}$ at 300 ng/ml, stimulated about 15% of the cells to initiate DNA synthesis within 28 hrs. Addition of EGF with $PGF_{2\alpha}$ at 30 or 300 ng/ml increases this value to 55% or 58%, respectively, which was further enhanced to 79% by insulin. The interaction of $PGF_{2\alpha}$ with EGF-stimulated cells was specific among other prostaglandins tested. PGE_1 or PGE_2 added at 30 ng/ml with EGF, or with EGF and insulin, did not increase the labelling index. Only a higher

TABLE 1. Effect of different combinations of Prostaglandins, EGF and insulin on the initiation of DNA synthesis in confluent Swiss 3T3 cells

Additions	Labelling without insulin	Index % with insulin
None	0.5	0.8
$PGF_{2\alpha}$ (300) ng/ml)	15.0	47.4
EGF (20 ng/ml)	13.2	45.0
EGF + $PGF_{2\alpha}$ (30 ng/ml)	55.0	79.0
EGF + $PGF_{2\alpha}$ (300 ng/ml)	58.0	79.5
EGF + PGE_1 (30 ng/ml)	15.0	−
EGF + PGE_1 (300 ng/ml)	22.2	48.0
EGF + PGE_2 (30 ng/ml)	13.2	50.3
EGF + PGE_2 (300 ng/ml)	33.4	68.6
Fetal Calf Serum (10%)	92.0	98.1

Labelling index was determined as indicated in Materials and Methods. Cultures were exposed to [methyl-^{3}H] thymidine from 0-28 hrs after additions and processed for autoradiography as in Fig. 2. Prostaglandins were dissolved in absolute ethanol and diluted so that the final concentration of ethanol in the culture medium was 0.01%. Insulin was added at 50 ng/ml. Reprinted from Jimenez de Asua et al. (26).

concentration of 300 ng/ml PGE_2, the prostaglandin most closely related in structure to $PGF_{2\alpha}$, increased the labelling index but to a lesser extent than $PGF_{2\alpha}$. Furthermore, PGE_1 or PGE_2 at low concentrations enhanced only the mitogenic effect of $PGF_{2\alpha}$, but not that of EGF. Together these results support the interpretation that EGF and $PGF_{2\alpha}$ are acting through different signals to stimulate cell proliferation[21,26, 27,38].

4. The biochemical events stimulated by Prostaglandin $F_{2\alpha}$, and E_1 or E_2

Which are the biochemical events stimulated by these prostaglandins, and what are their relationship to the mitogenic effect? According to their site and time of interaction and the type of pathways involved, it is possible to divide these events into a) surface membrane changes, and b) intracellular events. These events can be early events, occurring within minutes of mitogenic stimulation, and late events, which take place hours after cells have been stimulated (43). Furthermore, some of the early surface membrane changes may activate early intracellular events, and some intracellular changes can influence later events occurring at the level of the plasma membrane.

Addition of $PGF_{2\alpha}$ to quiescent Swiss 3T3 cells, rapidly increases $^{86}Rb^+$ uptake, a measurement of Na^+/K^+-ATPase activity (31,37). This event is blocked by ouabain but not by cycloheximide indicating that it does not depend on protein synthesis. $PGF_{2\alpha}$ also stimulates phosphate uptake. The phenomenon follows a biphasical pattern. The early phase which occurs within minutes is insensitive to cycloheximide while this inhibitor prevents the late phase of phosphate uptake indicating a dependance on protein synthesis (31). Furthermore, phosphate uptake can be partially blocked by ouabain indicating that both the activation of the Na^+/K^+-ATPase and phosphate uptake may have some mechanisms in common. $PGF_{2\alpha}$ also stimulates the phosphorylation of the ribosomal S_6 protein and polysome formation as well as incorporation of [^{3}H] leucine into acid precipitable material as a measurement of total protein synthesis (28,51). Although the exact timing of these events is not known, the phosphorylation of the S_6 ribosomal protein is believed to occur very rapidly after $PGF_{2\alpha}$ stimulation. Protein synthesis occurs about 2 hours and it has been suggested that phosphorylation of S_6 may be involved in controlling the initiation of protein synthesis (51).

Recent evidence from our laboratory (35) has shown that $PGF_{2\alpha}$ rapidly stimulates the turnover of phosphatidylinositol and increases the level of diacylglycerol within minutes of its addition to resting Swiss 3T3 cells (Fig. 3). In contrast, EGF which is mitogenic for these cells (26,35) did not increase phosphatidylinositol turnover (Fig. 3). The effect of $PGF_{2\alpha}$ was also selective when compared to other prostaglandins with closely related structures (Fig. 4). Furthermore, PGE_1 did not potentiate the effect of $PGF_{2\alpha}$ in stimulating phosphatidylinositol turnover, even though PGE_1 intacts with $PGF_{2\alpha}$ to synergistically increase DNA synthesis in Swiss 3T3 cells. This indicates that the synergistic interaction of $PGF_{2\alpha}$ and PGE_1 occurs at a biochemical event different from phosphatidylinositol turnover (35).

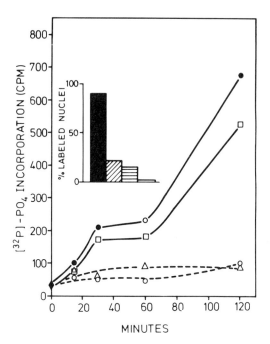

FIG. 3. Stimulation of phosphatidylinositol formation of EGF (100 ng/ml, PGF$_{2\alpha}$ (300 ng/ml) or Fetal Calf Serum (10% v/v). (O) control; (△) EGF; (□) PGF$_{2\alpha}$ and (●) FCS. Insert: Values of the labelling index for (□) control; (≣) EGF; (▨) PGF$_{2\alpha}$ and (■) Fetal Calf Serum. For determination of phosphatidylinositol formation and DNA synthesis cultures were prelabelled with [^{32}P]PO$_4$ and labelled for autoradiography as indicated in Materials and Methods. Reprinted from Macphee et al. (35).

Is there any known biochemical event at which PGE$_1$ and EGF express their synergistic effects with PGF$_{2\alpha}$? Evidence from our laboratory has shown that PGF$_{2\alpha}$ can stimulate glucose uptake (23,25). This phenomenon occurs at about 2 hours after PGF$_{2\alpha}$ addition and increases up to 6 hours. This phenomenon can be blocked by cycloheximide, indicating that it is dependent on protein synthesis (25,26,38). Addition of PGF$_{2\alpha}$ together with EGF, or of PGF$_{2\alpha}$ with PGE$_1$ or PGE$_2$ for 6 hr synergistically stimulated glucose uptake, indicating that the events induced by PGF$_{2\alpha}$, EGF, and PGE$_1$ or PGE$_2$ converge to this common biochemical event, which is protein synthesis-dependent and which occurs late in the prereplicative phase. Insulin further enhanced synergistically the stimulation of glucose uptake stimulated either by PGF$_{2\alpha}$ with EGF or by PGF$_{2\alpha}$ with PGE$_1$ or PGE$_2$ (26,38).

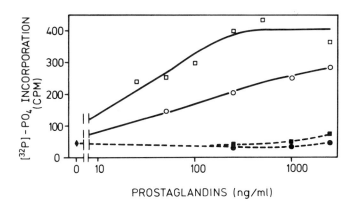

PROSTAGLANDINS (ng/ml)

FIG. 4.   Dose response curve of PGE_1, PGE_2, $PGF_{2\alpha}$ and $PGF_{2\beta}$ for the stimulation of phosphatidylinositol formation. (●) PGE_1; (O) PGE_2 (□) $PGF_{2\alpha}$ and (■) $PGF_{2\beta}$. Prelabelling with [^{32}P]PO_4 or labelling with [methyl-^3H]thymidine was in Fig. 3. Reprinted from Macphee et al. (35).

Other evidence obtained in our laboratory showed that tunicamycin an inhibitor of the synthesis of dolichol-pp-N-acetylglucosamine (the first metabolic step on the pathway of N-glycosylated proteins) also inhibits the initiation of DNA synthesis (28). This inhibition only occurs if tunicamycin is added within 0 to 9 hours after $PGF_{2\alpha}$ stimulation. When total proteins were labelled with [^{14}C]-mannose from 0 to 5 hours after $PGF_{2\alpha}$ stimulation, and separated by one dimensional gel electrophoresis, numerous proteins were labelled. Tunicamycin added at 500 ng/ml markedly reduced the incorporation of [^{14}C]-mannose, indicating that N-glycosylation was responsible for the labelling of the proteins. This indicates that the N-glycosylation of proteins early during prereplicative phase may be a prerequisite for the initiation of DNA synthesis in Swiss 3T3 cells (28).

A summary of the biochemical events known to occur upon mitogenic stimulation by $PGF_{2\alpha}$ in Swiss 3T3 cells in shown in Fig. 5.

5.   The relevance of mitogenic stimulation by Prostaglandins and other mitogens of Swiss 3T3 cells to the origin of malignant transformation

What is the relevance of prostaglandins in the control of normal cell proliferation and proliferation of transformed and cancer cells?

From the results outlined in the previous sections it is possible to conclude that there are different underlying mechanisms leading to the initiation of DNA replication. These mechanisms are controlled by growth factors (or mitogens), such as EGF or $PGF_{2\alpha}$, together with non-mitogenic substances, such as insulin, PGE_1 or PGE_2, which can modulate the effect of these growth factors in stimulating the

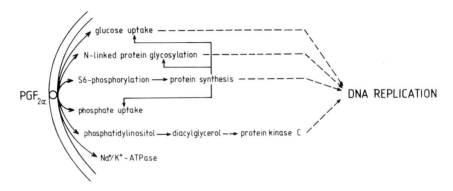

FIG. 5. Biochemical events stimulated by $PGF_{2\alpha}$ in Swiss 3T3 cells. Dotted lines indicate that it is not yet known how this event could regulate the initiation of DNA synthesis.

initiation of DNA synthesis. It can be postulated from the structural differences between EGF and $PGF_{2\alpha}$ that each has different cell surface binding sites. There is, in contrast to EGF, no direct evidence for $PGF_{2\alpha}$ receptors on the cell surface of Swiss 3T3 cells. However, the synergistic effect of $PGF_{2\alpha}$ and EGF on 2-deoxyglucose uptake further indicates that some of the early events are different for these two growth factors. This hypothesis is supported by the fact that PGE_1 or PGE_2 at low concentrations enhances the stimulatory effect of $PGF_{2\alpha}$ but not that of EGF. Interestingly, the synergy between $PGF_{2\alpha}$ and EGF, which can be enhanced by insulin, is not enhanced by PGE_1 or PGE_2. While it cannot be assumed that EGF and PGE_1 or PGE_2 act through identical pathways, since only EGF is by itself mitogenic, it could indicate that EGF and PGE_1 or PGE_2 share a common event for determining the rate of entry into S phase, or it could indicate that their signals for the putative regulatory event partially cancel each other.

Other results recently obtained by Hunter and his coworkers (9) and in our laboratory (21,26,35) further support the concept of different initial events stimulated by $PGF_{2\alpha}$ and EGF. In resting Swiss 3T3 cells EGF rapidly stimulates a tyrosine protein kinase leading to phosphorylation of two cellular proteins in the tyrosine group within 1 hr after stimulation. In the same cells $PGF_{2\alpha}$ does not stimulate tyrosine phosphorylation (9). On the other hand, $PGF_{2\alpha}$ stimulates phosphatidylinositol turnover in Swiss 3T3 cells, while EGF does not (35). The culture conditions used to study these two different biochemical events were the same and allowed both growth factors to stimulate initiation of DNA synthesis.

It has been recently reported that a phospholipid-dependent protein kinase C is activated by diacylglycerol, a product of stimulated phosphatidylinositol turnover (7). Since $PGF_{2\alpha}$ stimulates phosphatidylinositol turnover, and increases diacylglycerol level (35), it can be postulated that $PGF_{2\alpha}$ could subsequently also stimulate protein kinase C. It could thus be envisaged that part of the specificity of a growth factor for stimulating different biochemical events lies in the protein kinases activated. This view is summarized in Fig. 6.

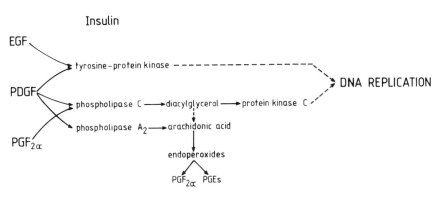

FIG. 6. A possible view of differential protein kinases activated by growth factors and hormones, which could regulate pathways leading to DNA replication.

The early stimulation of different protein kinases by different growth factors could generate some of the initial signals required to induce the events leading to the initiation of DNA synthesis. However, it is unlikely that the activation of protein kinase(s) is by itself a sufficient signal or event. Firstly, while tyrosine protein kinase activity obtains its peak within the first hour, EGF and $PGF_{2\alpha}$ are required for at least 8 hr in Swiss 3T3 cells to stimulate DNA synthesis. Secondly, insulin also stimulates tyrosine protein kinase activity (9) and yet by itself does not stimulate DNA replication. Thirdly, an analog of EGF, which can stimulate tyrosine phosphorylation, is not mitogenic in Swiss 3T3 cells (9).

Studies with platelet derived growth factor (PDGF) provide another line of evidence that different types of early biochemical events are relevant for regulating initiation of DNA synthesis. In Swiss 3T3 cells, low concentrations of PDGF alone stimulate 80% of the cells to enter S phase within 28 hr (Jimenez de Asua, unpublished results), a percentage obtained with $PGF_{2\alpha}$ only in combination with EGF and insulin or with PGE_1 or PGE_2 and insulin (26,38). Furthermore, PDGF stimulates tyrosine phosphorylation of at least 5 cellular proteins, and it also stimulates phosphatidylinositol turnover and diacylglycerol production (16). Whether these latter events increase the activity of protein kinase C remains to be shown.

What is the relevance of these results and interpretations for the understanding of transformation? The concept that multiple signalling systems operate in normal cells to regulate cell proliferation (20,24, 26,27), leads to the conclusions that there is no unique mechanism for transformation and constitutive proliferation. Furthermore, Vogt and Dulbecco (55) proposed the concept of neoplastic progression by graded alterations. Together these concepts imply that depending on the type of cancer, different signals and events may be changed.

These views are compatible with the studies on transforming growth factors (TGF)(10,11,36) and fibroblastic-derived growth factor (FDGF) (3-5,12) produced and secreted by sarcoma virus-transformed mouse cells and by SV-28 polyoma virus-transformed BHK cells, respectively. FDGF may be similar to PDGF, since they share chromatographic properties, and in Swiss 3T3 cells each stimulates the initiation of DNA replication with a labelling index of about 80% within 28 hr (12, Jimenez de Asua, unpublished results). Adding FDGF and PDGF together did not further enhance DNA synthesis (12). Certain transformed cells no longer require PDGF for proliferation, possibly because they may produce and release a similar growth factor (45). Furthermore, it has been shown in Swiss 3T3 cells that PDGF can stimulate the synthesis of $PGF_{2\alpha}$ and PGE_1 (46). However, inhibiting prostaglandin synthesis with indomethacin did not reduce [^{3}H]thymidine incorporation in PDGF-stimulated cells (46). This may indicate that the synthesis of $PGF_{2\alpha}$ or PGE_1 is not essential for DNA synthesis and that PDGF is operating sufficiently through other pathways. This is consistent with the proposition that PDGF may be activating several different signalling systems, some of which may be also shared by EGF, insulin and certain prostaglandins. If several signalling systems and intersecting pathways are simultaneously in operation, this could reduce the growth factor requirement and the sensitivity to inhibitors, which may act only on certain pathway(s).

The secretion of growth factors by cancer and transformed cells led to the hypothesis of ectopic autostimulation of cell proliferation. This hypothesis has now received support by the discovery that the product of simian sarcoma virus onc gene, p28 sis, shows a high degree of amino acid sequence homology to human PDGF (13,57). Even though the functional homology remains to be established, this observation suggests that virally-induced transformation properties can be of cellular origin. The increased synthesis and secretion of $PGF_{2\alpha}$ and PGE_1 observed in virally-transformed and in certain cancer cells could reflect one, or even both of these two phenomena: Cells producing $PGF_{2\alpha}$ could autostimulate themselves, and viral onc genes could change the spectrum of enzymatic activities for the synthesis of specific prostaglandins. Indeed, different lines of evidence indicate that the activity of phospholipase A_2 or other acylhydrolases are markedly increased in cells stimulated by PDGF or by TPA, a potent tumor promotor (6,32); this would lead to increased production of arachidonic acid, a precursor of prostaglandin synthesis. But other enzymes leading to the synthesis of certain classes of prostaglandins and leukotrienes may also be affected, for example cyclooxygenase and lipoxygenase (6).

The experimental evidences presented show that, using Swiss 3T3 cells as a model system, $PGF_{2\alpha}$ interacting with PGE_1, PGE_2 or other hormones, can induce properties which are considered to be characteristic of transformed cells, such as changes in morphology and arrangements, increase in glucose uptake and increase in the rate of cell proliferation. Even though this model cell system and the interaction of prostaglandins may be limited to certain signals and events leading to DNA replication, these may constitute targets for controlling cell proliferation.

ACKNOWLEDGEMENTS

We are extremely grateful to Dr. Michael Minks for stimulating discussions and criticisms on the manuscript. We also thank Ignacio Jimenez de Asua for helping with the searching and organization of the references and to Stanislava Poskocil for skillful technical assistance. A.M.O. is a Special Fellow of the Leukemia Society of America, Inc.

REFERENCES

1. Baserga, R. (1976): Multiplication and Division in Animal Cells, Marcel Decker, New York.
2. Bhana, D., Hillier, K. and Karim, S.M.M. (1971): Cancer, 27: 233-237.
3. Burk, R.R. (1973): Proc. Natl. Acad. Sci. U.S.A., 70: 369-372.
4. Burk, R.R. (1980): In: Control Mechanisms in Animal Cells, edited by L. Jimenez de Asua, R. Levi-Montalcini, R. Shields and S. Iacobelli, pp. 245-247, Raven Press, New York.
5. Burk, R.R. and Williams, C.A. (1971): In: Growth control in Cell Cultures, edited by G.E.M. Wolstenhome and Knight, J. pp. 107-125, Ciba Foundation Symp. Churchill Livingstone, London.
6. Bresnick, E. (1982): In: Prostaglandins and Cancer,Prostaglandins and Related Lipids, edited by T.J. Powles, R.S. Bockman, K.V.Honn and P. Ranwell, pp. 189-204.
7. Castagna, M., Takai, Y., Kalbuchi, K., Sano, K., Kikkawa, U. and Nishizuka, Y. (1982): J. Biol. Chem.,257: 7847-7851.
8. Carpenter, G. and Cohen, S. (1979): Ann. Rev. Biochem., 48:193-201.
9. Cooper, J., Bowen-Pope, D.F., Raines, E., Ross, R. and Hunter, T. (1982): Cell 31: 263-273.
10. DeLarco, J.E. and Todaro, G.J. (1978): Proc. Natl. Acad. Sci. U.S.A., 75: 4001-4005.
11. DeLarco, J.E. and Todaro, G.J. (1978): J. Cell Physiol., 84:335-342.
12. Dicker, P., Pohjanpelto, P., Pettican, P., and Rozengurt, E. (1981): Exp. Cell Res., 135:221-227.
13. Doolittle, R., Kunkapiller, M.W., Hood, L.E., Devare, S.G., Robbins, K.C., Aaronson, S.T. and Antoniades, H. (1983): Science, 221:275-276.
14. Dulbecco, R. (1969): Science, 166:962-968.
15. Goldyne, M.E., Lindgren, J.A., Claesson, H.E. and Hammarström, S. (1980): Prostaglandins, 19:155-164.
16. Habenicht, A.J.B., Glomset, J.A., King, W.C., Nist, C., Mitchell, C.D. and Ross, R. (1981): J. Biol. Chem., 256:12329-12335.
17. Hammarström, S. (1977): Eur. J. Biochem., 74:7-12.
18. Hammarström, S., Samuelson, B. and Bjursell, G. (1973): Nature New Biol., 243:50-51.
19. Hial, V., Horakova, Z., Shalf, R.E. and Beaven, M.A. (1976): Eur. J. Pharmacol., 37:367-376.
20. Holley, R.W. (1980): In: Control Mechanisms in Animal Cells, edited by L. Jimenez de Asua, R. Levi Montalcini, R. Shields and S. Iacobelli, pp. 15-25. Raven Press, New York.
21. Jimenez de Asua, L. and Otto, A.M. (1983): In: Proc. 1st European Conference on Serum-Free Cell Culture, edited by G. Brunner and G. Fischer, Springer Verlag, Heidelberg. (in press).

22. Jimenez de Asua, L., Clingan, D. and Rudland, P.S. (1975): Proc. Natl. Acad. Sci. U.S.A., 72:2724-2728.
23. Jimenez de Asua, L., O'Farrell, M.K., Bennett, D., Clingan, D. and Rudland, D.S. (1977): Nature, 265:151-153.
24. Jimenez de Asua, L., O'Farrell, M.K., Clingan, D. and Rudland, P.S. (1977): Proc. Natl. Acad. Sci. U.S.A., 74:3845-3849.
25. Jimenez de Asua, L., Richmond, K.M.V., Otto, A.M., Kubler, A.M., O'Farrell, M.K. and Rudland, P.S. (1979): In: Hormones and Cell Culture, edited by G. Sato and R. Ross, Cold Spring Harbor Conferences in Cell Proliferation, 6:403-424. Cold Spring Harbor.
26. Jimenez de Asua, Richmond, K.M.V. and Otto, A.M. (1981): Proc. Natl. Acad. Sci. U.S.A., 78:1004-1008.
27. Jimenez de Asua, L., Smith, C. and Otto, A.M. (1982): Cell Biol. Int. Rep., 6:791-797.
28. Jimenez de Asua, L., Foecking, M.K. and Otto, A.M. (1983): Cell Biol. Int. Rep., 7:499-500.
29. Jimenez de Asua, L., Otto, A.M., Lindgren, J.A. and Hammarström, S. (1983): J. Biol. Chem., 258:8774-8780.
30. Karim, S.M.M. (1972): The Prostaglandins, Progress in Research, Medical and Technical Publishing Co., Oxford.
31. Lever, J.E., Clingan, D. and Jimenez de Asua, L. (1976): Biochem. Biophys. Res. Comm., 71:136-143.
32. Levine, L. (1982): In: Prostaglandins and Cancer, prostaglandins and related Lipids, edited by T.J. Powles, R.S. Bockman, K.V. Honn and P. Ranwell, pp. 189-204.
33. Levine, L., Hinkle, P.M., Voelkel, E.F. and Tashjian, A.H. (1972): Biochem. Biophys.Res. Comm., 47:888-892.
34. Lindgren, J.A., Claeson, H.E. and Hammarström, S. (1979): Exp. Cell Res., 124:1-5.
35. Macphee, C., Drumond, A.H., Otto, A. and Jimenez de Asua, L. (1983) : J. of Cell Physiol., submitted to publication.
36. Marquardt, H. and Todaro, G.J. (1982): J. Biol. Chem., 257: 5220-5225.
37. Moroney, J.A., Smith, A., Thomel, D. and Wenner, C.E. (1978): J. Cell Physiol., 95:287-294.
38. Otto, A.M., Nilsen-Hamilton, M., Boss, B., Ulrich, M.O. and Jimenez de Asua, L. (1982): Proc. Natl. Acad. Sci. U.S.A., 79:4992-4996.
39. Plescia, O.J., Smith, A.H. and Grinwich, K. (1975): Proc. Natl. Acad. Sci. U.S.A., 72:1848-1851.
40. Pollard, M. and Luckert, P.H. (1981): Proc. Soc. Exp. Biol. Med., 167:161-164.
41. Powles, T.J., Bockman, R.S., Honn, K.V. and Ranwell, P. (1982): Prostaglandins and Cancer, Prostaglandins and Related Lipids, Alan R. Liss, Inc. New York.
42. Rodan, S.B., Rodan, G.A., Simmons, H.A., Walenga, R.W., Feinstein and Raisz, L.G. (1982): In: Prostaglandins and Cancer, Prostaglandins and Related Lipids, edited by T.J. Powles, R.S. Bockman, K.V. Honn and R. Ranwell, pp. 573-578. Alan R. Liss, New York.
43. Rozengurt, E. (1979): Hormones and Cell Culture, edited by G. Sato and R. Ross. Cold Spring Harbor Conferences in Cell Proliferation, 6:778-788, Cold Spring Harbor, New York.
44. Sammuelson, B., Goldyne, M., Granström, E., Hamberg, M., Hammarström, S. and Malmsten, C. (1978): Ann. Rev. Biochem.,47:997-1029.

45. Scher, C.D., Pledger, W.J., Martin, P., Antoniades, H. and Stiles, C.D. (1978): J. Cell Physiol., 97:371–374.
46. Shier, W.T. and Durkin, J.P. (1982): J. Cell Physiol., 112:171–182.
47. Steck, P.A., Voss, P.G. and Wang, J.L. (1979): J. Cell Biol., 83:562–575.
48. Strausser, J. and Humes, J. (1975): Int. J. Cancer, 15:724–730.
49. Tan, W.C., Privett, O.S. and Goldyne, M.E. (1974): Cancer Res., 34:3229–3231.
50. Tashjian, A.H., Voelkel, E.F., Goldhaber, P. and Levine, L. (1973): Prostaglandins, 3:515–524.
51. Thomas, G., Martin-Perez, J., Siegmann, M. and Otto, A.M. (1982): Cell, 30:235–242.
52. Todaro, G.J. and Green, H. (1963): J. Cell. Biol., 17:299–313.
53. Todaro, G.J., DeLarco, J.E. and Cohen, S. (1976) Nature, 264: 26–31.
54. Voelkel, E.F., Tashjian, A.H., Franklin, R., Wasserman, E., Levine, L. (1975): Metabolism, 24:973–978.
55. Vogt, M. and Dulbecco, R. (1963): Proc. Natl. Acad. Sci. U.S.A., 49:171–179.
56. Voss, P.G., Steck, P.A., Calamia, J. and Wang, J.L. (1982): Exp. Cell Res., 138:397–407.
57. Waterfield, M.D., Scrace, G.T., Whittle, N., Stroobant, P., Johnsson, A., Wasteson, A., Westermark, B., Heldin, C.H., Huang, J.S. and Devel, T.M. (1983): Nature, 304:35–39.

Icosanoids and Cancer, edited by H. Thaler-Dao, et al. Raven Press, New York © 1984.

Effects of Eicosatetraenoic Acids on Lymphocyte Proliferation *In Vitro*

*N. Gualde, *S. Mexmain, *J. C. Aldigier, **J. S. Goodwin, and *M. Rigaud

*Immunology and Biochemistry Research Unit-Medical School, 87032 Limoges, Cedex, France; and **University of New Mexico Medical School, Albuquerque, New Mexico*

There are two major pathways for arachidonic acid metabolism in the peritoneal mouse macrophages. The cyclooxygenase activity leads to primary prostaglandins E2, D2 and F2α as well as prostacyclin and thromboxane A2. The lipoxygenase pathway produces hydroperoxyeicosatetraenoic acids (HPETEs) which are subsequently reduced to hydroxyeicosatetraenoic acids (HETEs). (11). Inhibition of immune function by endogenous PGE2 represents a physiologic negative feedback mechanism initiated by antigen challenge (17). Thus this arachidonic acid metabolite acts as an important local regulator of immune reactions since the short half life of this compound limits its activity to the site of production.

Similarly HPETEs and HETEs are products of macrophage lipoxygenase with a short half life and they could also act on the lymphocyte activities.

In this paper we will describe the results we observed concerning the effects of some HPETEs and HETEs on lymphocyte proliferation in vitro.

MATERIAL AND METHODS

15.L.HPETE Synthesis

15 L HPETE was obtained by incubation of soybean lipoxygenase I with arachidonic acid according to the method of Hamberg and Samuelsson (7).

HETEs Synthesis

5-, 8-, 9-, 11-, 12- and 15-HPETEs were prepared from arachidonic acid by reaction with H_2O_2, in the presence of Cu^{2+}, as described
by Boeynaems et al (2). The reaction products were submitted to high-
pressure liquid chromatography performed with a Waters Associates
instrument. A µPorasil column was used. The eluent solvent was that
described by Porter et al (10). One aliquot of each separated HPETE
(detected at 235 nm) was reduced with triphenylphosphine at 0°C for
30 minutes. The identity of each HETE was assessed as methyl esters
trimethysilyl ethers, by high-efficiency glass capillary column chromatography prior to mass spectrometry.

Mice

C57Bl/6 (B6, $H-2^b$) and DBA/2 (D2, $H-2^d$) mice were all purchased
from the Iffa Credo laboratory. Splenocyte and thymocyte suspensions
were prepared by mincing spleen and thymi in RPMI 1640 medium.

In vitro activation of lymphocytes by mitogens

Mouse splenocytes, human T cells or T cell subsets, respectively
$2x10^6$ cells/ml or $1x10^6$ cells/ml were cultived in RPMI 1640 medium
(Flow laboratories) supplemented with 10 % inactivated fetal calf serum (FCS-Flow laboratories), 1 % hepes, $5x10^{-5}$M 2-mercaptoethanol, L
glutamine 10^{-4}M and antibiotics. The experiments were set up in flat-
bottomed Falcon microtest II plates. Each experiment (200 µl per well)
was set up in triplicate. Either concanavalin A (Con A) or phytohaemagglutinin (PHA) (Pharmindustrie) and HPETE or HETE were simultaneously
added at the initiation of the culture. At day three, 2 µCi of ^3H
thymidine (CEA France, specific activity 1 Ci/mmol) were added in each
well and the cultures continued for 6 hours. Thereafter cells were
harvested and adsorbed onto glass-fiber filters in an automatic cell
harvester, dried at 60°C and transferred to scintillation vials containing scintillation fluid.

In vitro activation of lymphocytes by mixed lymphocyte reactions

Mixed lymphocyte reactions (MLR) were performed in flat-bottomed Falcon microtest II. One hundred microliters of responding cells (C57B1/6 splenocytes - $5x10^3$/ml) were cocultived with 100 µl of irradiated DBA/2 stimulating cells ($5x10^3$/ml). The culture medium was RPMI 1640 completed as described for experiments with mitogens. Each tested HPETE and HETE was added at the beginning of the test. Each experiment was set up in triplicate. On the third day, 2 µCi of ^3H thymidine were added per well and then samples were processed as described for stimulation by mitogens.

In vitro generation of cytotoxic T lymphocytes

$7x10^6$ C57B1/6 splenocytes (H-2^b) were cocultived with $6x10^6$ irradiated DBA/2 splenocytes (H-2^d) in a 24-well tissue-culture plates (Linbro). Culture medium was RPMI 1640 completed as used for MLR. HPETEs and HETEs were added at the initiation of the coculture. Activated cells were harvested at day 5 and tested for cytotoxic activity. For the cytotoxicity assay, effector lymphocytes (E) were suspended to $1x10^7$ cells/ml in Eagle's minimum medium supplemented with 5 % FCS. One hundred microliters of this undiluted cell suspension and 3- and 9-fold dilutions thereof were added to 100 µl of ^{51}Cr-labelled P815 (H-2^d) target cells (T) (100 µl, $1x10^5$ cells/ml). The assays were then incubated for 4 hours at 37°C in an atmosphere of 5 % CO_2 in humidified air. Subsequently, the supernatant from each well was obtained with a supernatant harvester (Titertrek). The degree of ^{51}Cr release in test wells was compared with that of control target cells incubated with naïve splenocytes and with three times freezed/thawed target cells. The percentage of ^{51}Cr release was calculated according to the formula : A - C / FT - C x100 (A, assay ; C, control with naïve cells ; FT, freezed/thawed cells).

Isolation of human T cells and B cells

Peripheral blood mononuclear cells (PBMC) were isolated from heparinized blood of healthy adult donors on Ficoll-hypaque density gradients. Glass adherent cells were removed by incubation at 37°C for 1 hour on glass petri dishes in RPMI 1640 with 20 % FCS. T cells and B cells were separated by rosetting with aminoethylthiouranium (AET) treated sheep red blood cells followed by centrifugation over Ficoll-hypaque for 30 minutes at 300 g.

Isolation of human T cell subsets

The subsets were isolated by complement-mediated lysis after the procedure of Thomas et al (15) slighty modified. Briefly $5x10^7$ cells were suspended in 1/250 diluted OKT4 or OKT8 antibody in RPMI 1640 media containing 20 % FCS and were incubated 90 mn at room temperature. Low tox M rabbit complement (Cedarlane) was added at a final concentration of 1/20 and incubation was further carried out for 90 mn at 37°C. After that, less than 3 % of the living cells were still carrying the marker of the eliminated subset. The cells were treated before and/or after preincubation with 15 HPETE.

Human cell cultures

$2x10^5$ fresh B cells were combined with 10^5 preincubated T cells or T cell subsets and with or without 10^5 fresh T cells, all from the same donor. The cells were cultured at 37°C in 5 % CO_2 in 1 ml RPMI 1640 medium with 20 % FCS in 12x75 mm plastic culture tubes (Falcon 2054) stimulated with pokeweed mitogen (PWM) at a final concentration of 1/200. Cultures were stopped at 8 days and IgG and IgM concentrations were determined in the supernates by an ELISA method as previously described (3).

Monoclonal antibodies anti human T cell subsets

The monoclonal antibodies OKT4 and OKT8 were purchased from Ortho pharmaceuticals. OKT4 is a monoclonal antibody reacting with the helper/inducer subset of human T cells. OKT8 and Leu2 detect suppressor and cytotoxic T cells. Directly fluoresceinated Leu2 reacting with cytotoxic/ suppressor T cells was purchased from Becton–Dickinson ; $1x10^6$ cells were treated by 100 µl of this 1/2 diluted antibody before cytofluorograph analysis (Ortho 50).

Indirect immunofluorescence with monoclonal antibodies and cytofluorography analysis

Anti Lyt-1.2 and anti Lyt-2.2 monoclonal antibodies were purchased from New England Nuclear. Lyt-1.2 is a monoclonal antibody reacting with the helper/inducer subset of mouse T cells Lyt-2.2 reacts with the suppressor/cytotoxic cells.

Splenocytes or thymocytes ($2x10^6$) preincubated with 15 HETE (10^{-6} to 10^{-9} M final concentration) were incubated at 4°C for 60 mn in 200 µl of free serum RPMI 1640 with $1x10^{-3}$ dilution of a monoclonal antibody were then washed and incubated with $1x10^{-2}$ dilution of fluorescent goat Fab anti mouse Ig, incubated at 4°C for 60 mn and then washed. Fluorescent cells were analysed by a cytofluorograph (Ortho 50).

Flow microfluorometric analysis of nuclear DNA

It was performed as Vindelov (16). Briefly after preincubation with 15 HETE (10^{-6} to 10^{-9} final concentration) the cell's membrane were lysed by Nonidet P40 and DNA stained using ethidium bromide. Fluorescence due to fluorochrome binding to RNA was abolished by RNAse. The staining was studied by flow microfluorometry (Ortho 50).

RESULTS

Table 1 shows that the lymphocyte response to mitogens was tremendously decreased by HPETEs. These results were obtained using a final concentration for each HPETE of 10^{-5}M but a significant inhibitory effect on Con A and PHA stimulated lymphocytes was observed with concentration of HPETEs as low as 10^{-8}M.

TABLE 1. <u>Inhibition of lectins induced lymphocyte proliferation by</u>
<u>HPETEs. (Each result is the mean of 3 experiments)</u>[a]

	PHA 9 µg/ml	Con A 6 µg/ml
Controls	20233 ± 5136	41460 ± 17577
5 HPETE	3382 ± 2242	9299 ± 13379
8 HPETE	3230 ± 2406	2540 ± 684
9 HPETE	2253 ± 2151	1650 ± 1258
11 HPETE	2073 ± 840	2970 ± 2081
12 HPETE	1697 ± 1424	2145 ± 406
15 HPETE	2473 ± 1185	1949 ± 817

[a]Results are expressed as ^{3}H thymidine uptake in cpm ± SD

The non toxicity of the HPETEs towards the mouse lymphocytes was assessed by (i) trypan blue exclusion test (ii) measurement of ^{51}Cr released by radiolabelled and HPETEs treated lymphocytes.

Similarly the lymphocyte alloreactivity (studied by the mean of mixed lymphocyte reaction) was diminished by HPETEs. Thus when B6 lymphocytes were stimulated by irradiated D2 cells the thymidine uptake in
terms of cpm was 4750 ± 1000 (mean of 5 experiments) without HPETEs versus 525 ± 105 cpm with 5 HPETE, 710 ± 95 cpm with 8 HPETE, 1517 ± 125
with 9 HPETE, 978 ± 25 with 11 HPETE, 1214 ± 117 with 15 HPETE.

On the same way the effects of 15 HPETE and 15 HETE were also observed when the reactivity of B6 responders was estimated by the generation
of B6 (H-2^b) anti D2 (H-2^d) killer cells tested against P815 (H-2^d) target cells (table 2).

In some experiments B6 splenocytes were suspended into RPMI 1640
containing 10 % FCS and incubated during 18 hours with 15 HPETE or 15
HETE. At the end of the preincubation the cells were washed and combined

with fresh B6 splenocytes. 3.5×10^5 fresh B6 splenocytes were combined with 3.5×10^5 either 15 HPETE treated or 15 HETE treated B6 splenocytes. These cells were cocultived with irradiated D2 stimulators (splenocytes). It was observed that the response of fresh lymphocytes was partially inhibited by the addition of splenocytes preincubated with the lipoxygenase products (table3).

TABLE 2. <u>Inhibition of generation of killer cells by 15 HPETE and 15 HETE (mean of four experiments)</u>

Product added to cultures	Lysis of radiolabelled P815 cells[a]		
	100 : 1	33 : 1	11 : 1
medium	80	40	20
15 HPETE	10	5	2
15 HETE	30	20	15

[a]Lysis is percentage of specific release of ^{51}Cr at three effector to target cell ratios (E/T = 100:1 ; 33:1 ; 11:1).

TABLE 3. <u>Inhibition of MLR between fresh B6 splenocytes and D2 stimulators by either 15 HPETE or 15 HETE treated cells[a]</u>

No of experiment	cells preincubated with 15 HPETE (molar concentration)				
	10^{-6}	10^{-7}	10^{-8}	10^{-9}	10^{-10}
1	49	12	30	0	3
2	51	57	57	50	45
3	49	47	32	25	18

[a]Results are expressed as percent inhibition of the response of fresh cells plus cells preincubated with eicosanoids compared to fresh cells plus cells preincubated with medium alone.

The last experiments show that mouse lymphocytes incubated with HPETE or HETE acquired a suppressive activity, the same phenomenom was observed with human T cells. Human T cells preincubated with 15 HPETE for 18 hours no longer supported immunoglobulin production of fresh autologous B cells. In 6 experiments the IgG production was suppressed 75 % and the IgM production was suppressed 83 % by T cells preincubated with 15 HPETE compared to T cells preincubated in complete media. The suppressing effect of T cells preincubated with 15 HPETE was maintained when equal numbers of fresh autologous T cells were added to the preincubated T cells. The suppressive effect of the 15 HPETE treated T cells was almost lost if the cells were exposed to 2500 rads X-irradiation after incubation with the 15 HPETE (the reduction of IgG synthesis was only 20 %).

The above data suggested that 15 HPETE and 15 HETE induce a radio-sensitive suppressor cell from mouse splenocytes or human resting peripheral blood T cells. We then investigated the phenotypic nature of the eicosanoids induced suppressor cells. When splenocytes were incubated in vitro for 48 hours with 15 HETE (10^{-6} to 10^{-8} final concentration) it was noticed an increase of Lyt-1$^+$ and mostly Lyt-2$^+$ cells. This augmentation was more significant for a 10^{-7}M final concentration of 15 HETE (table 4). We observed the same results with thymocytes (data non shown).

TABLE 4. Modification of splenocyte Lyt markers by 15 HETE

preincubation	Lyt-1$^+$2$^-$cells	Lyt-1$^-$2$^+$cells
medium	30 ± 8	8 ± 3
15 HETE	35 ± 6 (+ 16 %)	14 ± 5 (+ 75 %)

In the same way we have observed that treatment of human T cells with OKT8 monoclonal antibody plus complement before preincubation with 15 HPETE did not influence suppressor cell generation (86 % inhibition of IgG production by cells preincubated with 15 HPETE versus 73 % inhibition by cells treated with OKT8 plus complement then preincubated with

15 HPETE), while the same treatment with OKT8 plus complement after preincubation with 15 HPETE eliminated the suppression of IgG production in the subsequent culture (33 % enhancement of IgG production by T cells preincubated with 15 HPETE and then treated with OKT8 plus complement). In addition, treatment of the T cells with OKT4 plus complement before preincubation with 15 HPETE caused a reduction in suppressor activity of these cells (28 % inhibition of IgG production by cells treated with OKT4 plus complement before preincubation with 15 HPETE).

One explanation for the above data is that 15 HPETE and 15 HETE induce a population of lymphocytes to become a population of suppressor cells. For example one possibility is that 15 HPETE induces an OKT8 (-) T cell to become an OKT8 (+) radiosensitive suppressor cell. This hypothesis is sustained by the following experiment. When T cells or OKT8 (-) T cells were incubated for 18 hours with or without 15 HPETE (1×10^6 cells/ml, 15 HPETE 10^{-6}M final concentration) and afterthat the percentage of cells bearing cytotoxic/suppressor surface markers determined by incubation with directly fluoresceinated Leu 2 followed by cytofluorograph analysis we observed a large increase in suppressor cells in the OKT8 (-) T cell population and a smaller one in the whole T cell population (table 5).

TABLE 5. <u>Increase in the percentage of T cells bearing suppressor cell marker after incubation with 15 HPETE</u>

cell population	preincubation	Percent Leu 2(+) cells			
		experiments			
		1	2	3	mean
T cells	media	29	24	31	28
T cells	15 HPETE	32	40	35	36
OKT8 (-) T cells	media	3	17	4	8
OKT8 (-) T cells	15 HPETE	27	37	29	31

The problem was to determine if the increase of percentage of cells car-

rying the suppressor/cytotoxic surface markers was merely a membrane phenomenon resulting from the expression or relocation of hidden OKT8 or
Lyt-2 antigens or if it was a mechanism related to a cell proliferation
and/or differenciation. Therefore the cell cycle of 15 HETE treated lymphocytes (thymocytes or splenocytes) was studied by ethidium bromide
staining and flow microfluorometric analysis of nuclear DNA. It was observed that 15 HETE increases the percentage of cell in G2 phase (after
41 hours of preincubation) and that this increment was preceded from
the 17th to the 22nd hour by an increase of cells in the S phase (table
6).

TABLE 6. Flow microfluorometric analysis of nuclear DNA.
Percentage of 15 HETE treated cells in S or G2 phases
(compared to the controls incubated with medium)

cell cycle phase	duration of preincubation (hours)					
	17	19	22	24	41	48
S	+38	+100	+95	-15	0	-10
G2	- 5	- 10	- 5	+10	+20	+ 3

DISCUSSION

There is a good deal of evidence that 15 HPETE and 15 HETE inhibit
many lymphocyte functions in vitro. We already described the inhibitory
capacity of eight HPETEs and HETEs on lymphocyte mitogenesis in vitro (4)
phenomenon which was also observed by Bailey et al with 15 HETE (1). We
later evidenced that 15 HPETE inhibits the rosette formation of human T
lymphocytes with sheep red blood cells and that this phenomenon was HLA-
linked (5). So far it seems that 15 HPETE and 15 HETE are strong immuno-
suppressor in vitro and in vivo (6), but the mechanism of this eicosanoid induced immunosuppression is not yet totally clear. In other words
it is not very well known how 15 HPETE and 15 HETE act for decreasing a
great number of activities of immune cells. It could be possible that
these metabolites are effective on the whole lymphocyte popu-

lation merely by an alteration of some lymphocyte physical property or by inducing a modification of the cells' metabolism. However it is likely that in regard of the experiments described in this report the eicosanoïds induced immunosuppression results from the induction of suppressor cells.

Bailey and al(1) described that 15 HETE (concentrations ranging from 5×10^{-6} to 2.5×10^{-5}M) added to PHA stimulated splenocytes blocked the thymidine uptake by the lectin pulsed T cells. They also observed that the effects of 15 HETE were maximal if added in the first 8 hours following mitogen addition. According to the authors the effect of 15 HETE on lectins stimulated splenocytes resulted from the inhibition of 12 HETE synthesis by immune cells. On the other hand 15 HETE and 5 HETE increase the level of intracellular cyclic guanylate monophosphate (cGMP) (8), this phenomenon is usually associated with an enhancement of cells activities such as lymphocyte proliferation. It is likely that the intracellular balance between cAMP an a cGMP is an important factor for the lymphocyte proliferation and differentiation (14) and since we observed that 15 HETE increases lymphocyte cGMP (data not shown) it seems that the effects of 15 HETE on lymphocyte metabolism are opposite, i.e. (i) augmentation of cGMP which give rise to a proliferation and (ii) inhibition of 5 HETE production which leds to an immunosuppression.

One may argue that 15 HPETE inhibits the synthesis of PGI_2 (12). Honn et al (9) admitted that the increase of tumor metastasis observed after intraveinous injections of 15 HPETE resulted from the decrease of PGI_2 synthesis which enhance the platelet aggregation.
However it is possible that the immunosuppression induced in vivo by 15 HPETE is an enhancing factor for tumor growth.

It should be pointed out that in vitro both 15 HPETE and 15 HETE dramatically modify the viscosity of the splenocytes' plasmatic membranes as we reported before (6). There is therefore a chance that 15 HPETE and 15 HETE are effective in vitro on lymphocyte activities by inducing a rigidity of the lymphocyte membranes thus blocking the mobility of the receptors and preventing them to cooperate, phenomenon which is necessary for the initiation of the mitogenesis.

However the modification of the physical state of the cell membranes cannot explain why the sensitivity of human lymphocytes to 15 HPETE is HLA-linked (5) and why, as we observed before, the OKT8 (+) cells are less sensitive to 15 HPETE than the OKT4 (+) T cell subset in regard of the mitogen induced thymidine uptake (NG. PhD thesis in immunology – Paris 1983). In other words, how could a simple modification of the physical state of the cells explain the HLA-linked and OKT-linked differences of sensitivity

The mechanism of eicosanoid induced immunosuppression is more complex than a simple modification of (i) the metabolism or (ii) the viscosity of the cells'membranes. For instance we observed some opposite phenomenons induced by 15 HPETE or 15 HETE such as an inhibition of the proliferative response to lectins (in term of thymidine uptake) and an augmentation of both intracellular cGMP and DNA. These modifications preceded an increase of the number of cells carrying the OKT8 or Lyt2 suppressor markers and these cells actually inhibit the immune response of fresh T cells or B cells.

Therefore we speculate that 15 HPETE and 15 HETE induce the proliferation and/or differenciation of a subset of presuppressor cells giving rise to suppressor OKT8 (+) or Lyt2 (+) lymphocytes.

According to this hypothesis the increase of cGMP and the synthesis of DNA may be related to the proliferation of the suppressor subset which could be more sensitive to one or more of the following factors : (i) HPETEs and HETEs (ii) increase of the intracellular cGMP (iii) balance between lipoxygenase and prostaglandin synthetase activities.

Finally one should keep in mind that aspirin and indomethacin are not exclusively inhibitors of PGs synthesis (13) and that experiments or therapeutics which include this kind of drugs deal with blockade of both prostaglandins and 15 HPETE synthesis.

Our results confirm that oxygenated arachidonic acid metabolites other than PG_s are important regulator of the immune response. As PG_s these metabolites, mainly produced by activated macrophages, are probably cells to cells (macrophages to lymphocytes) messengers for an inhibiting feed-back.

It should be noticed that HPETES and HETES are also synthetised by tumor cells suggesting that tumors may be able to escape to immunosurveillance by the mean of an eicosanoid induced immunosuppression and one may suggest the use of both lipoxygenase and cyclooxygenase inhibitors as antitumoral therapy.

ACKNOWLEDGMENTS

Supported in part by Institut National de la Santé et de la Recherche Médicale (PCR 127013) and by Centre National Interprofessionnel de l'Economie Laitière.

The authors wish to thank Marie-Hélène Ratinaud for her expert technical assistance (Service Commun de Cytofluorographie de l'Université de Limoges).

REFERENCES

1. Bailey, J.M., Bryant, R.W., Low, C.E., Pupillo, M.B., Vanderhoek, J.Y. (1982) : Cell Immunol., 67 : 112

2. Boeynaems, J.M., Brash, A.R., Oates, J.A., Hubbard, W.C. (1980) : Anal Biochem., 104 : 259

3. Ceuppens, J.L., Gualde, N., Goodwin, J.S. (1982) : Cell Immunol., 69 : 150

4. Gualde, N., Rigaud, M., Rabinovitch, H., Durand, J., Beneytout, J.L., Breton, J.C. (1981) : C R Acad Sci Paris., 293 : 359

5. Gualde, N., Rabinovitch, H., Fredon, M., Rigaud, M. (1982) : Eur J Immunol., 12 : 773

6. Gualde, N., Chable-Rabinovitch, H., Motta, C., Durand, J., Beneytout, J.L., Rigaud, M. (1983) : Biochim Biophys Acta., 750 : 429

7. Hamberg, M., Samuelsson, B. (1967) : J. Biol. Chem., 242 : 5329

8. Harbon, M., Leiber, D., Vesin, M.F. (1983) : In : Advances in Prostaglandin, Thromboxane and Leukotriene Research Vol. 12, edited by B. Samuelsson, R. Paoletti and P. Ramwell, pp 423-428. Raven Press, New-York

9. Honn, K.V., Busse, W.D., Sloane, B.F. (1983) : Biochem. Pharmacol., 32 : 1

10. Porter, N.A., Wolf, R.A., Yarbro, E.M., Weenen, H. (1979) : Biochem. Biophys. Res. Commun., 89 : 1058

11. Rabinovitch, H., Durand, J., Gualde, N., Rigaud, M. (1981) : Agents Actions., 11 : 580

12. Salmon, J.A., Smith, D.R., Flower, R.J., Moncada, S., Vane, J.R. (1978) : Biochim. Biophys. Acta., 523 : 250

13. Siegel, M.I., Mc Connel, R.T., Porter, N.A., Selph, J.L., Truax, J.F., Vinegar, R., Cuatrecasas, P. (1980) : Biochem. Biophys. Res. Commun., 92 : 688

14. Strom, T.B., Lundin, A.P., Carpenter, C.B. (1977) : In : Progress in Clinical Immunology, edited by R.S. Schwartz, pp 115-153. Grune and Straton, New York

15. Thomas, Y., Sosman, J., Irigoyen, O., Friedman, S.M., Kung, P.C., Goldstein, G., Chess, L. (1980) : J Immunol., 125 : 1283

16. Vindelov, L.L. (1977) : Virchows Arch B Cell Path., 24 : 277

17. Webb, D.R., Osheroff, P.L. (1976) : Proc. Natl Acad Sci USA., 43 : 1300

Icosanoids and Cancer, edited by H. Thaler-Dao, et al. Raven Press, New York © 1984.

Disordered Prostaglandin Production and Cell Differentiation/Proliferation in Cancer

R. Bockman, A. Bellin, and N. Hickok

Memorial Sloan-Kettering Cancer Center, New York, New York 10021

1. Augmented Prostaglandin Production, a Cancer Induced Disorder.

Enhanced prostaglandin synthesis is frequently noted in the cancer bearing host. Many tumor cell lines constituitively release more prostaglandin product than the parent tissues from which they were derived[30]. Interestingly, non-malignant tissues (e.g., monocytes) from tumor bearing hosts, including man, may also show augmented arachidonate metabolism compared to appropriate, non-cancer bearing controls[23]. It is enhanced metabolism of arachidonate that results in abnormal levels of biologically active prostaglandins, thromboxane, and leukotrienes in the cancer bearing host. These bioactive lipids may directly modulate the growth and differentiation of host and tumor cells. In addition, these prostaglandins can alter host-tumor cell interactions that can affect host immunocompetance, indirectly facilitating tumor growth and spread. Preliminary experiments exploring the possible mechanisms responsible for disordered prostaglandin production and its consequences will be presented following a brief review.

Early experiments carried out in our laboratory demonstrated augmented prostaglandin synthesis by macrophages from tumor bearing animals[23]. Resident peritoneal macrophages from C57Bl/6 mice bearing a transplantable fibrosarcoma (MC-16) released more PGE than non-tumor bearing littermates. Following challenge with inflammatory stimuli, the macrophages from tumor bearers showed a several-fold enhancement of PGE release and continued to show enhanced production with restimulation. Cells derived from non-tumor bearing littermates showed less of an initial release of PGE after exposure to stimuli and little or no response with restimulation. The data clearly showed that macrophages from tumor bearing animals had a markedly augmented capacity to metabolize arachidonate. However, it is not known whether the monocytes from tumor

169

bearing mice had more PG-synthase, a more stable PG-synthase, or greater substrate availability, perhaps through altered handling (traffic) of substrate.

In monocytes from mice and man PGE and thromboxane were found to be the major arachidonate products. It was striking that the pattern of PG-synthase products was, in part, a function of the in vitro culture conditions, e.g., time in culture, and species studied[4]. From these studies, it was evident that in order to understand cell regulation of PG synthesis (i.e., enzyme activation, synthesis, and substrate availability) we needed a defined model. Specifically, we required a human cell line, preferably with a single active PG-synthase, that produced large amounts of enzyme and product. We are fortunate to have recently established such a cell line, Lu-65.

A large and ever growing body of literature argues that disordered arachidonate metabolism plays a central role in the initiation and propagation of the malignant state. The enzymes involved in arachidonate metabolism have been shown to have a direct role in carcinogensis[20,28,35] as well as a facilitative role on tumor implantation, growth and metastasis[14]. In the latter two processes, altered host immunocompetence induced by disordered prostaglandin synthesis may be a mechanism by which tumor growth and spread is favored. In general, cell regulation of bioactive lipid production can be effected at three levels: (1) enzyme activity, (2) new enzyme synthesis, and (3) substrate availability. To date, the small amount of available data on cellular regulation of arachidonate metabolism comes largely from animal systems; essentially no information is available on the human enzyme systems. Recently, we have established a cell line (Lu-65) derived from a human giant cell cancer of the lung. This tumor produces large amounts of prostaglandin E providing us with the opportunity to isolate and purify a single active prostaglandin synthase. Protein isolation and purification of PG-synthase have been carried out. In addition we have achieved a preliminary isolation of PG-synthase mRNA by immunoprecipitation. The data derived from these studies should contribute significantly to our understanding of cell regulation of arachidonate metabolism. Eventually, it should be possible to rationally manipulate product formation by specifically inducing or inhibiting select enzyme pathways. Pharmacological modulation of arachidonate metabolism with the goal of favorably altering the levels of these potent biological modifiers may one day prove to be an important adjunct to cancer therapy.

2. Biological Consequences of Excess Prostaglandins.

Immune cell dysfunction and depressed immunocompetence are frequently associated with cancer and may contribute to its morbidity and mortality. The mec-

hanisms that are responsible for these phenomena are
poorly understood. In certain malignant conditions (of
which Hodgkin's Disease serves as a prime example),
immunodepletion and multifunctional immune cell disorders are found to progress with advancing stage of
disease[31]. In such patients, excessive monocyte synthesis of prostaglandin E, a potent modulator of immune
cell function, has been shown to occur[3,11]. As prostaglandins can exert their immunomodulatory effects at
both the stem and mature T cell levels, it seems reasonable to speculate that augmented synthesis of
arachidonate metabolites may contribute to the disorders of T cell ontogeny and mature T cell function
seen in patients with Hodgkin's Disease. Indeed, the
progressive loss of committed T stem cells could be
shown to be significantly correlated with the increased
levels of endogenous prostaglandins that occurs with
advancing stage of disease. Our recent data impli-
cating prostaglandins in the pathophysiology leading to
depressed immunocompetence in cancer patients is discussed.

B. PRELIMINARY STUDIES ON CELL REGULATION OF PROSTAGLANDIN PRODUCTION

The prostaglandins are synthesized from arachidonic acid via a three-step process utilizing the
membrane-bound enzyme complex, PG synthase. The first
two steps are common to the synthesis of all PG classes
with the third step determining the final PG product.
Controls on the enzyme complex and hence PG synthesis
can be exerted at three levels: (1) induction of PG
synthase synthesis, (2) alteration of existing PG synthase activity, and (3) changes in the concentration of
available substrate, arachidonic acid.

1. Establishment and Characterization of Lu-65.

Factors that affect PG production are legion; however, the level at which this control is effected is,
in general, unknown. To begin to study the question of
cell regulation of PG synthesis we have examined the
newly established human cell line, Lu-65. This unique
cell line was derived from a patient with a large cell
anaplastic lung cancer and represents one of three such
cell lines ever described[2]. To establish the line,
minced tumor was initially injected in a nude mouse and
then adapted to tissue culture. The isoenzyme pattern
and cytogenetics of Lu-65 indicate that the line is of
human origin, and is a new, i.e., non-contaminated
line[2]. A number of biological activities associated
with the cell line are sufficient to explain the clinical syndromes presented by patients[5]. Coincidentally,
the Lu-65 cell line produces nanogram amounts of PGE
with less that 6% of other arachidonate metabolites

produced[5].

2. Initial Studies on Enzyme Isolation and Purification.

To date, our studies have shown the PG synthase complex in the Lu-65 cell line to be membrane-bound and localized to the microsomal fraction, as it is in other species[21,32]. The enzyme complex can be differentially solubilized from the PGE synthase-rich microsomes with Tween-20, yielding, initially, the cyclooxygenase/hydroperoxidase (PGH synthase) activity. Upon further treatment with Triton X-100 the PGE isomerase activity can be solubilized. Subsequently, the PGH synthase is purified by gel filtration, Sephadex isoelectric focusing, and a further gel filtration step.

The active protein fraction from Lu-65 has a molecular weight of 60,000-80,000 as measured by gel filtration, a pH maximum of 7.5-8.0, and consumes oxygen upon addition of arachidonic acid. Peroxidase activity can be demonstrated. The enzyme showed enhanced activity in the presence of heme, phenol or hydroquinone. In the presence of cofactors, the enzyme was resistant to attack by trypsin. Aspirin and indomethacin inhibit conversion of arachidonic acid as measured by oxygen consumption. These properties are in agreement with those we and others have observed in purified ram seminal vesicle (RSV) PGH synthase[21,32]. Further purification of the enzyme complex from this human cell line is still in progress. Using purified enzyme the numerous endogenous factors that may regulate enzyme activity in vivo will be examined. Concurrently, total mRNA has been extracted and purified in an effort to identify PG-synthase specific message. Preliminary identification of mRNA translation product has been achieved by immunoprecipitation using a polyvalent antibody to RSV. Such studies will allow us to follow cell regulation of prostaglandin production at the level of enzyme synthesis.

3. Substrate Traffic in Tumor Cells and Normal Monocytes.

Many mechanisms may operate to move and accumulate arachidonate (C20:4) within cells and thereby modulate C20:4 availability to PG synthase. For example, cells may differ in the amount of C20:4 contained in membrane phospholipids (PL) due to alterations in absolute amounts of C20:4 or the relative ratio of C20:4 to other fatty acids (FA). Alternatively, cells may differ in their ability to mobilize C20:4 from PL, perhaps as a consequence of the cells' endowment of specific transacylases and phospholipases, the enzymes responsible for trafficking FA. Since any one or a combination of these factors may regulate the cells ability to synthesize PG, we have attempted to measure absolute levels of C20:4 as well as, the relative ratio

of C20:4 to other key FA (notably linoleic, C18:2).
Further we have looked at the ability of cells to move
radiolabeled FA. In all cases we have tried to compare
the data obtained in malignant human cell lines with
that derived from human monocytes. These results are
briefly summarized.

    a. Measurement and Manipulation of Arachidonate
       Content.

Several permanent tumor cell lines, originally
derived from patients with renal cell adenocarcinoma
were studied for their ability to release PGE. Tumor
cells (1-2x10^6) were placed into cell culture and incubated with various amounts of C20:4, (0-25 ug/ml). As
can be seen in Figure 1, a dose dependent increase in
PGE production was noted for some cases, for other cell
lines, little change was seen.

An attempt was made to correlate prostaglandin production with the relative and absolute amounts of PL
bound FA, particularly C20:4 and C18:2. Following cell
culture in the presence and absence of added C20:4, the
cell pellets were washed and then membrane PL extracted
with chloroform: methanol (3:1). Free FA was prepared
by alkaline hydrolysis and extracted into acidified
chloroform:methanol. The individual, underivatized FA
were separated and quantified by reverse phase high
performance liquid chromatography (HPLC), (Figure 2).
For the renal cell lines studied, the levels of C20:4
were initially very low (< 0.01 and 0.02 ug/10^6 cells
for SKRC-29 and SKRC-7 respectively), and increased
when the cells were cultured in the presence of 25 ug
C20:4 (0.5 and 0.09 ug/10^6 cells, respectively). No
consistent change in the level of C18:2 was found. An
absolute increase in C20:4 content and PGE production
was achieved by incubating the cells with relatively
high levels of C20:4. However, the cell line (SKRC-7)
which showed greater accumulation of C20:4, had lower
levels of PGE production, thus it appears that C20:4
metabolism does not depend simply on the absolute
amount of FA present in PL.

    b. Arachidonate Traffic.

For many cell systems, in order for C20:4 metabolism
to occur, FA is moved into and subsequently out of
membrane PL. This movement of FA is poorly understood
and depends on complex transacylation steps regulated
in part by a variety of phospholipases and lipases that
have yet to be isolated or characterized. We have
attempted to follow C20:4 turnover in the membrane PL
in select tumor cell lines and normal monocytes to look
for differences in metabolism of C20:4 and movement
within PL. Lu-65 cells that were original derived
from human lung cancer and which we know to incorporate
and convert C20:4, were allowed to adhere to glass
coverslips. The cells were exposed to ^{3}H-C20:4 for 2h
by which time incorporation has reached a plateau; the
cells and supernatant media were then tested for 20:4

content and PG activity following extraction with chloroform: methanol. The major PL classes were separated using one dimension thin layer chromatography (TLC) developed with chloroform:methanol:acetic acid: water 50:25:8:4 (v/v) [4]. Zones that coeluted with authentic phosphatidyl choline (PC), phosphatidyl ethanolamine (PE) and phosphatidyl inositol (PI) were visualized, scraped, and the tritiated lipids were counted in a Beta-scintillation counter. Tritiated prostaglandins released into the supernatant media were extracted by the method of Folch and analyzed by 2-D TLC as previously described[4]. The majority of ^{3}H-C20:4 was found in PI (17,490 $\pm$ 1915 CPM) with lesser amounts in PC and PE (7661 $\pm$895 and 3872 $\pm$1882 CPM, respectively); Figure 3. The phosphate content of the three PL classes was analyzed to assess the relative proportion of each PL class in Lu-65. PC, PE and PI showed 0.93, 0.40 and 0.05 ug $PO_4/10^6$ cells respectively. Thus, while PC and PE were the most abundant PL, ^{3}H-C20:4 was preferentially esterified to PI. Following the 2h labelling of Lu-65 cells with ^{3}H-C20:4; the Lu-65 cells were cultured for 4 hrs during the time the cells constituitively produced ^{3}H-PGE$_2$, Figure 3. After the 4 h of culture, extraction of cellular lipids showed that the amount of radiolabel in PI was decreased while PC and PI had increased slightly. However, changes in radiolabel between the initial and after 4h incubation were not significant for any of the PL classes. No consistent change in the distribution of ^{3}H-C20:4 amongst the PL classes was noted when the incubation was carried out in the presence of structurally unrelated inhibitors of cyclooxygenase. These inhibitors profoundly inhibited ^{3}H-PGE$_2$ release but had no effect on ^{3}H-C:20:4 release into the media, Figure 3.

Similar studies of ^{3}H-C:20:4 turnover were carried out using monocytes from normal human subjects. Peripheral blood monocytes were isolated by density centrifugation and adherence as previously described[4,15]. After culture overnight the cells were allowed to incorporate ^{3}H-C 20:4. Tritiated PL in cell membrane and ^{3}H-PGE$_2$ release were followed as previously described for Lu-65. After 2h of ^{3}H-C 20:4 incorporation, the distribution of radiolabel in PC, PE and PI was 2514 $\pm$ 700, 1696 $\pm$655 and 3223 $\pm$1126, respectively. As with Lu-65 there appeared to be preferential uptake of label into PI though PI accounted for the smallest concentration of PL in monocytes. After 4h of cell culture, the total radioactivity in all PL classes decreased, 634 $\pm$ 71, 446 $\pm$60 and 853 $\pm$336 CPM/10^6 cells for PC, PE and PI respectively, figure 4. During this time period 2125 $\pm$285 CPM were released as ^{3}H-PGE$_2$. The addition of zymosan, an inflammatory stimulus, to the cell cultures caused a marked stimulation of ^{3}H-PGE$_2$ release and a greater decline in the radioactivity of all 3 PL classes. It is worth noting the subtle but consistent

difference between Lu-65 and monocyte handling of [3]H-
C20:4. The Lu-65 showed greater incorporation of [3]H-
C20:4 into PL and consistent loss of CPM from PI. The
monocytes studied one day after isolation incorporate
less label and show the same percent loss of counts
from all three PL classes, rather than a preferential
loss from PI as did Lu-65 cells. Platelets have been
reported to preferentially utilize C20:4 from PI via
phospholipase C and diglyceride lipase[24]. The
mechanism by which there is highly specific labelling
of the smallest PL class in Lu-65 and monocytes is
unknown nor is the pathway of C20:4 release for either
cell known. It is highly speculative but conceivable
that in a malignant cell like Lu-65 with a high consti-
tuitive rate of PG synthesis, C20:4 is rapidly trafficked through the major PL source for its cyclooxygenase, i.e., PI. By contrast, in the stimulus-coupled
secretion of PG by the monocyte, C20:4 is more widely
distributed amongst the PL classes. Wide distribution
of substrate would require a more complicated sequence
of phospholipase activation to occur in order to
release C20:4 thereby providing more control over cell
production. Finally both Lu-65 and the monocyte
release similar amounts of ^{3}H-PGE during the 4h incubation; however, the Lu-65 turned over nearly 5 times
more ^{3}H-C20:4 than the monocyte. We can speculate that
this represents more efficient metabolism of available
substrate by the monocyte. It is not known whether
monocytes can modulate the efficiency of utilizing
available substrate. In fact if ^{3}H-C20:4 released from
prelabelled cells is an indicator of C20:4 turnover,
then our early data would argue that the increased PGE
release seen after stimulation is not due to increased
efficiency of substrate utilization. By contrast the
increased PGE release seen with monocytes from patients
with Hodgkin's Disease (HD) appears due to increased
efficiency of utilizing free C20:4. These conclusions
are based on our observations that with zymosan stimulation, monocytes from normal subjects release much
more C20:4 than PGE_2 compared to what they release in
the basal state. However, monocytes from patients with
HD release proportionately more PGE than C20:4 compared
with monocytes from control subjects[3]. One possible
explanation is that there is more efficient utilization
of C20:4 by monocytes from patients with HD.

It is evident from such studies that we have much to
learn about cell regulation of arachidonate metabolism.
Virtually nothing is known regarding controls of enzyme
activity or enzyme synthesis in any cell system. A
large amount of information exists on substrate
handling of cells. Yet, little is known about the
exact mechanisms by which C20:4 is trafficked through
cell phospholipids and ultimately made available for
cyclooxygenase or lipoxygenase. Even less is known
about alteration of C20:4 turnover in those malignant

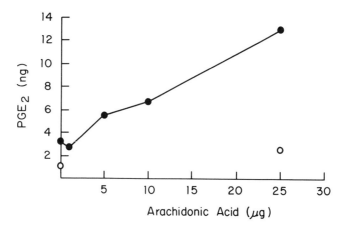

FIG. I.   Prostaglandin E levels in media conditioned
for 24h by 2×10^6 cells from renal adenocarcinoma
cell lines SKRC-29, closed circles; and SKRC-7 open
circles as a function of C 20:4 concentration in the
media.

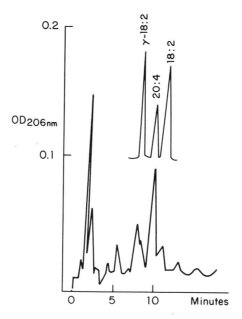

FIG. 2.   HPLC elution pattern of underivatized free
fatty acids from chloroform-methanol, alkaline hydrolyzed extractions of renal adenocarcinoma cells.
C 20:4 and C 18:2 levels were quantified by comparisons
with external standards, see insert. Reverse phase
chromatography was carried out on a Waters Associates
C18 column eluted with acetonitrile and water (80:20,
v/v) acidified with phosphoric acid and monitoring UV
absorption at 206 nm.

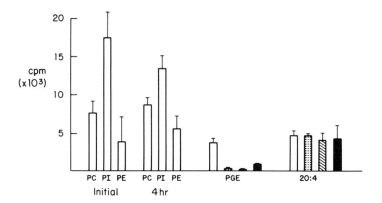

FIG. 3. Distribution of ^{3}H-C 20:4 into the membrane phospholipids (PC = Phosphatidyl choline, PI = Phosphatidyl inositol and PE = phosphatidyl ethanolamine) of Lu 65 after 2h exposure (initial) to 1 uCi ^{3}H-C 20:4. The cells from parallel cultures were washed to remove all non-incorporated ^{3}H-C 20:4, cultured for 4h in fresh media before C20:4 distribution in phospholipid was checked. ^{3}H-PGE$_2$ release into the media was measured after the 4h incubation in plain media (open bars) or in the presence of uM amounts of indomethacin (stippled), flurbiprofen (crosshatched) and 10 uM aspirin (solid).

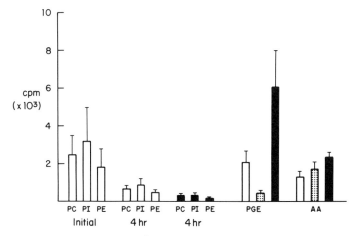

FIG. 4. Distribution of ^{3}H-C20:4 into membrane phospholipids of human monocytes after a 2h exposure (initial) of 10^6 cells to 1uCi of ^{3}H-C20:4. Parallel cell cultures were cultured for an additional 4h after unincorporated label was removed and ^{3}H-C20:4 distribution examined (4h) for cells cultured in plain media (open bars) or in the presence of 50 ug/ml zymosan (solid bars). ^{3}H-PGE$_2$ release into the media was measured after the 4h incubation in plain media, in the presence of uM indomethacin or zymosan (open, stippled and solid bars respectively).

states associated with augmented arachidonate metabolism. Nevertheless, disordered prostaglandins production is frequently associated with cancer and probably profoundly influences tumor-host interaction.

C. Biologic Consequences of Augmented Prostaglandin Production

1. Prostaglandins & CFU-TI.

A circulating precursor T lymphocyte (CFU-TI) has been described which undergoes clonal expansion to form colonies in soft agar[25,33,10,8,27,6]. Early studies presented evidence that monocytes and macrophages released factors, some of which inhibited others facilitated clonal T lymphocyte expansion in soft agar[8,34]. In previous studies from our laboratory with the clonable granulocyte/macrophage precursor (CFU-c), we were able to show balanced regulation of cell proliferation/differentiation involving PGE_2[16-18]. Suspecting that there might be a parallelism between the CFU-C and CFU-TI systems, the effects of prostaglandins and monocytes on T colony formation were examined[6]. In a soft agar system, T colonies were shown to arise from a small subset of phytohemagglutinin responsive T lymphocytes found in peripheral blood and lymph nodes[6]. The mature cells, when pooled from many colonies, could be shown to have functional activity[6]. The addition of PGE_2 caused a dose dependent inhibition of T colony formation with the 50% point of inhibition occurring at 0.18 uM PGE_2. Prostaglandin E_1 was as potent as PGE_2, whereas PGD_2 was without effect at up to 10.0 uM concentration[6], suggesting that the stereochemistry of the isomerically distinct pentane ring was critical for biologic effect. Low concentrations of $PGF_{2\alpha}$ ($<$10uM) appeared to augment colony numbers, whereas higher concentrations of $PGF_{2\alpha}$ ($\geq$10uM) were inhibitory[6]. The addition of small numbers of normal monocytes mimicked the effect seen with PGE_2. When prostaglandin synthase inhibitors were added with the monocytes, inhibition mediated by small numbers of monocytes was abolished. Finally, a highly significant correlation between endogenous levels of PGE, as measured by radioimmunoassay and T colony numbers, was demonstrated[6]. These data suggested that monocytes, through their synthesis of PGE_2, could regulate the clonal expansion of circulating T cell precursors[6]. Although PGE is a physiologically relevant regulator of stem cell proliferation, it is clearly, not the only inhibitory agent. Indeed, other macrophage derived factors have been postulated to be key regulators[8,27,6,34]. Furthermore, our own studies demonstrated the inability of cyclooxygenase inhibitors to block the inhibitory activity seen when large numbers of macrophages were added to the test system[6]. Nevertheless, prostaglandin

production by physiologically relevent numbers of monocytes appears to be an important mechanism for regulation of T cell ontogeny.

2.   Prostaglandins & Hodgkin's Disease.
     Impaired cell mediated immunity is a well reported
occurrence in patients with Hodgkin's
disease[1,7,12,13,19,].   Prostaglandins caused inhibition
of T cell function as measured in in vitro assays used
to assess mature T lymphocyte function[9,29].   Marked
elevation of PGE levels have been measured in immune
cell cultures from patients with Hodgkin's disease[3].
The addition of a prostaglandin synthase inhibitor to
lectin-activated lymphocyte cultures augmented thymidine incorporation to control levels[11].   Monocytes have
been shown to be prime immune cell producers of prostaglandins[4,15,22] and have also been identified as sup-
pressors of T cell function in Hodgkin's
disease[13,11,26,3].   It is plausible that monocytes may
mediate immune cell suppression, in part, through their
synthesis of prostaglandins;   however, the mechanism(s)
by which monocytes effect the profound and progressive
immunosuppression seen in Hodgkin's Disease has yet to
be elucidated.
     T colony formation by the peripheral blood and
spleen mononuclear cells from 36 previously untreated
patients with Hodgkin's Disease was examined[3].   Progressive reduction in colony number was evident with
advancing stage of disease, whether peripheral blood or
spleen cells were examined.   The negative correlation
of colony number with stage of disease was significant.
The addition of indomethacin (2 uM) caused a significant increase in T colony formation, thereby distin-
guishing the Hodgkin's Disease patients from normal
subjects.   While colony number increased with the addition of a prostaglandin-synthase inhibitor to the cultures, colony numbers could not be restored to normal
levels in the patients with advanced stages of disease.
These data suggest that a progressive immunodepletion
occurs at a stem cell level with advancing stage of
disease and that prostaglandins may, in part, be causative.
     Measurement of immune cell synthesis of prostaglan-
dins showed augmented PGE levels which increased with
advancing stage of disease.   Cell separation experiments gave evidence that adherent monocyte and macrophage synthesis of PGE could account for the augmented
levels measured.   When PG levels were examined by tritiated arachidonic acid conversion[3,4] and separation by
2-D thin layer chromatography, PGE_2 was the major prostaglandin class synthesized.   Changes in lipoxygenase
products could not be examined by this technique.
     While there was a strong correlation between mono-
cyte synthesis of PGE and depressed T colony counts,
this does not mean that depressed T colony formation

was caused by the increased PGE production. Nevertheless, there appears to be sufficient evidence to suggest that excessive host production of PGE could suppress CFU-TI colony formation leading to a multiclass
T-cell depletion. As an extrapolation of this latter
conclusion, we currently are testing the premise that
persistently elevated PGE levels may result in the
progressive attrition of CFU-TI to a point sufficient
to result in depressed immunocompetence. Patients with
newly diagnosed Hodgkin's Disease are currently under
long-term follow-up protocols to explore this premise.

D. Conclusion:

Disordered arachidonate metabolism has been reported
in patients with cancer. Coincident with enhanced or
altered prostaglandin synthesis, various pathophysiological conditions thought to favor cancer growth and
spread are noted to occur. Specifically, depressed
immunocompetance can result from prostaglandin mediated
suppression of committed stem cell or mature immune
cells proliferation or function. The mechanisms
leading to altered tumor or host cell metabolism of
arachidonate in cancer patients are unknown. This lack
of information is compounded by the virtual absence of
data concerning cell regulation of arachidonate metabolism in vitro and in vivo. Using a newly isolated
human cell line (Lu-65) we have begun to study cell
regulation (of arachidonate metabolism) at the levels
of enzyme control, mRNA translation, and substrate
availability. To our knowledge these are the first
studies to be carried out in a human tumor cell system
in this detailed manner. From our preliminary experiments with ^{3}H-C20:4 we found rapid incorporation of
label into membrane PL. Further, the label was preferentially accumulated in PI. During cell culture,
^{3}H-PGE$_2$ release and loss of ^{3}H-C20:4 from PI were
coincident. Monocytes showed a similar preferential
labelling of PI. Interestingly, the monocytes were
more efficient with regard to the percentage of ^{3}H-PGE$_2$
compared to the amount of free ^{3}H-C20:4 they released.
Stimulation with inflammatory agents such as zymosan
resulted in a similar and coincident rise in ^{3}H-PGE$_2$
and ^{3}H-C20:4 release. Strikingly, monocytes from
patients with Hodgkin's Disease release similar levels
of ^{3}H-C20:4 as normal subjects, but significantly more
^{3}H-PGE$_2$. The mechanism responsible for this more efficient conversion of ^{3}H-C20:4 is not known.

Coincident with the disordered arachidonate metabolism seen in cancer patients, multiple defects in
immune cell function have been reported. To date these
two phenomena are merely correlated findings. No
direct evidence has been presented showing that the
first is responsible even in part for the second, nor
has it been disproved.

REFERENCES

1. Aisenberg, A.C. (1965): Nature (Lond.), 205:1233-1235.

2. Anger, B., Bockman, R.S., Andreef, M., Erlandson, R., Jhanwar, S., Kameya, T., Saigo, P., Wright, W., Beattie, E.J., Jr., Oettgen, H., and Old, L.J. (1982): Cancer, 50:1518-1529.

3. Bockman, R.S. (1980): J. Clin. Invest., 66:523-531.

4. Bockman, R.S. (1981): Prostaglandins, (21)1:9-31.

5. Bockman, R.S., Bellin, A., Repo, M.A., Hickok, N.J., and Kameya, T. (1983): Cancer Res., 43:4571-4576.

6. Bockman, R.S., and Rothschild, M. (1979): J. Clin. Invest., 64:812-819.

7. Case, D.C., Hansen, J.A., Corrales, E., Young, C.W., Dupont, B., Pinsky, C.M, and Good, R.A. (1976): Cancer (Phila.), 38:1807-1815.

8. Claesson, M.H., Rodger, M.B., Johnson, G.R. Whittingham, S., and Metcalf, D. (1977): Clin. Exp. Immunol., 28:526-534.

9. Droller, M.J., Schneider, M.U., and Perlman, P. (1978): Cell. Immunol., 39:165-177.

10. Fibach, E., Gerassi, E., and Sachs, L. (1976): Nature (Lond.), 259:127-129.

11. Goodwin, J.S., Messner, R.P., Bankhurst, A.D., Peake, G.T., Saiki, J.H., and Williams, Jr. R.C. (1977): N. Engl. J. Med., 297:963-968.

12. Graze, P.R., Perlin, E., and Royston, I. (1976): J. Natl. Cancer Inst., 56:239-243.

13. Hillinger, S.M. and Herzig, G.P. (1978): J. Clin. Invest., 61:1620-1627.

14. Honn, K.V. (1982): In: Prostaglandins and Cancer: First International Conference, edited by T. Powles, R. Bockman, K. Honn International Conference, edited by T. Powles, R. Bockman, K. Honn and P. Ramwell, pp 733-752. Alan R. Liss, Inc., New York

15. Kurland, J.I., and Bockman, R.S. (1978): J. Exp. Med., 147:952-957.

16. Kurland, J., Bockman, R.S., Broxmeyer, H., and Moore, M.A.S., (1978): Science, 199:552-555.

17. Kurland, J., Broxmeyer, H., Bockman, R.S., Pelus, L., and Moore, M.A.S. (1978): Blood 52:388-407.

18. Kurland, J.I., Pelus, L., Ralph, P., Bockman, R.S., and Moore, M.A.S (1979): Proc. Natl. Acad. Sci. (U.S.A.), 76:2326-2330.

19. Levy, R., and Kaplan, H.S. (1974): N. Engl. J. Med., 290:181-186.

20. Marnett, L.J., Reed, G.A., and Johnson, J.T. (1977): Biochem. Biophys. Res. Comm., 79:569-576.

21. Miyamoto, T., Ogino, N., Yamamoto, S., and Hayaishi, O. (1976): J Biol Chem, 251:2629-2636.

22. Morley, J., Bray, M.A., Jones, R.W., Nugteren, N.H., and Van Dorp, D.A. (1970): Prostaglandins, 17:730-736.

23. Pelus, L.M., and Bockman, R.S. (1979): J. Immunol., 123:2118-2125.

24. Rittenhouse-Simmons, S. (1979): J. Clin. Inv., 63:580-587.

25. Rozenszajn, L.A., Shoham, D., and Kalecham, I. (1975): Immunology, 29:1041-1055.

26. Schecter, G.P. and Soehnlen, F. (1978): Blood, 52:261-271.

27. Shen, J., Wilson, F. Shifrine M., and Gershwin, M.E. (1977): J. Immunol., 119:1299-1305.

28. Sivarajah, K., Anderson, M.W., and Eling, T.E. (1978): Life Science, 23:2571-2578.

29. Smith, J.W., Steiner, A.L., Newberry Jr, W.M., and Parker, C.W. (1971): J. Clin. Invest., 50:432-441.

30. Thomas, D.R., Philpott, G.W., and Jaffe, B.M. (1974): Expt'l. Cell Res., 84:40-46.

31. Twomey, J.J., Laughter, A.H., Farrow, S., and Douglass, C.C. (1975): J. Clin. Invest., 56:467-475.

32. Van der Ouderaa, F.J., Buytenhek, M., Nugteren, D.H., and Van Dorp, D.A. (1977): Biochim. Biophys. Acta, 487:315-331.

33. Wilson, J.D., and Dalton, G. (1976): Aust. J. Exp. Biol. Med. Sci., 54:27-34.

34. Zeevi, A., Goldman, I., and Rozenszajn, L.A. (1977): Cell Immunol., 28:235-247.

35. Zenser, T.V., Mattamal, M.B. Ambrecht, H.J., and Davis, B.B. (1980): Cancer Res., 40:2839-2845.

Icosanoids and Cancer, edited by H. Thaler-Dao, et al. Raven Press, New York © 1984.

Modulation of Normal and Leukemic Human Hemopoietic Cell Differentiation by Prostaglandin E

Louis M. Pelus

Department of Developmental Hematopoiesis, Sloan Kettering Institute,
New York, New York 10021

In vitro agar culture methodologies which quantitate and measure the proliferation and maturation of human hemopoietic stem cells have improved our insight into mechanisms which control normal and leukemic cell differentiation. Increased understanding of the biology of cellular differentiation, particularly the nature of humoral and microenvironmental imbalances, may ultimately lead to the development of new therapeutic strategies for hematologic diseases. Bone marrow culture systems that support the proliferation and differentiation of marrow progenitor cells which give rise to granulocytes and monocytes-macrophages (CFU-GM), erythrocytes (BFU-e) and megakaryocytes (CFU-M) offer one means for investigating mechanisms which control blood cell proliferation and maturation (5,15). The magnitude of the regulatory networks which control these systems can be appreciated by the fact that the production rate for granulocytes and monocytes alone has been estimated to be greater than 10^9 cells/kg/day under homeostatic conditions. This communication will describe recent studies on the control of myeloid cell differentiation, particularly as they relate to cell cycle kinetics and expression of HLA-DR (Ia-like) antigens, and newly defined prostaglandin E (PGE) mediated mechanisms for modulating cell cycle and Ia-antigen expression as a mean to control normal and abnormal granulocyte and monocyte-macrophage production.

HUMORAL CONTROL OF CFU-GM PROLIFERATION

Granulocyte-monocyte progenitor cell proliferation is controlled by diffusible factors (3,4) and aberrations in these normal regulatory networks may play a role in the pathophysiology of leukemia by providing a growth advantage to the leukemic clone (2-4,11-14). Prostaglandins of the E series (12,14) and acidic isoferritins (AIF) (1,4) have been implicated in the normal physiological regulation of CFU-GM proliferation, but are essentially ineffective in controlling CFU-GM proliferation in many patients with acute and chronic leukemia and myeloproliferative disorders. The loss of sensitivity of leukemic progenitor cells to normal regulatory factors permits the unhindered clonal expansion of the abnormal clone at the expense of normal cells which remain under the influence of normal regulatory control mechanisms. Furthermore, in some forms of leukemia overproduction of normal

regulatory factors occurs as a compensatory mechanism aimed at controlling rising cell numbers (3). However, this serves only as an additional constraint upon normal cells.

TABLE 1. CFU-GM sensitivity in normal marrow and in patients with
leukemia and preleukemia.

Source of marrow	Number of cases	Prostaglandin E sensitivity, M		
		ID_{50}	ID_{70}	ID_{90}
Normal	36	10^{-7}	10^{-9}	10^{-11}
Acute myeloid leukemia	34	10^{-5}	10^{-6}	10^{-6}
Chronic myeloid leukemia	30	10^{-5}	10^{-5}	10^{-5}
Preleukemia	13	10^{-6}	10^{-6}	10^{-8}
(RAEB) BR$_a$ BR^a		10^{-7} 10^{-5}	10^{-8} 10^{-5}	10^{-10} 10^{-5}
(CMMS) MA$_b$ MA^b		10^{-6} 10^{-5}	10^{-7} 10^{-5}	10^{-8} 10^{-5}
" GA$_b$ GA^b		10^{-8} 10^{-5}	10^{-9} 10^{-5}	10^{-11} 10^{-5}

RAEB=refractory anemia with excess of blasts; CMMS=chronic myelomono-
cytic syndrome.
a. For each marrow sample, the ID_{50}, ie, the concentration of PGE at
which inhibition was 50% of the control value was calculated. Similarly, each ID_{70} and ID_{90} was determined.
b. Patient progressed to acute leukemia. Note loss of PGE inhibition.
**Reprinted with permission from "Regulation of the Immune Response",
S. Karger, 1983.

Prostaglandins of the E series inhibit the clonal expansion of
normal human CFU-GM in a dose dependent fashion over a concentration
range of 10^{-5} through 10^{-12}M (Table 1)(11,12,14), with an
$ID_{50}=10^{-7}$M. Clone analysis has established that the effects of PGE
on total CFU-GM result from a preferential effect on
monocyte-macrophage colony forming cells, with an $ID_{50}=5 \times 10^{-9}$M.
The overall dose dependent effect of PGE observed in agar culture
studies is deceiving and results as a consequence of chemical
degradation of the PGE molecule. Recent evidence using the 16,16
dimethyl PGE_2 analog likewise indicates an identical dose dependent
effect when tested in vitro, since this analog is equally chemically
unstable. However, a plateau inhibitory effect on CFU-GM was observed

over a concentration range of 10^{-5} through 10^{-11}M when tested in intact mice (7). Specificity analysis by comparison to a number of primary prostaglandins, thromboxane, prostacyclin and 6-keto-PGF$_{2\alpha}$ indicates that the E series prostaglandins (PGE$_1$ and PGE$_2$) are at least 10 times more potent in inhibiting human CFU-GM proliferation than any other members of the prostaglandin family (14). Acidic isoferritins also inhibit normal CFU-GM in a plateau fashion over a concentration range of 10^{-6} through 10^{-17}M (4). The plateau inhibition curves normally observed for these regulators (approximately 50%) suggests an action restricted to a subpopulation of CFU-GM.

Analysis of PGE and AIF sensitivities of CFU-GM from patients with leukemia indicate that abnormal regulatory responses characterize most forms of leukemia (Table 1)(2,10,11). In patients with preleukemia a heterogeneity of response was observed, ranging from near normal to overt leukemic phenotype. In 3 patients who displayed normal or near normal sensitivity to PGE, serial analysis showed loss of sensitivity to PGE associated with progression to acute leukemia. In these patients, loss of sensitivity to growth regulation preceeded clinical onset of acute leukemia by 1.2, 2.5 and 2.8 months (8).

SELECTIVE ACTION OF PGE AND AIF ON SUBPOPULATIONS OF CFU-GM

Analysis of the possible subpopulation specificities of PGE and AIF indicated that the effects of both of these compounds are selective for CFU-GM that are in S-phase of the cell cycle and express Ia-like HLA-DR antigen (1,10,11)(Table 2). Treatment of marrow cells with high specific activity tritiated thymidine (^{3}H-Tdr) or monoclonal mouse anti-human HLA-DR antibody plus complement (αIa+C') removes that population of CFU-GM sensitive to inhibition by PGE and AIF. The facts that these regulators are specific for CFU-GM which are in S-phase as well as for CFU-GM which express Ia-antigen suggested that perhaps CFU-GM Ia-antigen was expressed relative to S-phase of the cell cycle. This hypothesis was tested by consecutive treatments with ^{3}H-Tdr and Ia+C' (Table 2). Consecutive treatments with both agents produced no further reduction in total CFU-GM than either agent used alone, and in both cases those CFU-GM surviving treatment were insensitive to the inhibitory effects of PGE and AIF. These studies indicated that the target cell for both AIF and PGE was a subpopulation of CFU-GM which expressed Ia-antigen or at least an Ia-antigen epitope, perhaps at higher density, relative to S-phase of the cell cycle.

The expression of Ia-antigen appears necessary for growth regulation of CFU-GM, at least in vitro. This requirement is particularly significant with respect to patients with chronic myeloid leukemia where in 50 patients tested to date, CFU-GM Ia-antigen expression was absent or greatly diminished (12,13) in spite of a quantitatively normal S-phase population of CFU-GM (13) and correlated with hyporesponsiveness of leukemic CFU-GM to inhibition by both PGE and AIF (Table 3). In two patients, higher levels of Ia-antigen were detected and occurred coincident with considerable, albeit abnormal, regulatory sensitivity (12). The regulatory sensitivity observed, however, was no longer detected following treatment with αIa+C'.

Table 2. Selective effects of PGE and AIF on CFU-GM in S-phase or expressing Ia-antigenic determinants.

| Treatment | CFU-GM/10^5 bone marrow cells Percent of Control | | |
	Media	+PGE (10^{-7}M)	+AIF (10^{-9}M)
Media	100	52	53
Tdr	100	52	52
^{3}H-Tdr	54	54	52
Tdr+^{3}H-Tdr	98	53	54
C'	97	51	53
Ia+C'	53	52	51
^{3}H-Tdr + Ia+C'	56	53	54
Ia+C' + ^{3}H-Tdr	52	52	51

Table 3. Altered Ia-antigen expression by CFU-GM from patients with CML.

| Source of bone marrow | Mean percentage Ia$^+$ CFU-GM Antibody Dilution | | | |
	1:100	1:250	1:500	1:1000
Normal (n=14)	52±2*	46±3*	49±3*	47±2*
CML (n=13)	18±5	10±5	18±4	4±2

*p< 0.0005

MODULATION OF CFU-GM Ia-ANTIGEN EXPRESSION

In situ, the marrow CFU-GM population is in a dynamic process of differentiation and at any given time only a small population of the total cells which have the capacity to ultimately enter S-phase and express Ia-antigen will be detected by in vitro methods which rely on pulse exposure treatments to assess these parameters. In agar culture, the onset of colony formation is asynchronous, however all CFU-GM and their progeny which proliferate must enter S-phase, presumably express Ia-antigen, and therefore should respond to the inhibitory effects of PGE and AIF. This however is not the case, and the final degree of inhibition by these regulators which can be observed is usually equivalent to the proportion of CFU-GM which can be demonstrated to be Ia$^+$ and in S-phase at culture initiation. This effect might be explained in two ways: 1) the regulatory compounds are inactivated shortly after culture initiation, or 2) the CFU-GM populations lose regulatory sensitivity in culture. Delayed and/or multiple addition experiments indicated that regulator metabolism was not responsible. With respect to loss of CFU-GM sensitivity it could be shown that CFU-GM lost their ability to express Ia-antigen within 3-6 hrs when maintained in suspension culture at 37°C prior to culture in soft agar (1,10). No loss of Ia-antigen was observed on cells maintained at 4°C or 22°C. In all cases, Ia-antigen expression was associated with the equivalent lack of reponsiveness of these cells to PGE and AIF. These data indicate that CFU-GM Ia-antigen expression is transient, at least in vitro, and may explain the subpopulation effects of PGE and AIF. Furthermore, membrane turnover/shedding of CFU-GM Ia-antigen may represent a mechanism whereby clonal expansion of myeloid cells can be limited only if inhibitory regulators are present at precise times, or maintained in elevated amounts for extended time periods.

The transitory nature of CFU-GM Ia-antigen expression and its association with the regulation of progenitor cell proliferation by PGE and AIF led us to ask if antigen expression could be modulated, and would this coincide with equivalent changes in CFU-GM sensitivity to negative growth regulation in vitro. Several studies have demonstrated that short pulse exposure to PGE elevates the fraction of murine and human stem cells which can be shown to be in S-phase of the cell cycle (6,18). The cycle related expression of CFU-GM Ia-antigen suggested to us that PGE might be used to modulate antigen expression as a consequence of its effect on cell cycle. We therefore developed a culture system which permitted analysis of cell cycle kinetics, Ia-antigen expression and regulatory sensitivity of CFU-GM during a defined time in suspension culture prior to culture in soft agar. This suspension culture system permits the modulation of events associated with the loss of CFU-GM Ia-antigen and regulatory reponsiveness, and allows for reinduction under appropriate conditions. In addition, it is possible to study modulation of cell cycle related events associated with antigenic expression. In this system the proportion of marrow CFU-GM which are in S-phase and express Ia-antigen are quantitated. The sensitivity of these cells to PGE and AIF is also determined. These parameters are measured by appropriate treatment of cells, ie, thymidine suicide (S-phase) and cytotoxic antibody treatment (αIa+C'), and subsequently culturing in soft agar with or without PGE and AIF to determine changes in CFU-GM cloning efficiency as a consequence of the treatments performed and culture in agar with the growth regulators. Replicate groups of cells are placed into suspension culture (1.5-3 million cells per 1.0 ml) in the absence or presence of PGE for 3-24 hrs (usually 24 hrs). Following suspension culture each group is retreated to determine the proportion of S-phase and Ia[+] CFU-GM and their response to PGE and AIF. This protocol offers the advantage of cell analysis during the first 24 hrs in culture which is not possible in direct agar culture.

Bone marrow cells were exposed to PGE in suspension culture for 0, 3, 6 and 24 hrs and CFU-GM Ia-antigen and cycle status quantitated at the end of the suspension culture period. The data from these studies reflect the effects of PGE present during the suspension culture on the parameters investigated. In these studies, PGE did not prevent the loss of Ia-antigen detection normally observed within 3-6 hrs but resulted in the capacity to detect Ia[+] CFU-GM after 24 hrs (10). The loss of Ia-antigen detection observed did not result from loss of S-phase clone forming cells. The detection of Ia^+ CFU-GM following suspension culture in the presence of PGE could have occurred as a result of Ia-antigen reexpression by those Ia^-, S-phase CFU-GM detected in cultures maintained without PGE, or could have resulted from expression of new S-phase CFU-GM induced by PGE. In order to determine which mechanism occurred, marrow cells were treated with ^{3}H-Tdr and $\alpha Ia+C'$ before and after suspension culture (Table 4).

Table 4. <u>Cell cycle status, Ia-antigen expression and response to inhibition by PGE and AIF of CFU-GM after suspension culture.</u>

Treatment prior to suspension culture	Present throughout suspension culture	% CFU-GM		% Inhibition CFU-GM	
		S-phase	Ia^+	PGE, 10^{-7}M	AIF, 10^{-9}M
Media	media	38±1	4±3	0±0	3±1
	$+10^{-8}$M PGE	57±2	55±2	40±1	40±1
^{3}H-Tdr	media	4±1	0±0	0±0	0±0
	$+10^{-8}$M PGE	33±1	32±1	34±1	34±1
Ia + C'	media	2±1	3±1	4±1	4±1
	$+10^{-8}$M PGE	39±2	35±1	36±1	36±2

Total CFU-GM in S-phase or Ia^+ prior to suspension culture: S-phase=40±2%; Ia^+=44±3%. Average inhibition of CFU-GM prior to suspension culture: PGE=44±2%; AIF=42±2%.

In those groups of CFU-GM treated to remove S-phase and Ia^+ CFU-GM prior to suspension culture, neither S-phase nor Ia^+ nor regulatory sensitive CFU-GM could be detected in cultures maintained in media alone. However, Ia^+ and S-phase CFU-GM sensitive to inhibition by PGE and AIF could be detected in a 1:1 relationship when cultured with PGE. This suggested that the mechanism of action of PGE was to induce new S-phase, Ia^- CFU-GM from a population of noncycling Ia^- cells which give rise to CFU-GM. In control cultures which were untreated prior to suspension culture with PGE, a rise in the proportion of S-phase CFU-GM was observed in comparison to control cultures incubated without PGE (Table 4).

The number of Ia^+ CFU-GM detected was equal to the number of S-phase colony forming cells observed, and the degree of restoration of responsiveness to PGE and AIF was directly proportional to the percentage of S-phase and Ia^+ CFU-GM. The majority of cycling and antigen positive CFU-GM detected in these cultures were probably derived from noncycling cells induced into cycle by PGE. However, since no Ia^+ CFU-GM were detected in control cultures despite the presence of S-phase CFU-GM, whereas after culture with PGE both are present to an equivalent degree, it appears that Ia-antigen was reexpressed on those Ia⁻ S-phase CFU-GM detected in control cultures. Thus, the mechanism of action of PGE appears twofold (see Figure 1): 1) to induce differentiation of new Ia⁺ S-phase CFU-GM from a noncycling Ia⁻ cell compartment, and 2) to restore antigen expression to Ia⁻ S-phase CFU-GM. the capacity of PGE to mediate these effects was observed to occur in plateau fashion over the concentration range of 10^{-6} through 10^{-10}M and to a lesser but still significant degree with as little as 10^{-12} to 10^{-14}M concentration (10). Kinetic investigations have indicated that PGE must be and need only be present during the first 3 hrs of the suspension culture to initiate these events.

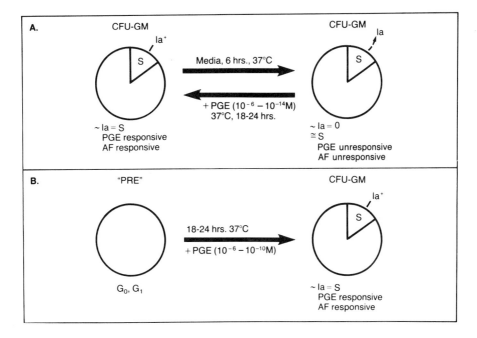

FIG. 1. Mechanisms of action of PGE on CFU-GM Ia-antigen expression.

MODULATION OF Ia-ANTIGEN ON CFU-GM FROM PATIENTS WITH CML. ASSOCIATION WITH RESTORATION OF NORMAL REGULATORY CONTROL.

The lack of or diminished expression of Ia-antigens on CFU-GM from patients with chronic myeloid leukemia has been linked with the lack of regulatory sensitivity observed in these patients. To further define the role of Ia-antigen as a principal factor responsible for the abnormal growth regulatory phenotype observed in these patients, the capacity to modulate CML CFU-GM Ia-antigen expression as a mechanism to restore growth regulation was investigated (Figure 2 and Table 5). As described previously, those leukemic CFU-GM tested prior to suspension culture were essentially unresponsive to PGE and AIF, as compared to normal CFU-GM, (Figure 2) and displayed a diminished capacity for Ia-antigen expression (Table 5). However following suspension culture with PGE for 24 hours, CFU-GM from patients with CML displayed normal regulatory responsiveness to PGE and AIF equivalent to that reinduced on normal CFU-GM (Figure 2). Furthermore, the pattern of Ia-antigen expression on patient CFU-GM was restored to the plateau detection usually observed on normal cells (Table 5). Thus, following suspension culture with PGE, CML-CFU-GM can no longer be distinguished from normal CFU-GM by their in vitro growth regulatory phenotype. However, this leads to the question of whether or not those CFU-GM from patients with CML detected after culture with PGE are leukemic CFU-GM or represent a

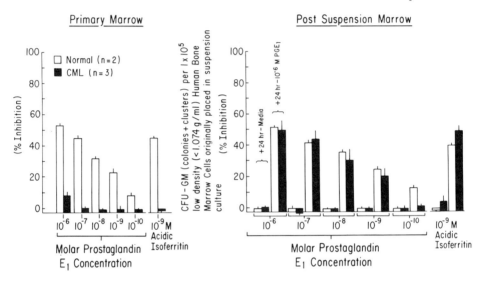

FIG. 2. Sensitivity of CFU-GM from normals and patients with CML before and after suspension culture with PGE.

population of residual normal colony forming cells. Several studies have suggested that under conditions of aggressive chemotherapy non-clonal and presumably non-neoplastic hematopoietic cells can be detected (9,17). We therefore performed cytogenetic analysis of pooled proliferating colonies. Cytogenetic analysis indicated that all metaphases detected both before and after suspension culture with PGE were Philadelphia (Ph[1]) chromosome positive, and therefore members of the neoplastic clone (13). The detection of only Ph[1]-positive CFU-GM agrees with the majority of studies by others which find little evidence for residual normal hematopoiesis in patients with CML (16). These studies also agree with our earlier studies which demonstrated overt leukemic growth regulatory phenotypes in those patients treated with agressive chemotherapy who temporarily had reverted to a Ph[1]-negative bone marrow cytogenetic profile (11). Overall, these data indicate that the abnormal phenotype expressed by CML CFU-GM can be altered and restored to normal and represents a phenotypic reversion of a malignant cell. Furthermore these studies support a direct regulatory association between expression of CFU-GM Ia-antigen and hemopoietic regulation.

Table 5. Quantitation of CFU-GM Ia-antigen before and after suspension culture with PGE.

Time of assay	Anti-HLA-DR antibody dilution	Mean percentage Ia^+ CFU-GM	
		Normal	CML
Primary	1:100	48±2	24±8
	1:250	47±2	7±4
	1:500	43±1	4±2
	1:1000	43±1	1±1
Postsuspension Media alone	1:100	5±1	7±3
	1:250	5±1	3±2
	1:500	2±1	1±1
	1:1000	5±1	1±1
Plus 10^{-6}M PGE_1	1:100	51±1	47±3
	1:250	48±1	44±3
	1:500	46±1	42±3
	1:1000	47±2	40±4

CONCLUSION

Experimental evidence indicates that Ia-antigen expression or events associated with antigen expression may define a state of progenitor cell responsiveness to regulatory control by prostaglandin E (PGE) and acidic isoferritins (AIF) in vitro. In support of this hypothesis we have shown that: 1) in vitro, human CFU-GM Ia-antigen expression is transient, and loss of antigen expression occurs coincident with loss of CFU-GM responsiveness to inhibition by PGE and AIF; 2) in patients with chronic myeloid leukemia, CFU-GM Ia-antigen expression is absent or greatly diminished and correlates with hyporesponsiveness of leukemic colony forming cells to growth inhibition; 3) in suspension preculutre, PGE has the capacity to modulate CFU-GM responsiveness to regulatory control as a consequence of induction of CFU-GM Ia-antigen reexpression; 4) suspension preculture of CFU-GM from patients with chronic myeloid leukemia with PGE results in the induction of a normal pattern of Ia-antigen expression on Philadelphia (Ph[1]) chromosome positive CFU-GM and their progeny, and restoration of normal responsiveness of these CFU-GM to inhibition by PGE and AIF in agar culture.

With respect to myeloid leukemia, no single phenotypic change unequivocally explains neoplastic transformation of hematopoietic cells. Collectively the data described define an abnormal CFU-GM

phenotype characterized by altered expression of cell surface anti-
gen(s) associated with hyporesponsiveness to normal regulatory control
mechanisms. The ability to modulate antigen expression and restore
growth regulatory control, at least in vitro, indicates that the
behavior of leukemic cells can be altered, and may represent an alternative to cytoreductive therapy.

Lastly, it is apparent that the effects of PGE on hematopoiesis are
biphasic. At low as well as high concentrations, PGE promotes CFU-GM
differentiation by modulating cell cycle kinetics and coincident growth
regulation as a consequence of Ia-antigen expression. The insensitivity
of CFU-GM to inhibition by levels of PGE found in human plasma combined
with the ability of these same concentrations of PGE to augment CFU-GM
cell cycle and modulate Ia-antigen expression support the CFU-GM
differentiating role of PGE. At higher PGE levels, normally associated
with infection and inflammation, at which CFU-GM are sensitive to
inhibition, clonal CFU-GM expansion can be limited without compromising
the differentiation of earlier stem cells into the CFU-GM compartment.

ACKNOWLEDGEMENTS

This work was supported by grant CA-33225 awarded by the National
Cancer Institute, DHHS, and The Gar Reichman Foundation. Dr. Pelus is
a Scholar of the Leukemia Society of America.

REFERENCES

1. Broxmeyer, H.E. (1982): J. Clin. Invest., 69: 632-642.
2. Broxmeyer, H.E., Bognacki, J., Dorner, M.H., deSousa, M.
    (1981): J. Exp. Med., 153: 1426-1444.
3. Broxmeyer, H.E., Grossbard, E., Jacobsen, N., Moore, M.A.S.
    (1979): New Engl. J. Med., 301: 346-351.
4. Broxmeyer, H.E., Jacobsen, N., Kurland, J., Mendelsohn, N., and
    Moore, M.A.S. (1978): J. Natl. Cancer Inst., 60: 497-512.
5. Burgess, A.W., and Metcalf, D. (1980): Blood, 56: 945-958.
6. Feher, I., and Gidali, J. (1974): Nature (Lond.), 247: 550-551.
7. Gentile, P., Byer, D. and Pelus, L.M., in press.
8. Gold, E., Conjalka, M., Pelus, L.M., Jhanwar, S.C., Broxmeyer,
    H.E., Middleton, A., Clarkson, B.D., Moore, M.A.S., in press.
9. Goto, T., Nishikori, M., Arlin, Z., Gee, T., Kempin, S.,
    Burchenal, J., Strife, A., Wisniewski, D., Lambek, C., Little,
    C., Jhanwar, S., Chaganti, R., Clarkson,B. (1982): Blood, 59:
    793-806.
10. Pelus, L.M. (1982): J. Clin. Invest., 70: 568-578.
11. Pelus, L.M., Broxmeyer, H.E., Clarkson, B.D., and Moore, M.A.S.
    (1980): Cancer Res., 40: 2512-2525.
12. Pelus, L.M., Broxmeyer, H.E., Moore, M.A.S. (1981): Cell Tissue
    Kinet., 14: 515-526.
13. Pelus, L.M., Gold, E., Saletan, S., Coleman, M. (1983): Blood,
    62: 158-165.
14. Pelus, L.M., Saletan, S., Silver, R., Moore, M.A.S. (1982):
    Blood, 59: 284-292.
15. Quesenberry, P., and Levitt, L. (1979): New Engl. J. Med., 301:
    819-823.
16. Singer, J.W., Fialkow, P.J., Steinmann, L., Najfeld, V., Stein,
    S.J., Robinson, W.A. (1979): Blood, 53: 264-268.

17. Singer, J.W., Arlin, Z., Najfeld, V., Adamson, J.W., Kempin, S.J., Clarkson, B.D., and Fialkow, P.J. (1982): Blood, 56: 356-360.
18. Verma, D.S., Spitzer, G., Zander, A.R., McCredie, K.B., and Dicke, K.A. (1981): Leukemia Res., 5: 65-71.

Icosanoids and Cancer, edited by H. Thaler-Dao, et al. Raven Press, New York © 1984.

Eicosapolyenoic Acid Metabolites Formed by Mastocytoma and Basophilic Leukemia Cells

Sven Hammarström

Department of Physiological Chemistry, Karolinska Institutet, S-104 01 Stockholm, Sweden

Previous investigations have shown that polyoma virus transformed 3T3 and BHK fibroblasts produce greater quantities of prostaglandins E_2, $F_{2\alpha}$, E_1, and 6-keto $F_{1\alpha}$ than non-transformed cells. This alteration is secondary to increased basal release of precursor fatty acids (arachidonic and 8,11, 14-eicosatrienoic acid). When the transformed cells grow in culture, prostaglandins (predominantly prostaglandin E_2) accumulate in the growth medium. Prostaglandin E_2 stimulates cyclic AMP biosynthesis and decreases the rate of cell division in culture. The adenylate cyclase of these tumor cells, however, requires higher prostaglandin concentrations than the adenylate cyclase of many normal cells for comparable stimulatory effects. Thus, in mixed cultures or in <u>vivo</u>, prostaglandins produced by tumor cells may inhibit proliferation of normal cells markedly without affecting the growth of the producing tumor cells. This may facilitate the establishment and spreading of tumor cells, e.g. if the proliferation of cells belonging to the immune system are affected (for review, see 4, 5).

STRUCTURE OF A SLOW REACTING SUBSTANCE (SRS) FORMED BY MASTOCYTOMA CELLS (LEUKOTRIENE C_4)

A smooth muscle contracting factor was originally detected in perfusates from lungs treated with snake venoms. The factor, called "slow reacting substance", is a potent stimulator of bronchial smooth muscle. It also enhances vascular permeability to macromolecules (reviewed in 16). During attempts to determine the chemical structure of SRS, we observed that a murine mast cell tumor (CXBGABMCT-1) was a good source of SRS, following stimulation with the calcium ionophore A23187 (15). The structural work (see Fig. 1) showed that the compound is a tripeptide derivative of a 20 carbon fatty acid with four double bonds (three of which are conjugated) and a hydroxyl group. The peptide part is linked to the fatty

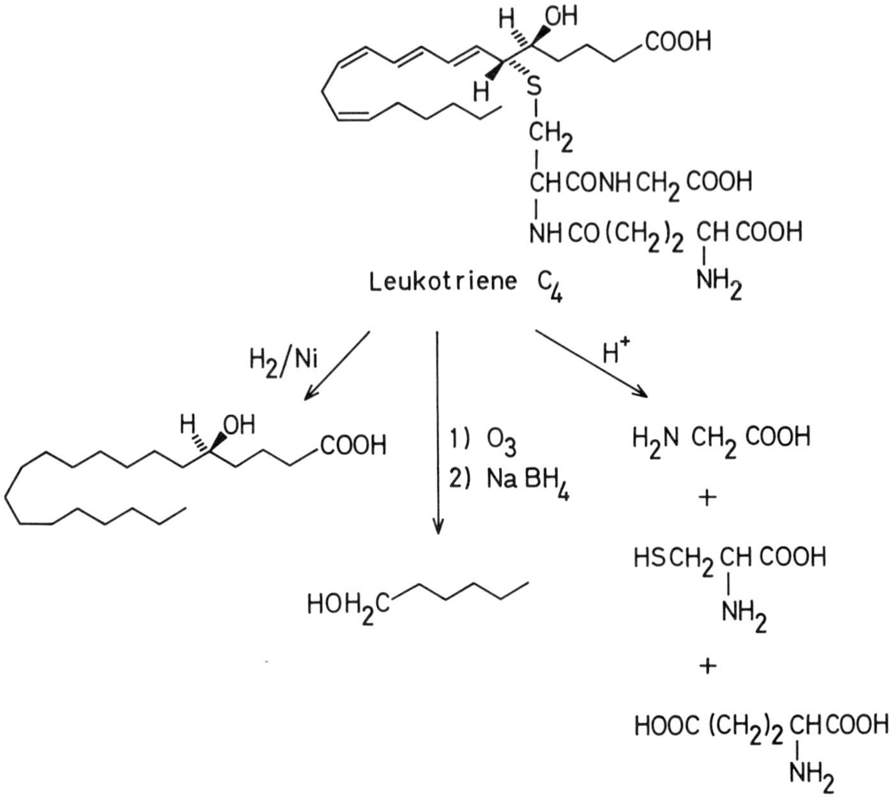

Fig. 1 Reactions used for the characterization of
     leukotriene C_4

acid as a thioether, derived from the sulfhydryl group of
glutathione (11, 15).

STRUCTURE OF A LEUKOTRIENE C_4 METABOLITE (LEUKOTRIENE D_4)
        FORMED BY RAT BASOPHILIC LEUKEMIA CELLS

    Another tumor cell, rat basophilic leukemia cells, had been
shown to produce SRS in response to ionophore A 23187 (13).
The compound in question was isolated and characterized (18).
The structure was similar to that of leukotriene C_4 but the
peptide part consisted of cysteinylglycine rather than glutathione. This suggested that the compound produced by RBL cells
was formed by metabolism of leukotriene C_4. The structure of
the metabolite (leukotriene D_4) is shown in Fig. 2. Involvement of γ-glutamyl transpeptidase in the biosynthesis of leukotriene D_4 has been demonstrated using a specific transition
state inhibitor of the enzyme (17).

CONVERSION OF POLYUNSATURATED FATTY ACIDS TO LEUKOTRIENES BY
      MASTOCYTOMA AND BASOPHILIC LEUKEMIA CELLS

    In addition to arachidonic acid, 5,8,11-eicosatrienoic,
8,11,14-eicosatrienoic , and 5,8,11,14,17-eicosapentaenoic

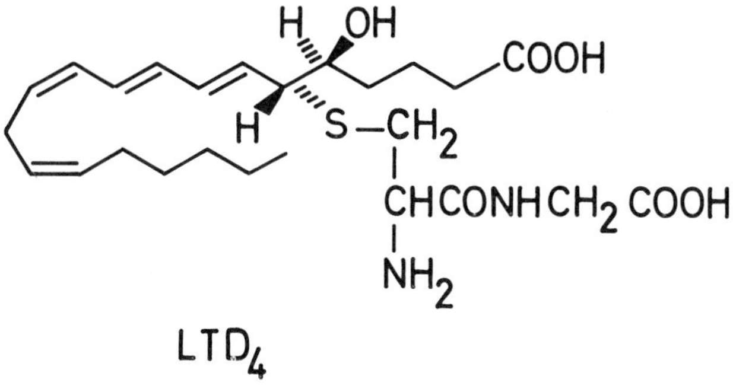

Fig. 2   Structure of leukotriene D_4

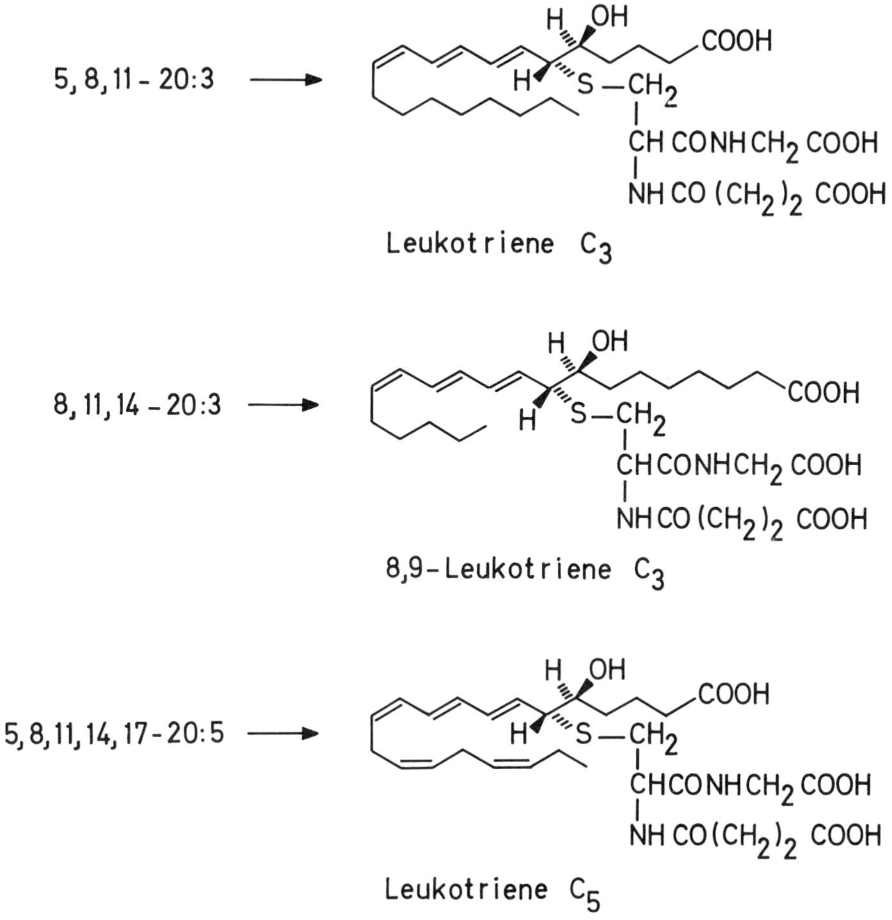

5,8,11 - 20:3 $\longrightarrow$

Leukotriene C_3

8,11,14 - 20:3 $\longrightarrow$

8,9-Leukotriene C_3

5,8,11,14,17 - 20:5 $\longrightarrow$

Leukotriene C_5

Fig. 3   Conversion of 5,8,11- and 8,11,14-eicosatrienoic
acids (preceeding page) and 5,8,11,14,17-eicosapen-
taenoic acid to leukotrienes C_3, 8,9-C_3, and C_5.

acid are converted to leukotrienes C by mastocytoma cells and
to leukotrienes C, D, and E (the cysteine analog of leukotriene D) by basophilic leukemia cells (6 , 7 , 8 ,19). The first
and last mentioned acids give products differing structurally
from leukotriene C_4 by the presence of one less or one additional double bond, respectively (leukotrienes C_3 and C_5).
8,11,14-Eicosatrienoic acid is converted by mastocytoma cells
to a positional isomer of leukotriene C_3 (8,9-leukotriene C_3)
as shown in Fig. 3.

A pathway for the biosynthesis of leukotriene C_4 from
arachidonic acid and glutathione was proposed in the papers
describing the chemical characterization of the molecule (11,
15). In this pathway, arachidonic acid is first converted to
a hydroperoxy acid and then to an epoxy acid which is conjugated with glutathione to the leukotriene C_4 (Fig. 4). Experimental evidence supporting this pathway has subsequently been
obtained. The proposed epoxy acid intermediate was synthesized
chemically (1). It is labile and reacts with alcohols at
acid pH to form a pair of diastereoisomeric 5-hydroxy-12-al-
koxy-6,8,11,14-eicosatetraenoic acids. These derivatives were
demonstrated to be transiently formed during ionophore induced leukotriene biosynthesis in mastocytoma and basophilic
leukemia cells (10).

Evidence for the formation of a hyproperoxy acid intermediate was obtained using eicosapentaenoic acids labeled with
tritium at C-10 and with ^{14}C at the carboxyl group (9). The
label at C-10 was introduced stereospecifically by $LiAl^3H_4$
reduction of optically active O-tosyl, methyl ester derivatives of 8-hydroxystearic acids. The [8-^3H] stearic acids obtained by CrO_3 oxidation were transformed into [10-^3H] eicosapentaenoic acids by the marine fungus Saprolegnia parasitica.
After addition of [1-^{14}C] eicosapentaenoic acid, the mixtures
of tritium and ^{14}C labeled substrates were incubated with
mastocytoma cells in the presence of L-cysteine and ionophore
A 23187. Leukotriene C_5 and 5-hydroxy-6,8,11,14,17-eicosapen-
taenoic acid were formed. Analyses of the $^3H/^{14}C$-ratios showed
that substantial loss (91%) of tritium occurred during the
conversion of the [10D_S-^3H] labeled eicosapentaenoic acid to
leukotriene C_5 and that tritium was largely retained (94%)
when the [10L_R-^3H] labeled eicosapentaenoic acid was the substrate. In the former case, 5-hydroxy-6,8,11,14,17-eicosapen-
taenoic acid was markedly enriched with tritium (273% compared
with the precursor acid) whereas no isotope enrichment was
observed in 5-hydroxy-eicosapentaenoic acid formed from
[10L_R-^3H] labeled eicosapentaenoic acid. The results indicate
that the conversion of eicosapentaenoic acid to leukotriene
C_5 involves stereospecific loss of the 10-pro-S hydrogen. The
substrate for this enzyme catalyzed elimination is 5-hydrope-

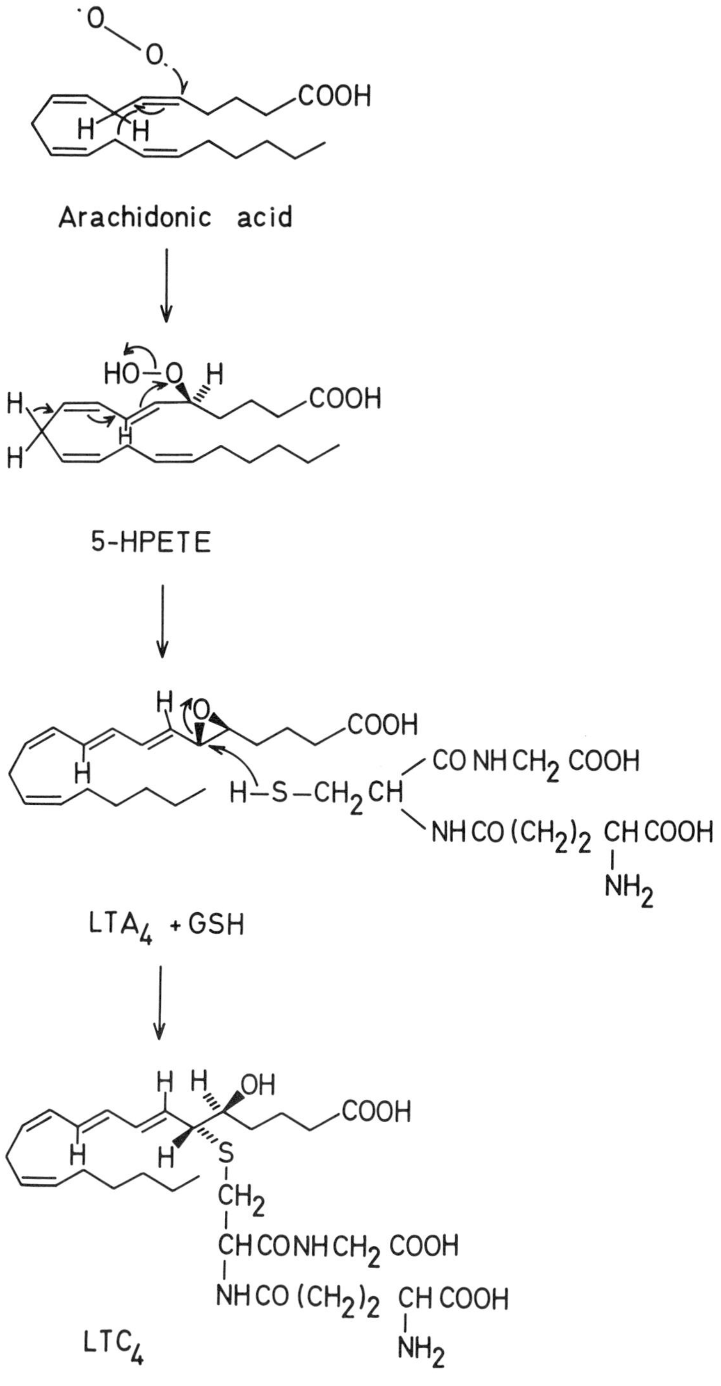

Fig. 4 Pathway for the conversion of arachidonic acid to leukotriene C_4

roxy-6,8,11,14,17-eicosapentaenoic acid because of the observed isotope accumulation in the corresponding hydroxy acid.
The breaking of the C-H bond at C-10 in the hydroperoxy acid
is also the rate-limiting step of this transformation (Fig.5).

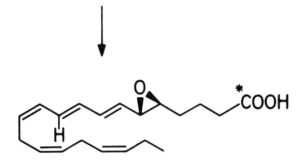

5-hydroperoxy-6,8,11,14,17-20:5

Leukotriene A$_5$

Fig. 5   Mechanism of leukotriene A$_5$ biosynthesis

The reaction shown in Fig. 5 is analogous to a lipoxygenase
reaction but oxygen of the hydroperoxy group at C-5 serves
as the nucleophile rather than molecular oxygen (cf. (14)).
It is of interest to note that the conversion of arachidonic
acid to leukotriene C$_4$ is inhibited by 5,8,11-eicosatriynoic
acid (17), a selective inhibitor of platelet 12-lipoxygenase
(3). The presumed mechanism of inhibition involves conversion of the acetylenic acid to an allenic acid by hydrogen

abstraction from C-10 which occurs during the reaction catalyzed by platelet lipoxygenase (9).

BIOLOGICAL EFFECTS OF LEUKOTRIENES

Prior to the structural work on leukotrienes, several biological effects of partially purified preparations of SRS-A
had been observed (16). In addition to the eliciting of con-
tractions of bronchial smooth muscle, permeability effects
had been observed in guinea pig skin. These effects have been
confirmed and further investigated using chemically pure leu-

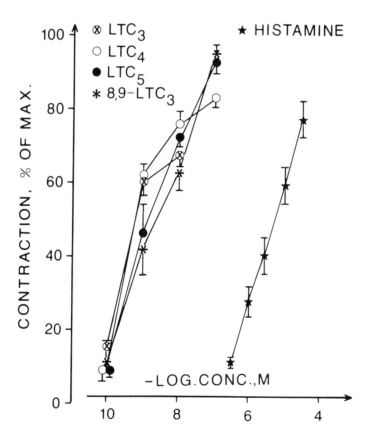

Fig. 6   Dose-response curves for the effects of leukotrienes
and histamine on guinea pig lung strips.

kotrienes. Characteristic features of leukotriene induced
airway smooth muscle responses are long duration of the con-
tractions and a higher potency of leukotrienes compared to
histamine (3-4 orders of magnitude, see Fig. 6). Peripheral
airways are more sensitive to leukotrienes than are central
airways (12). This is compatible with in vivo observations
that leukotriene C_4 reduces pulmonary dynamic compliance
without markedly affecting the pulmonary resistance (20).

   The effects of leukotrienes on the permeability of micro
blood vessels to macromolecules have been investigated using
the hamster cheek pouch model. Intravital microscopy of the
cheek pouch of animals preinjected with fluorescein-isothio-
cyanate conjugated dextran showed that topical application
of leukotrienes C_4, D_4, or E_4 resulted first in a transient
constriction of arterioles and terminal arterioles. The vaso-
constriction was maximal ca. 1 min after the application and
had ceased 5 min after application. At the latter time, leakage of FITC labeled dextran occurred at multiple sites around
postcapillary venules. The number of leakage spots per unit
area was proportional to the logarithm of leukotriene concentration (Fig. 7). Histamine induced a similar permeability
effect but the concentrations needed were 1000 fold greater
than those of leukotriene D_4. The difference compared with
leukotriene C_4 was even greater (2).

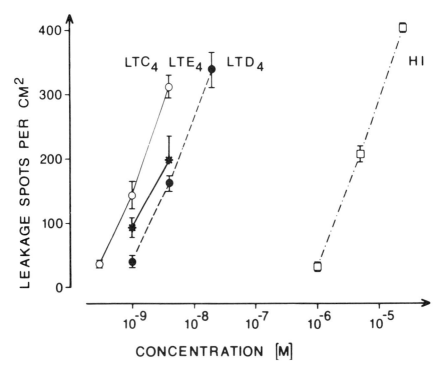

Fig. 7   Dose response curves for leukotrienes and histamine
          as stimulators of vascular permeability.

REFERENCES

1. Corey, E.J., Clark, D.A., Goto, G., Marfat, A., Mioskow-ski, C., Samuelsson, B., and Hammarström, S. (1980): <u>J. Amer. Chem. Soc.</u>,102, 1436-1439; correction 3663

2. Dahlén, S.-E., Björk, J., Hedqvist, P., Arfors, K.-E., Hammarström, S., Lindgren, J.Å., and Samuelsson, B. (1981): <u>Proc. Natl. Acad. Sci. U S A</u>, 78:3887-3891.

3. Hammarström, S. (1977): <u>Biochim. Biophys. Acta</u> 487, 517-519.

4. Hammarström, S. (1982): In: <u>Proc. Int. Congr. on Prosta-glandins and Cancer</u>, edited by T.J. Powles, R.S.,Bockman, K.V. Honn, and P. Ramwell, pp. 297-308, Allan Liss, New York.

5. Hammarström, S. (1982): <u>Arch. Biochem. Biophys</u>. 214, 431-445.

6. Hammarström, S. (1980): <u>J. Biol. Chem</u>. 255, 7093-7094.

7. Hammarström, S. (1981): <u>J. Biol. Chem</u>. 256, 2275-2279.

8. Hammarström, S. (1981): <u>J. Biol. Chem</u>. 256, 7712-7714.

9. Hammarström, S. (1983): <u>J. Biol. Chem</u>. 258, 1427-1430.

10. Hammarström, S. and Samuelsson, B. (1980): <u>FEBS Lett.</u>, 122, 83-86.

11. Hammarström, S., Murphy, R.C., Samuelsson, B., Clark, D. A., Mioskowski, S., and Corey, E.J. (1979): Biochem. Biophys. Res. Commun. 91, 1266-1272

12. Hedqvist, P., Dahlén, S.E., Gustavsson, L., Hammarström, S. and Samuelsson, B. (1980): <u>Acta Physiol. Scand</u>. 110, 331-333.

13. Jakschik, B., Falkenhein, S., and Parker, C.W. (1977): <u>Proc. Natl. Acad. Sci. U S A</u>, 74, 4577-4581.

14. Maas, R.L. and Brash, A.R. (1983): <u>Proc. Natl. Acad. Sci. U S A</u>, 80, 2884-2888.

15. Murphy, R.C., Hammarström, S., and Samuelsson, B. (1979): <u>Proc. Natl. Acad. Sci. U S A</u>, 76, 4275-4279.

16. Orange, R.P. and Austen, K.F. (1969): <u>Adv. Immunol</u>. 10, 105-144.

17. Örning, L. and Hammarström, S. (1980): <u>J. Biol. Chem</u>. 255, 8023-8026.

18. Örning, L., Hammarström, S., and Samuelsson, B. (1980): Proc. Natl. Acad. Sci. U S A, 77, 2014-2017.

19. Örning, L., Bernström, K., and Hammarström, S. (1981): Eur. J. Biochem., 120, 41-45.

20. Smedegård, G., Hedqvist, P., Dahlén, S.E., Revenäs, B., Hammarström, S., and Samuelsson, B. (1982): Nature, 295, 327-329.

Icosanoids and Cancer, edited by H. Thaler-Dao, et al. Raven Press, New York © 1984.

Fatty Acid Metabolism and Cell Proliferation. VI. Properties of Antithrombotic Agents that Influence Metastasis

David G. Cornwell, Jenifer A. Lindsey, Hanfang Zhang, and Nobuhiro Morisaki

Department of Physiological Chemistry, The Ohio State University, Columbus, Ohio 43210

ABSTRACT

Studies from many laboratories show that polyunsaturated fatty acids are involved in the control of cell proliferation. Fatty acids are oxidized by a variety of free radical reactions to cyclic endoperoxides (prostanoid pathways) and to acyclic hydroperoxides (lipid peroxide pathways). The different peroxides, their derivatives and radicals formed during their synthesis and metabolism generate either positive or negative signals for cell proliferation. Agents may be divided into 4 general classes according to their effects on prostanoid and lipid peroxide pathways, and cell proliferation. The antiaggregatory compounds dipyridamole and nafazatrom belong to agent classes with characteristics that help to explain their very different effects on cell proliferation and metastasis.

INTRODUCTION

Platelet aggregation is induced by tumors, and aggregating platelets elaborate growth factors that promote tumorigenesis (38,40). A number of investigators have suggested that antiaggregatory compounds will break this cycle and inhibit tumor metastasis (10,15,16,19,38,40). Indeed, prostacyclin (PGI_2), the naturally occuring antiaggregatory prostanoid, was shown to be a potent anti-metastatic agent (15,17,19). Many antiaggregatory agents promote PGI_2 synthesis or prolong the activity of PGI_2. However, the anti-metastatic effect of an antiaggregatory agent is not always a simple function of its effect on PGI_2. The problem is demonstrated by the antiaggregatory agents dipyridamole, 2,6-bis(diethanol-amino)-4,8-dipiperidinopyrimido-[5,4-d]pyrimidine, and nafazatrom, or Bay g 6575, 1-[2-(β-napthyloxy)ethyl]-3-methyl-2-pyrazolin-5-one.

Dipyridamole (2,34,37) and nafazatrom (4,9,39) both stimulate the release or prolong the activity of PGI_2. Both agents appear to be antioxidants. Dipyridamole blocks intracellular lipid peroxidation (34) while nafazatrom inhibits lipoxygenase (18) and blocks co-oxidation reactions during prostanoid synthesis (9). Nevertheless, these agents have very different effects on cell proliferation and metastasis. Dipyridamole promotes cell proliferation (8,14,24,34) and has little effect on metastasis (13,16) while nafazatrom inhibits both cell proliferation and metastasis (1,15,18,19). We suggest that the differences between dipyridamole and nafazatrom are related to their effects on fatty acid metabolism in specific cells.

Essential fatty acids are metabolized by a number of free radical reactions to cyclic endoperoxides (prostaglandin pathways) and acyclic hydroperoxides (lipid peroxide pathways). Various peroxides, their metabolites, and radicals formed during their synthesis and metabolism give both positive and negative signals for cell proliferation. Studies from our laboratory and elsewhere describing the direct effects of prostanoids and lipid peroxides on cell proliferation are summarized by us in a recent review (6). Prostanoids and lipid peroxides also have indirect effects on cell proliferation which involve biological processes such as immunosurveillance or cellular differentiation (6). These secondary effects are beyond the scope of this paper.

Several prostanoids show a concentration-dependent stimulation and a concentration-dependent inhibition of cell proliferation (6). These effects and their relationship to fatty acid metabolism are described in a schematic diagram (FIG. 1). Prostanoid synthesis increased as

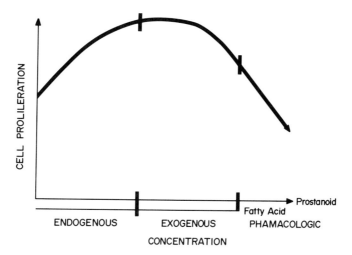

FIG. 1. A schematic diagram relating prostanoid synthesis with fatty acid concentration, and showing the concentration-dependent stimulatory and inhibitory effects of prostanoids on cell proliferation.

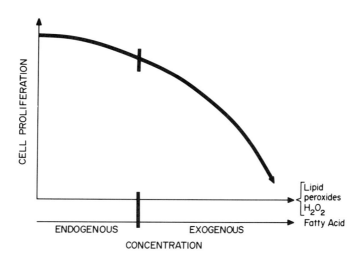

FIG. 2. A schematic diagram relating lipid peroxide synthesis with fatty acid concentration and showing the concentration-dependent inhibitory effect of lipid peroxides on cell proliferation.

the fatty acid concentration is increased both through fatty acid
release (Endogenous fatty acid effect) and the addition of
extracellular fatty acid (Exogenous fatty acid effect). Prostanoid
levels provided by biosynthesis eventually plateau because the
cyclooxygenase complex is saturated with substrate (6,33). Very high
prostanoid levels are achieved by the direct addition of a specific
prostanoid (Pharmacologic prostanoid effect).

Lipid peroxides show only a concentration-dependent inhibition of
cell proliferation (6). This effect and its relationship to fatty
acid metabolism are described in a schematic diagram (FIG. 2). Lipid
peroxides are generated by several pathways involving lipoxygenase,
co-oxidation, during prostanoid synthesis, and the microsomal P_{450}
system (6). Lipid peroxide levels are greatly increased by the
addition of extracellular fatty acids probably through the stimulation
of peroxisomal metabolism and the generation of H_2O_2 by fatty acid
oxidation in these organelles (3).

TABLE 1. Agent classification scheme based on prostanoid and/or
          lipid peroxide synthesis, and cell proliferation in the
          presence of low and high fatty acid levels

AGENT	PROSTANOIDS	PEROXIDES	PROLIFERATION	
			LOW F.A.	HIGH F.A.
I	↑[a]	O	↑	O
II	↑	↓	↑	↑
III	O	↓	O–↑	↑
IV	↓	↓	O	↑

[a] ↑, Increased; O, Unchanged; ↓, Decreased

Agents that alter the cellular levels of prostanoids and/or lipid
peroxides have profound effects on cell proliferation. Our studies
(6) show that these agents may be divided into 4 general classes

(Table 1). Class I agents only stimulate prostanoid synthesis. These agents only promote cell proliferation in the presence of low fatty acid levels. Class II agents stimulate prostanoid synthesis and block lipid peroxide synthesis. These agents promote cell proliferation in the presence of both low and high fatty acid levels. Class III agents only block lipid peroxide synthesis. These agents sometimes promote cell proliferation when the fatty acid level is low and these agents always promote cell proliferation when the fatty acid level is high. Class IV agents inhibit both prostanoid and lipid peroxide synthesis. These agents only promote cell proliferation in the presence of high fatty acid levels. We provide examples of each agent class in this paper and we show that dipyridamole and nafazatrom belong to agent classes which explain their different effects on cell proliferation and metastasis.

MATERIALS AND METHODS

Materials

Arachidonic acid [20:4 (n-6)] was purchased from Nu-Chek (Elysian, MN.) and used only when a test for lipid peroxides (21) was negative. Other reagents were obtained from the following sources: vitamin E, α-naphthol (α-N) and propyl gallate (PrGa) (Eastman, Rochester, N.Y.); dipyridamole (Boehringer Ingelheim, Ridgefield, CT.); hydralazine HCl (Sigma, St. Louis, MO.); nafazatrom (Miles, West Haven, CT.); HEPES buffer (GIBCO, Grand Island, N.Y.); gentamycin sulfate (Schering, Kenilworth, N.J.); amino acids (Microbiological Associates, Walkersville, MD.); fetal bovine serum (Sterile Systems, Logan, UT.; Hyclone lots 100331 and 100348). Antiserum for the radioimmunoassay (RIA) of 6-keto-PGF$_{1\alpha}$ was kindly supplied by Dr. L. Levine.

Tissue Culture

Primary cultures of smooth muscle cells were established from the dissected medial layer of guinea pig aorta from prepubertal males (20,21). Growth Medium was prepared from 1X Eagle's minimum essential medium containing Hank's salts and 25 mM HEPES buffer supplemented with 50 µg/ml of gentamycin sulfate, 2 mM glutamine, 1X non-essential amino acids, 1 mM sodium pyruvate, 1.3 mg/ml of sodium bicarbonate, and 10% fetal bovine serum. Experimental Medium for lipid peroxidation and prostanoid studies with confluent cells consisted of Growth Medium supplemented with 20% fetal bovine serum, 1X essential amino acids, and 1X essential vitamins. Cloning Medium contained 10% fetal bovine serum and the same supplements as Experimental Medium. Fatty acids and other agents were dissolved in 95% ethanol and diluted with Experimental Medium or Cloning Medium. Control cultures were treated with medium containing the same amount of 95% ethanol. Cells were used at passage levels 4 to 6.

Cell Proliferation

Cells 3 to 5 days post confluent were seeded at low densities (40 to 200 cells/cm^2) in Falcon single-well (60 by 15 mm) plates. Cells were allowed to attach to the plastic plates for 1 day before initial treatment. Cells were retreated with a media change at day 5 of the incubation period. After an 8-10 day incubation period, cells were fixed in 3.7% phosphate-buffered formalin and stained with filtered Giemsa.

In some experiments, a frequency distribution of colonies based on colony number and colony size was obtained with an image analysis system (Optomax, Wallis, N.H.) equipped with an automatic chord sizing module (12). Image analysis generated the complement of a cumulative distribution for the number of colonies (f) as a function of increasing colony diameter (d). The total number of colonies in the culture (f_T) was provided by the colony frequency at the initial minimum colony diameter. The average number of cells per colony (N) in each segment of the distribution curve was calculated from the average colony d for the segment using the relationship:

$$\log N = 1.98 \log d - 3.469$$

The number of cells in each segment of the distribution curve was then obtained by multiplying N and the average f for the segment. These data, expressed as a cumulative distribution function, yielded the total number of cells (N_T) in the culture. The average colony size

(N_A) was obtained by dividing N_T by f_T and the number of population doublings (PD) was then expressed as $\log_2 N_A$.

In other experiments, a relative cell count was obtained from the total cell area on the Falcon plate (12,33). Cell area was measured by image analysis (Optomax). Cells from the same primary culture and the same batch of growth medium were compared in each treatment group.

Lipid Peroxidation

Lipid peroxidation in tissue cultures was measured with cells seeded at 1.3×10^4 cells/cm^2 in flasks containing 4 ml of Experimental Medium. Cells were grown to confluency before treatments were initiated. The incubation conditions and the thiobarbituric acid (TBA) assay for lipid peroxides are described elsewhere (11). As reported previously, TBA reactive material was found in cells but not culture media.

Prostaglandin Biosynthesis

Smooth muscle cells synthesize PGE_2 and PGI_2. These prostanoids are further metabolized in cultures. The end product of PGI_2 metabolism, 6-keto-PGF$_{1\alpha}$, was measured in this study. 6-Keto-PGF$_{1\alpha}$ in media was estimated by a standard RIA procedure (26). The cross-reactivity of the 6-keto-PGF$_{1\alpha}$ antibody was: PGE_2, 0.15%; PGD_2, 0.002%; PGF$_{2\alpha}$, 0.10%; 20:4 (n-6), 0.005%.

Statistics

Data are reported as mean ± SEM. The significance of differences in a treatment series was determined by a one-way analysis of variance (F ratio and F probability). Individual treatments were compared with the control by the Tukey-HSD test.

RESULTS AND DISCUSSION

Class I Agents (Hydralazine)

Compounds such as hydralazine (32) and cyclosporin A (28) display the properties of Class I agents (Table 1). Since hydralazine has been studied more extensively in our laboratory, it is selected here as an example of this class. Hydralazine stimulated the synthesis of both PGE_2 and PGI_2 (measured as 6-keto-PGF$_{1\alpha}$) when it was added to cultures that contained media alone (low fatty acid level). Data from

several incubation experiments are summarized in Figure 3. Hydralazine
(32) evidently stimulated fatty acid release since it had little
effect on prostanoid synthesis when the medium was enriched with 20:4
(n-6) (high fatty acid level). Furthermore, hydralazine (FIG. 3) had
only a small effect on lipid peroxide levels, measured as MDA, when
cultures were enriched with 20:4 (n-6).

Hydralazine had, as predicted, a significant effect on cell
proliferation when cells were grown in media alone (FIG. 4). The
total number of colonies (f_T) and the total number of cells (N_T) were
both increased significantly in culture treated with hydralazine. The

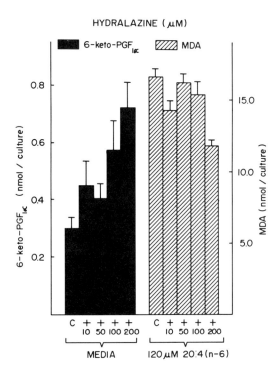

FIG. 3. Effects of hydralazine on fatty acid metabolism in
confluent smooth muscle cells showing the concentration-
dependent stimulatory effect on prostanoid synthesis
(6-keto-PGF$_{1\alpha}$) when cells were incubated for 24 h with media
alone, and the absence of a significant inhibitory effect on
lipid peroxidation (MDA) when cells were incubated for 24 h with
20:4 (n-6).

number of population doublings during an 8 day incubation period
increased from 6.7 in the control to 7.7 in the treated cultures.
Indomethacin blocked both prostanoid synthesis and enhanced cell
proliferation in treated cultures (32). Finally, hydralazine had
little effect on cell proliferation when the medium was enriched with
20:4 (n-6) (data not shown). These experiments show clearly that
Class I agents stimulate prostanoid synthesis and as a consequence
cell proliferation when cells are grown in media alone.

Class III Agents (Vitamin E)

The naturally occuring antioxidants, vitamin E and vitamin E
quinone, are highly effective inhibitors of lipid peroxidation in
cultures incubated either with media alone or media enriched with 20:4
(n-6) (11,27,33,34). However, the natural antioxidants have very

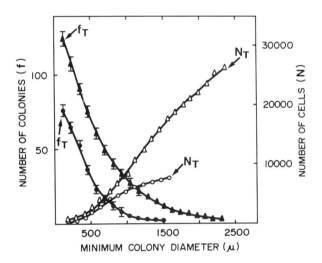

FIG. 4. Colony frequency-size distribution for smooth
muscle cells seeded at 200 cells/cm^2 and grown for 8 days
with and without 20 µM hydralazine. Frequency (f) and
cell number (N) data are plotted as described in the text.
Control f, ●; control N, O; hydralazine f, ▲; hydralazine N, Δ.

little effect on prostanoid synthesis in these cultures. Data for
vitamin E are presented in Figure 5. These properties place vitamin E

and vitamin E quinone in Class III of our classification scheme (Table 1). Class III agents always enhance cell proliferation when the medium is enriched with 20:4 (n-6). Vitamin E fulfills this criterion for a Class III agent (5,11,12,27,21,34). Class III agents sometimes enhance cell proliferation when cells are grown in media alone. This effect, which depends on the growth promoting properties of specific lots of fetal bovine serum (6), is demonstrated in Figure 5.

Early studies with vitamin E, particularly the experiments of Juhász-Schäffer (22) with explant cultures, led Mason (29) in 1933 to the hypothesis that vitamin E was a factor necessary both for cell growth and for cell differentiation. We have confirmed his hypothesis by demonstrating in this and other studies that vitamin E enhances the proliferation of a number of cell lines in culture (5,6,11,12,27,31,34). Furthermore, we have shown that cryoprotective agents also function as antioxidants and their ability to induce erythroleukemic cell

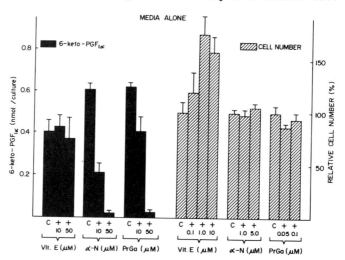

FIG. 5. Effects of the natural antioxidant, vitamin E, and the synthetic antioxidants, α-naphthol (α-N) and propyl gallate (PrGa), on prostanoid synthesis and cell proliferation showing prostanoid synthesis (6-keto-PGF$_{1\alpha}$) in confluent cultures incubated for 24 h with media alone and relative cell number [(treatment/control) x100] in cloning experiments (see text).

differentiation varies directly with their ability to scavenge oxygen centered radicals (30).

Class IV Agents (α-Naphthol and Propyl Gallate)

Naturally occuring antioxidants block lipid peroxidation without blocking prostanoid synthesis to a significant extent. A number of synthetic antioxidants show concentration-dependent inhibitory effects on both lipid peroxidation and prostanoid synthesis (35,36). For example, α-naphthol (α-N) and propyl gallate (PrGa) both block prostanoid synthesis when smooth muscle cells are incubated in media alone (FIG. 5). These compounds are designated as Class IV agents in our classification scheme (Table 1) and they have, as predicted, no effect on proliferation when cells are grown in media alone (FIG. 5).

Dipyridamole and Nafazatrom: Class II and Class IV

Agents Compared

The antiaggregatory agent dipyridamole functions as an antioxidant in model systems which use agents such as cumene hydroperoxide to oxidize 20:4 (n-6) (34). Nafazatrom also serves as an antioxidant in systems using cumene hydroperoxide as the oxidizing agent. For example, 400 μM nafazatrom inhibited the oxidation of 1 mM 20:4 (n-6) by cumene hydroperoxide (0.2 μl per ml) in the presence of 41 μM Fe^{3+}. Lipid peroxidation, estimated by the absorbance at 532 nm (TBA test), decreased from 0.166 ± 0.003 to 0.132 ± 0.003 (p<0.001) in this model system.

We suggested in a previous study that dipyridamole functioned as an antioxidant in stimulating the release of PGI_2 from aorta (34). Nafazatrom probably acts in the same manner. We found that 100 μM nafazatrom increased the PGI_2 yield from 40 to 100% when slices of guinea pig aorta were incubated with 30 μM 20:4 (n-6), a substrate level high enough to generate significant amounts of lipid peroxides (33). Nafazatrom had little effect on the PGI_2 yield when aorta slices were incubated in the absence of 20:4 (n-6). Other studies have shown that nafazatrom (4) acted like vitamin E (23,35) in stimulating vascular PGI_2 synthesis by aorta of diabetic rats.

Dipyridamole and nafazatrom both function as antioxidants which block lipid peroxidation when cells are incubated with 20:4 (n-6) for various time intervals (Fig. 6). The inhibitory effects of these

agents are concentration-dependent and there is very little difference
between the 2 agents in their ability to block lipid peroxidation.

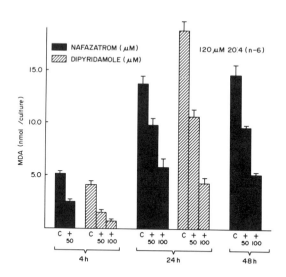

FIG. 6. Effects of dipyridamole and nafazatrom on lipid
peroxidation (MDA) in confluent smooth muscle cells
incubated for 4 h, 24 h and 48 h with 20:4 (n-6).

An earlier study from our laboratory (34) showed that dipyridamole,
like many antioxidants, initially inhibited prostanoid synthesis but
this agent evidently protected the enzyme complex allowing prostanoid
synthesis to continue for a longer time period. As a consequence,
prostanoid synthesis was diminished when cells were incubated for only
4 h and prostanoid synthesis was enhanced when the incubation period
was extended to 24 h. Data for cells incubated with media alone and
cells incubated with 120 µM 20:4 (n-6) are summarized in Figures 7 and
8.
    Nafazatrom like dipyridamole blocked prostanoid synthesis when
cells were incubated for 4 h (FIG. 7 and 8). However, nafazatrom
unlike dipyridamole continued to inhibit prostanoid synthesis when the
incubation period was extended to 24 h and 48 hr. The inhibitory
effect of nafazatrom like the stimulatory effect of dipyridamole was
most pronounced when the cells were incubated with media alone (FIG.
7).

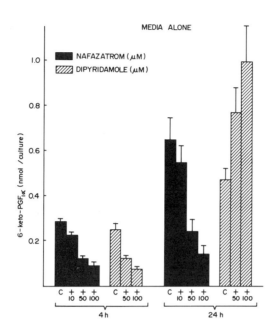

FIG. 7. Effects of dipyridamole and nafazatrom on prostanoid synthesis (6-keto-PGF$_{1\alpha}$) in confluent smooth muscle cells incubated for 4 and 24 h with media alone.

Prostanoid and lipid peroxidation data place dipyridamole and nafazatrom in different classes according to our classification scheme (Table 1). Dipyridamole, a Class II agent, should promote proliferation when cells are incubated either in media alone or in media enriched with 20:4 (n-6). Nafazatrom, a Class IV agent, should have its most significant effect on proliferation when cells are incubated in media enriched with 20:4 (n-6). These differences are demonstrated in Figure 9. Dipyridamole stimulated proliferation when cells were grown either in media alone (F ratio 14.903, F prob. 0.0001) or media enriched with 20:4 (n-6) (F ratio 18.613, F prob. 0). Nafazatrom had a marginal effect when cells were grown in media alone (F ratio 4.663, F prob. 0.021) and a significant effect when cells were grown in 20:4 (n-6) (F ratio 7.715, F prob. 0.003). Furthermore, dipyridamole had a greater effect than nafazatrom when these agents

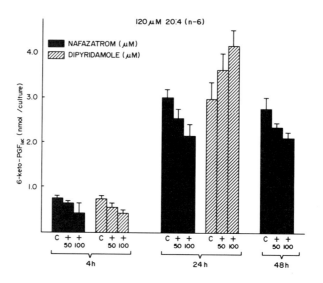

FIG. 8. Effects of dipyridamole and nafazatrom on
prostanoid synthesis (6-keto-PGF$_{1\alpha}$) in confluent smooth
muscle cells incubated for 4 h, 24 h and 48 h with
20:4 (n-6).

were compared at the same concentrations (FIG. 9).

Aggregating platelets release a growth factor that stimulates 20:4
(n-6) release and prostanoid biosynthesis (6,7,25). We suggest that
dipyridamole functions directly as an antioxidant that protects cyclooxygenase and causes both increased PGI$_2$ synthesis and increased cell
growth. Nafazatrom apparently acts indirectly as an antioxidant that
protects PGI$_2$ synthetase in tissues, such as aorta, containing cells
that are accessible to lipoxygenase products. Thus, dipyridamole and
nafazatrom both serve as antiaggregatory agents. However,
dipyridamole unlike nafazatrom, is itself an effective growth factor.
Dipyridamole enhances plaque formation (smooth muscle cell
proliferation) in aortas of rabbits and monkeys maintained on
atherogenic diets (8,14,24). This property of dipyridamole may
explain why dipyridamole is not an effective antimetastatic agent.

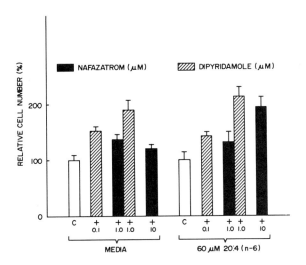

FIG. 9. Effects of dipyridamole and nafazatrom on cell proliferation in smooth muscle cells grown in media alone or media enriched with 20:4 (n-6); relative cell number [treatment/control) x100] in cloning experiments (see text).

ACKNOWLEDGEMENTS

This study was supported in part by a grant from the Central Ohio Heart Chapter, Inc. #82-4. We appreciate the support of Dr. George Milo, statistical analyses by Dr. Larry Sachs, technical assistance by Mrs. Judith Stitts, and the secretarial assistance of Mrs. Dorothy Ferguson.

REFERENCES

1. Ambrus, J.L., Ambrus, C.M., Gastpar, H., and Williams, P. (1982): J. Med., 13:35-47.
2. Blass, K.E., Block, H.U., Förster, W., and Pönicke, K. (1980): Brit. J. Pharmacol., 68:71-73.

3. Böck, P., Kramer, R., and Pavelka, M. (1980): <u>Peroxisomes and Related Particles in Animal Tissues</u>, pp. 33-37. Springer-Verlag, Wien.

4. Carreras, L.O., Chamone, D.A., Klerckx, P., and Vermylen, J. (1980): <u>Thromb. Res.</u>, 19:663-670.

5. Cornwell, D.G., Huttner, J.J., Milo, G.E., Panganamala, R.V., Sharma, H.M., and Geer, J.C. (1979): <u>Lipids</u>, 14:194-207.

6. Cornwell, D.G., and Morisaki, N. (In press): In: <u>Free Radicals in Biology</u>, Vol. VI, edited by W.A. Pryor, Academic Press, Inc., New York.

7. Coughlin, S.R., Moskowitz, M.A., Antoniades, H.N., and Levine, L. (1981): <u>Proc. Natl. Acad. Sci. USA</u>, 78:7134-7138.

8. Dembinska-Kiec, A., Rücker, W., and Schönhöfer, P.S. (1979): <u>Atherosclerosis</u>, 33:315-327.

9. Eling, T.E., Honn, K.V., Busse, W.D., Seuter, F., and Marnett, L.J. (1982): In: <u>Prostaglandins and Cancer: First International Conference</u>, Vol. 2, edited by T.J. Powles, R.S. Bockman, K.V. Honn, and P. Ramwell, pp. 783-787. Alan R. Liss, Inc., New York.

10. Gastpar, H., Ambrus, J.L., and Ambrus, C.M. (1982): In: <u>Interaction of Platelets and Tumor Cells</u>, edited by G.A. Jamieson, pp. 63-82. Alan R. Liss, Inc., New York.

11. Gavino, V.C., Miller, J.S., Ikharebha, S.O., Milo, G.E., and Cornwell, D.G. (1981): <u>J. Lipid Res.</u>, 22:763-769.

12. Gavino, V.C., Milo, G.E., and Cornwell, D.G. (1982): <u>Cell Tissue Kinet.</u>, 15:225-231.

13. Hilgard, P. (1982): In: <u>Interaction of Platelets and Tumor Cells</u>, edited by G.A. Jamieson, pp. 143-158. Alan R. Liss, Inc., New York.

14. Hollander, W., Kirkpatrick, B., Paddock, J., Colombo, M., Nagraj, S., and Prusty, S. (1979): <u>Exp. Mol. Pathol.</u>, 30:55-73.

15. Honn, K.V. (1982): In: <u>Prostanglandins and Cancer: First International Conference</u>, Vol. 2, edited by T.J. Powles, R.S. Bockman, K.V. Honn and P. Ramwell, pp. 733-752. Alan R. Liss, Inc., New York.

16. Honn, K.V., Bockman, R.S., and Marnett, L.J. (1981): <u>Prostaglandins</u>, 21:833-864.

17. Honn, K.V., Cicone, B., and Skoff, A. (1981): Science, 212: 1270-1272.

18. Honn, K.V., and Dunn, J.R. (1982): FEBS Lett., 139:65-68.

19. Honn, K.V., Meyer, J., Neages, G., Henderson, T., Westly, C., and Ratanatharathorn, V. (1982): In: Interaction of Platelets and Tumor Cells, edited by G.A. Jamieson, pp. 295-331. Alan R. Liss, Inc., New York.

20. Huttner, J.J., Cornwell, D.G., and Milo, G.E. (1977): T.C.A. Manual, 3:633-639.

21. Huttner, J.J., Gwebu, E.T., Panganamala, R.V., Milo, G.E., Cornwell, D.G., Sharma, H.M., and Geer, J.C. (1977): Science, 197:289-291.

22. Juhász-Schäffer, A. (1931): Arch. Pathol. Anat. Physiol., 281: 35-45.

23. Karpen, C.W., Pritchard, K.A., Jr., Arnold, J.H., Cornwell, D.G., and Panganamala, R.V. (1982): Diabetes, 31:947-951.

24. Koster, J.K., Jr., Tryka, A.F., H'Doubler, P., and Collins, Jr., J.J., (1981): Artery, 9:405-413.

25. Levine, L. (1982): In: Prostaglandins and Cancer: First International Conference, Vol. 2, edited by T.J. Powles, R.S. Bockman, K.V. Honn, and P. Ramwell, pp. 189-204. Alan R. Liss, Inc., New York.

26. Levine, L., Gjtierrez-Cernosek, R.M., and Van Vunakis, H. (1971): J. Biol. Chem., 246:6782-6785.

27. Liepkalns, V.A., Icard-Liepkalns, C., and Cornwell, D.G. (1982): Cancer Lett., 15:173-178.

28. Lindsey, J.A., Morisaki, N., Stitts, J.M., Zager, R.A., and Cornwell, D.G. (1983): Lipids, 18:566-569.

29. Mason, K.E. (1933): Am. J. Anat., 52:153-239.

30. Miller, J.S., and Cornwell, D.G. (1978): Cryobiology, 15:585-588.

31. Miller, J.S., Gavino, V.C., Ackerman, G.A., Sharma, H.M., Milo, G.E., Geer, J.C., and Cornwell, D.G. (1980): Lab. Invest., 42:495-506.

32. Morisaki, N., Lindsey, J.A., Milo, G.E., and Cornwell, D.G. (1983): Lipids, 18:349-352.

33. Morisaki, N., Sprecher, H., Milo, G.E., and Cornwell, D.G. (1982): Lipids, 17:893-899.

34. Morisaki, N., Stitts, J.M., Bartels-Tomei, L., Milo, G.E., Panganamala, R.V., and Cornwell, D.G. (1982): Artery, 11:88-107.

35. Panganamala, R.V., and Cornwell, D.G. (1982): Ann. N.Y. Acad. Sci., 393:376-390.

36. Panganamala, R.V., Miller, J.S., Gwebu, E.T., Sharma, H.M., and Cornwell, D.G. (1977): Prostaglandins, 14:261-271.

37. Serneri, G.G., Masotti, G., Poggesi, L., Galanti, G., and Morettini, A. (1981): Eur. J. Clin. Pharmacol., 21:9-15.

38. Steiner, M. (1982): In: Interaction of Platelets and Tumor Cells, edited by G.A. Jamieson, pp. 383-403. Alan R. Liss, Inc., New York.

39. Wong, P., Y-K., Chao, P., H.-W., and McGiff, J.C. (1982): J. Pharmacol. Exp. Therap., 223:757-760.

40. Zacharski, L.R. (1982): In: Interaction of Platelets and Tumor Cells, edited by G.A. Jamieson, pp. 113-129. Alan R. Liss, Inc., New York.

Icosanoids and Cancer, edited by H. Thaler-Dao, et al. Raven Press, New York © 1984.

Prostaglandins and Tumour Metastasis

Alan Bennett

Department of Surgery, King's College Hospital Medical School, Rayne Institute, London, SE5 9NU England

Many studies attest to the fact that malignant tumours usually form more prostaglandins (PGs) than do the normal tissues in which they arise (1). There are also a few studies that have examined primary tumour PGs in relation to metastasis and postoperative survival. This chapter concerns mainly studies in our laboratory on human mammary and lung cancer and mouse NC carcinoma.

Our research into breast cancer started in 1974, and at that time radioimmunoassays and mass spectrometry were in their infancy and not widely available. We therefore chose to use our pharmacological experience of bioassays, employing the rat stomach strip which responds to many PGs but is most sensitive to PGE compounds. For the purpose of comparison, and for the various advantages of bioassay, we have continued this type of measurement, combining it more recently with radioimmunoassay and mass spectrometry. We have now formally identified many eicosanoids in extracts of the human breast and lung carcinomas, which contain arachidonate, TXB_2, PGD_2, PGE_2, $PGF_{2\alpha}$, 6-keto-$PGF_{1\alpha}$, 6,15-diketo-13,14 dihydro-$PGF_{1\alpha}$, 6,15-diketo-$PGF_{1\alpha}$, 15-keto-13,14-dihydro-TXB_2 and 12-HETE (9,17). No PGE_1 was detected by the rather insensitive qualitative mass spectrometry, in contrast to the breast tumour radioimmunoassay results of Karmali et al (11). At present, only our bioassay results of primary tumour PGs are suitable for analysing tumour recurrence and patient survival. Some interesting relationships have emerged, particularly with regard to postoperative survival in breast cancer, but the results must be interpreted cautiously in view of the many problems of PG source, measurement and other factors discussed later.

BREAST CANCER

Evidence of breast cancer metastasis near the time of surgical removal of the primary tumour was examined by clinical and pathological staging and by skeletal scintigraphy following the injection of ^{99}Tc-ethanehydroxy-diphosphonate (5). The median amount of PG-like material (PG-lm) extracted from the primary tumours was higher in patients with positive bone scans near to the time of surgery than in those with negative scans. However, this was because tumours yielding low amounts of PG ($\leqslant$16ng PGE_2 equivalents/g tissue after homogenization in Krebs

solution) had negative bone scintiscans. Above this value, the incidence of positive bone scans was not related to the tumour PG yield (3).
Thus a high production of PG-lm by the primary tumours is not necessa-
rily associated with bone metastasis, a conclusion borne out by other
evidence. Tumour recurrence in the follow-up period was, if anything,
lower in bone than locally: the primary tumour median values of PG-lm
(obtained from homogenates in Krebs solution) for a recurrence at a
single site were (ng PGE_2 equivalents/g): local recurrence 76, bone
54, visceral metastasis 29ng. However, there was considerable overlap,
and the differences in amounts of primary tumour PGs were likely to
have arisen by chance with bone metastasis compared to the other 2
sites (P>0.14 for both comparisons). However, there was more likeli-
hood of a recurrence locally rather than viscerally with a high tumour
PG-lm yield (P=0.048). Results from a second study on another 98
patients also showed no clear relationship of primary tumour PG-lm to
recurrence in bone (unpublished). Nor was there any detected relationship between tumour oestrogen receptors and PG-lm (19).

   Indomethacin had no obvious effect on hypercalcaemia in breast cancer
(6), and benorylate, a relatively weak inhibitor of PG synthesis, did
not affect the incidence of bone metastasis in breast cancer patients
(14). Nevertheless, breast tumour PGs may play a part in metastasis.
They can release PG-lm into the blood (18) thus possibly affecting
platelet aggregation and the dispersion of malignant cells. Results
previously reported on some tumours (5) showed histological evidence
of a correlation between tumour PG-lm and the numbers of malignant cells
in blood vessels and lymphatics in primary breast tumours. Because of
discrepancies of interpretation by histologists we have not re-examined
this possible relationship in all the tumours from that study. However, Rolland et al (15) considered that the malignancy of breast correlated with the ability of microsomal enzyme to form PGE_2 from added
arachidonic acid. Our patient survival data show an inverse correlation with tumour PG-lm, at least up to 3 years postoperatively (P<0.0001)
but this relationship may not hold for longer survival periods. The
ratio of thromboxane:PGI_2 production by the mouse tumours described by
Donati et al (7) may be important in determining metastasis; greater
metastatic spread is thought to result from TXA_2-induced platelet aggregation. This might also be important in human mammary cancer (11).

HUMAN LUNG CANCER

   When it became apparent from our breast cancer study that PGs might
contribute to the disease, we decided to see if this was so in other
human malignancies. Lung cancer was chosen because it is also a common malignancy which metastasizes to the skeleton. Obvious differences
from breast cancer are the appalling prognosis (only about 20% of lung
cancer patients being operable and almost all being dead within 5 years
of diagnosis), and the different histological types of lung tumours.
The studies were done in the same way as in breast cancer, with bioassay of extracted tissue homogenates which prebably measures mainly
PGE_2.

   The relationship of tumour types to prognosis is not clearly established, but postoperative survival probably approximates to the following ascending order: small-cell undifferentiated carcinoma, large-

cell undifferentiated, poorly differentiated adenocarcinoma = poorly differentiated squamous, well differentiated adenocarcinoma = well differentiated squamous carcinoma. Median amounts of PG-lm produced by lung carcinomas were in the following ascending order: small-cell carcinomas, large-cell undifferentiated, well-differentiated squamous, poorly differentiated adenocarcinomas, poorly differentiated squamous and well-differentiated adenocarcinomas (4). It is therefore evident that small-cell carcinomas have the worst prognosis, and they produce the lowest amounts of PG-lm. However, taking all lung tumour types together, PG-lm production does not correlate with survival (P>0.3) (unpublished).

The reason for the different relationship of primary tumour PG-lm to survival in breast cancer compared with lung cancer is not understood, and is likely to be complex. Is it a function of the different types of cancer? Is it related to the advanced growth of lung tumours by the time they are diagnosed, compared with breast tumours which are often more easily detected? However, we found no obvious relationship of lung tumour size to PG-lm, whereas the size of breast tumours shows an inverse relationship to PG production (15). To what extent do measurements of PG-lm from excised primary tumours reflect their past metastatic activity? There are numerous problems in relating tumour PGs to metastasis and survival. The tumour produces many eicosanoids, some of which may act to produce one type of effect, and other PGs which may act differently. Responses to the same PG may even vary with its local concentration. The assay measures only some of the eicosanoids, and it does not determine whether they are produced by both the malignant and the host cells. There is an unknown time period between primary tumour metastasis and tumour excision. Experimentally, there is an inevitable delay between tumour resection and extraction which may alter the tumour PG content and the synthetic activity of the tissues. Furthermore, patients may have received various drugs that can influence PG metabolism.

MOUSE NC ADENOCARCINOMA

The NC tumour arose spontaneously in the mammary gland of a WHT/Ht mouse and has been transplanted in the same strain for several years. The tumour, which metastasizes principally to the lungs and mediastinum, was apparently of low immunogenicity (10), an important point in view of the influence of PGs on the immune system. In the NC tumour model, flurbiprofen or indomethacin alone slightly prolonged survival, and the effect was greater when the chemotherapeutic drugs methotrexate and melphalan were given simultaneously (2). Usually there was only an increase of the interval between tumour excision and extensive metastasis, but a few mice treated with the combined drugs were free of disease; no disease-free mice occurred in the control groups. The incidence of local recurrence at the excision site of the primary tumour was also less in groups given the combined therapy. Thus the PG synthesis inhibitors help retard the development of NC metastases, and may increase the chance of a cure with cytotoxic chemotherapy.

The mechanism of this action has not been elucidated. A theoretical possibility is that the PG synthesis inhibitors might increase bio-

availability of the chemotherapeutic drugs (eg by displacement from
plasma protein binding sites) but some of the evidence obtained so far
argues against this.   If there is a generally increased bioavaila-
bility of chemotherapeutic drugs, the PG synthesis inhibitors would
presumably give simultaneous protection to normal tissues, since flurbiprofen does not increase chemotherapeutic toxicity in normal mice
(2).   Indomethacin protects mice against gut and bone marrow damage
from methotrexate (13).   Evidence for a pharmacokinetic explanation is
that PGE_2 decreased the rate at which L1210 cells took up methotrexate
(8).   Since two unrelated PG synthesis inhibitors are effective on the
NC carcinoma, it seems likely that PGs are involved.   However, the
drugs may have other actions, such as an effect on cell calcium.   The
effect may be selective for methotrexate/melphalan since preliminary
results indicate that indomethacin does not increase the survival of
mice also given cyclophosphamide after NC tumour excision (unpublished).

THE USE OF PROSTAGLANDIN SYNTHESIS INHIBITORS IN HUMAN CANCERS

   Most studies in animals show a beneficial effect of giving PG synthesis inhibitors.   A few show no effect on the cancer, and even fewer
report a deleterious effect (1).   The question arises as to the benefit
of giving PG synthesis inhibitors to patients with cancer.   The drugs
seem to be of value in treating hypercalcaemia associated with some
"solid" tumours (16), and in treating diarrhoea caused by pelvic ir-
radiation (12).

   Furthermore, anti-inflammatory steroids which inhibit the release of
PG precursors are often given in chemotherapy regimes.   However, the
only reported study of a non-steroidal PG synthesis inhibitor on the
survival of patients shows that benorylate, a relatively weak inhibitor
of PG synthesis, had no effect in breast cancer (14).   Our double
blind trial with the more potent drug flurbiprofen in breast cancer is
still in progress, and the code will not be broken until the end of
1984.   In view of the complex interactions of PGs with various aspects
of cancer, and of apparent differences in the relationship of breast
and lung tumour PGs to patient survival, the effects of PG synthesis
inhibitors might vary with different cancers.   Perhaps the effects
even vary in the same type of cancer at different stages of its development.   It is therefore important to determine whether PG synthesis
inhibitors have a role in cancer therapy, and whether they can be safely
taken by cancer patients to treat the side effects of therapy, or to
treat other diseases.

References

1.   Bennett, A. (1982).   Prostaglandins and inhibitors of their synthesis in cancer growth and spread.   In: Endocrinology of Cancer, Vol
3.   Ed D.P. Rose, CRC Press Inc., Florida, pp 113.

2.   Bennett, A., Berstock, D.A. & Carroll, M.A. (1982).   Increased
survival of cancer-bearing mice treated with inhibitors of prostaglandin synthesis alone or with chemotherapy.   Br. J. Cancer 45, 762.

3.   Bennett, A., Berstock, D.A., Carroll, M.A., Stamford, I.F. &

Wilson, A.J. (1983). Breast cancer, its recurrence, and patient survival in relation to tumor prostaglandins. Adv. in Prostaglandin,
Thromb. and Leukotriene Res., Vol 12. (Eds. B. Samuelsson, R. Paoletti
and P. W. Ramwell). Raven Press, New York, pp 299.

4. Bennett, A., Carroll, M.A., Stamford, I.F., Whimster, W.F. &
Williams, F. (1982). Prostaglandins and human lung carcinomas. Br.
J. Cancer, 46, 6, 888.

5. Bennett, A., Charlier, E.M., McDonald, A.M., Simpson, J.S., Stamford, I.F. & Zebro, T. (1977). Prostaglandins and breast cancer.
Lancet, 2, 624.

6. Coombes, R.C., Neville, A.M., Bondy, P.K. & Powles, T.J. (1976).
Failure of indomethacin to reduce hydroxyproline excretion or hypercalcaemia in patients with breast cancer. Prostaglandins, 12, 1027.

7. Donati, M.B., Borowska, A., Bottazzi, B., Dejana, E., Giavazzi, R.,
Rotilio, D. & Mantovani, A. (1982). Metastatic potential correlates
with changes in the thromboxane-prostacyclin balance. Abstracts, 5th
International Prostaglandin Conference, p136.

8. Henderson, G.B., Zevely, E.M. & Huennekens, F.M. (1978). Cyclic
adenosine 3':5'-monophosphate and methotrexate transport in L1210
cells. Cancer Res. 38, 859.

9. Hensby, C.N., Carroll, M.A., Stamford, I.F., Civier, A. & Bennett,
A. (1982). Identification of arachidonate metabolites in normal and
malignant human lung. J. Pharm. Pharmac. 34, 811.

10. Hewitt, H.B., Blake, E.R. & Walder, A. (1976). A critique of the
evidence for active host defence against cancer, based on personal
studies of 27 murine tumours of spontaneous origin. Br. J. Cancer,
33, 241.

11. Karmali, R.A., Welt, S., Thaler, H.T. & Lefevre, F. Prostaglandins in breast cancer: relationship to disease stage and hormone
status. Br. J. Cancer, in press.

12. Mennie, S.A.T., Dalley, V., Dinneen, L.C. & Collier, H.O.J. (1975).
Treatment of radiation-induced gastrointestinal distress with acetyl-
salicylate. Lancet, ii, 942.

13. Powles, T.J., Alexander, P. & Millar, J.L. (1978). Enhancement of
anti-cancer activity of cytotoxic chemotherapy with production of normal
tissues in inhibition of prostaglandin synthesis. Biochem. Pharmacol.,
27, 1389.

14. Powles, T.J., Dady, P.J., Williams, J., Easty, G.C. & Coombes, R.
C. (1980). Use of inhibitors of prostaglandin synthesis in patients
with breast cancer. In: Advances in Prostaglandin and Thromboxane
Research, Vol 6, p 511 (B. Samuelsson, P.W. Ramwell and R. Paoletti,
Eds). Raven Press, New York.

15. Rolland, P.H., Martin, P.M., Jacquemier, J., Rolland, A.M. &

Toga, M. (1980).   Porstaglandin in human breast cancer: evidence suggesting that an elevated prostaglandin production is a marker of high metastatic potential for neoplastic cells.   J. Nat. Cancer Inst., 64, 1061.

16. Seyberth, H.W., Hubbard, W.C., Oelz, O., Sweetman, B.J., Watson, J.T. & Oates, J.A. (1977).   Prostaglandin mediated hypercalcemia in the VX_2 carcinoma-bearing rabbit.   Prostaglandins, 14, 319.

17. Stamford, I.F., Carroll, M.A., Civier, A., Hensby, C.N., Bennett, A. (1983).   Identification of arachidonate metabolites in normal, benign and malignant human mammary tissues.   J. Pharm. Pharmac. 35, 48.

18. Stamford, I.F., MacIntyre, J. & Bennett, A. (1980).   Human breast cancers release prostaglandins into the blood.   In: Advances in Prostaglandin and Thromboxane Research, Vol 6.   Ed B. Samuelsson, P. W. Ramwell and R. Paoletti.   Raven Press, New York, pp 571.

19. Wilson, A.J., Baum, M., Bennett, A., Griffiths, K, Nicholson, R.I. & Stamford, I.F. (1980).   Lymph node status, prostaglandins and oestrogen receptors are independent prognostic variables in human primary breast cancer.   Clin Oncol 6, 379.

Icosanoids and Cancer, edited by H. Thaler-Dao, et al. Raven Press, New York © 1984.

5-Lipoxygenase Inhibition in Relation to Cell Movement and Cancer

W. Dawson, J. R. F. Corvalan, E. Ann Kitchen, and M. G. Parry

Lilly Research Centre Limited, Windlesham, Surrey, GU20 6PH United Kingdom

The invasion of tumours by inflammatory cells is a common phenomenon (Gauci and Alexander, 1975) but the process by which this occurs has been less well documented. Recent work demonstrating the formation of a range of potent pharmacological agents from arachidonic acid by lipoxygenase attack has suggested that these agents may have a mechanistic role. The effects of three inhibitors of the 5-lipoxygenase enxzyme (5-LPO) on chemotaxis have been compared and a further series of studies looked at the effect of one of them, benoxaprofen, on tumour systems in vitro and in vivo. Benoxaprofen appears to have selective activity against 5-LPO whilst BW755c and nordihydroguaretic acid (NDGA) also inhibit 12- and 15-lipoxygenases (Harvey et al., 1983).

CELL MOVEMENT

A preparation of 60-70% rat mononuclear cells was harvested 24 hr after the intraperitoneal injection of glycogen. Rat poly morphonuclear cells (PMN, 70-80%) were obtained, again from the peritoneal cavity 4 hr after an injection of homologous rat serum. Guinea pig mononuclear cells were obtained 72 hr after the i.p. injection of glycogen (85-90%) and guinea pig PMN 17 hr after casein i.p. injection. All cells were centrifuged at 1000 r.p.m. for 5 min and resuspended in Gey's buffered salt solution (Gey's BSS).

The method used to examine chemotaxis was essentially that described by Wilkinson (1974) using polycarbonate membranes of 5.0 µm pore size and zymosan activated serum (ZAS) as the chemotaxin. Cells were checked for viability by a dye exclusion method. The assay period was 120 min for mononuclear cells and 90 min for PMN, after which the membranes were fixed, stained with Mayers haematoxylin, cleared in 2-ethoxyethanol and mounted for evaluation by the lower surface counting method. Numbers of leucocytes migrating per microscope field were counted at a magnification of 630x, in 10 fields per filter. Between 4-6 filters were used for each estimation and statistical analyses of the data were carried out using Student's 't' test. Leucocytes detaching from the filter were quantitated using a Coulter counter.

The chemotactic response of rat peritoneal mononuclear cells towards ZAS was significantly reduced following preincubation and resuspension of the cells in NDGA, BW755c and benoxaprofen (Table 1), whilst guinea pig mononuclear cell movement was only reduced by benoxaprofen and BW 755c.

TABLE 1.   Effect of lipoxygenase inhibitors on the chemotactic response
of mononuclear cells towards ZAS

Treatment	Conc^n (M)	Cell species	Mononuclear cells per field Mean ± s.e.m.		% change	p<
Controls		Rat	54.3	1.5		
BW755c	10^{-4}		15.5	1.2	71 ↓	0.001
Controls		Rat	43.3	3.0		
Benoxaprofen	10^{-4}		14.8	1.8	67 ↓	0.001
Controls		Rat	84.3	4.1		
NDGA	7.5×10^{-6}		44.9	4.7	47 ↓	0.001
Controls	10^{-4}	Guinea Pig	70.5	1.8		
BW755c			8.1	0.6	89 ↓	0.001
Controls		Guinea Pig	151.1	4.9		
Benoxaprofen	10^{-4}		89.1	8.0	41 ↓	0.001
Controls		Guinea Pig	138.6	8.8		
NDGA	7.5×10^{-6}		145.7	6.6	5 ↑	N.S.

In other experiments, the effects of all three compounds on rat
mononuclear cells and of benoxaprofen and BW755c on guinea pig cells
were shown to be dose dependent.

BW755c and benoxaprofen over the concentration range 10^{-5} to 10^{-4} M
did not modify chemotactic movement of rat PMN. NDGA at lower
concentrations decreased cell detachment from the filter with no effect
on total migration but at higher concentrations reduced both detachment
and migration (Table 2)

TABLE 2.   Effects of NDGA on the chemotaxis and adherence of rat PMN

Treatment	Conc^n (M)	PMN detaching per field Mean	s.e.m.	% change	p<	Total migration PMN per field Mean	s.e.m.	% change	p<
Controls		203	15			320	11		
NDGA	2.5×10^{-6}	293	14	45	0.01	343	18	7 ↑	N.S.
NDGA	2.5×10^{-5}	65	10	68	0.001	65	10	80 ↓	0.001
Controls		285	41			383	36		
NDGA	7.5×10^{-6}	321	21	13	N.S.	358	21	7 ↓	N.S.

When the compounds were tested on the chemotactic response of guinea
pig PMN, BW 755c and NDGA increased both detachment and total migration
whilst benoxaprofen had no significant effect on either parameter
(Table 3).

TABLE 3.   Effects of lipoxygenase inhibitors on the chemotaxis and adherence of guinea pig PMN

Treatment	Conc^n (M)	PMN detaching per field				Total migration PMN per field			
		Mean	s.e.m.	% change	p<	Mean	s.e.m.	% change	p<
Controls		80	10			256	10		
BW 755c	10^{-4}	112	5	40↑	0.05	330	19	29↑	0.05
Controls		29	10			297	54		
NDGA	7.5×10^{-6}	340	50	↑	0.02	595	33	100↑	0.02
Benoxaprofen	10^{-4}	21	4	27↓	N.S.	322	5	8↑	N.S.

IMMUNE AND TUMOUR SYSTEMS

Antigen specific T cell proliferation assay

Lymphocytes obtained from the draining lymph nodes (periaortic and inguinal) of rats 11 days after subcutaneous injection of 100 µg ovalbumin (in complete Freund's adjuvant) at the base of the tail were separated by SG-10 column filtration. The eluted cells were added to flat-bottomed microtitre plates at a concentration of 2×10^5 cells/cap. Rat spleen cells (0.25–2×10^5 cells/cap) treated with mitomycin C, following lysis of red cells, from syngeneic animals, were added to the lymphocytes. The lymphocyte proliferation response to ovalbumin was assessed after 3 days in culture by ^{3}H-Tdr (tritiated thymidine) incorporation. The effects of drugs (added at the beginning of the culture period) are shown in Table 4.

TABLE 4.   Drug effects on antigen specific proliferation

Cells	Drug	Conc^n (M)	^{3}H-Tdr incorporation		
			cpm	±s.e.m.	p<
lymphocytes 2×10^{-5})			17,067	1840	–
spleen cells 2×10^{-5})Benoxaprofen		10^{-4}	2,208	542	0.001
ovalbumin)Penicillamine		10^{-3}	6,108	1198	0.001
Indomethacin		10^{-5}	14,179	2558	N.S.

Benoxaprofen markedly suppressed the response and in other experiments (data not shown), the effect was shown to be dose dependent over the range 10^{-5}–10^{-4} M. Indomethacin had no significant effect at concentrations up to 10^{-5}M, whereas at high concentrations penicillamine suppressed the response.

In vitro tumour studies

The antigen proliferation assay can not differentiate between an effect on antigen processing and an anti-proliferative response and so the effect of benoxaprofen was examined on the growth of a number of tumour cell lines in culture (Table 5). Benoxaprofen, at a concentration of 10^{-4}M suppressed growth in all lines tested, whilst indomethacin demonstrated an inconsistent and variable activity in the same systems.

TABLE 5. Effect of benoxaprofen on growth of various tumour cell lines

Tumour designation	Species	Tumour type	Benoxaprofen effect[a] (10^{-4} M)
NS 1	Mouse	B myeloma	+
EL 4	Mouse	T lymphoma	++
RAJI	Human	B myeloma	++
MOLT 4	Human	T lymphoma	+
RPMI 5966	Human	Melanoma	+
NB_{100}	Human	Neuroblastoma	++

[a] + = 25-40% inhibition   ++ = 40-70% inhibition

In vivo tumour studies

Two in vivo models were established to extend the in vitro observations described in the previous section. The first was one of survival of C57Bl/6 mice injected intraperitoneally with 2×10^{-5} EL4 cells. Benoxaprofen was given orally for the first 11 days and the control animals survived 14 days. Benoxaprofen (10 mg/kg/day) increased the survival time by a mean of 2 days (groups of 10 mice) which was significant ($p < 0.002$). This model is inherently variable and a second model, injecting the EL4 cells subcutaneously was developed. A defined tumour formed, readily excisable by day 15. Benoxaprofen was again administered orally for the first 11 days following tumour inoculation and markedly suppressed tumour weight in a dose dependent fashion (Table 7).

TABLE 6. Effect of benoxaprofen on EL4 tumour weights in C57BL/6 mice (day 15) in groups of 10 mice

Treatment		Tumour weight (g)	p<
Control		0.459 ± 0.142	−
Benoxaprofen	10 mg/kg/day	0.320 ± 0.119	0.01
	30 mg/kg/day	0.167 ± 0.075	0.001
	60 mg/kg/day	0.181 ± 0.096	0.001

DISCUSSION

Depletion of intracellular levels of 5- and 11-HETEs by inhibitors of the lipoxygenase enzyme pathway has been shown to reduce cellular chemotactic response (Goetzl, 1980). Inhibition of PMN chemotaxis by ETYA, but not by indomethacin (Malmsten et al., 1980) and by NDGA (Showell et al., 1980) also suggests that the lipoxygenase pathway of arachidonic acid metabolism may be important in cell locomotion. The present studies clearly differentiate the effects of three lipoxygenase inhibitors, NDGA, BW755c and benoxaprofen on PMN and monocytes derived from rats and guinea pigs. The compounds had similar effects on rat monocyte chemotaxis but were different on guinea pig monocyte chemotaxis and on PMN chemotaxis when the cells derived from either species. These effects, or lack of them in the case of PMN chemotaxis are obtained at concentrations which are known to inhibit the synthesis and release of intracellular lipoxygenase-derived products of arachidonic acid from PMN in vitro (Harvey & Osborne, 1983).
It would seem unlikely that these effects were being modulated by a common mechanism, namely inhibition of 5-lipoxgenase enzyme activity. Clearly, further work must characterise the enzyme from each cell type and then examine the effect of each compound on it but the qualitative differences in response seen would suggest that different mechanisms of action are involved. The selective action of benoxaprofen on the 5-lipoxygenase enzyme may be important, allowing substrate diversion to 12- or 15- lipoxygenase pathways. BW755c and benoxaprofen are both "dual enzyme" inhibitors, affecting the cyclooxygenase pathway as well as the lipoxygenase route of arachidonic acid metabolism and this may be of great relevance. However, it is clear that caution must be used in the interpretation of data achieved with these compounds.
The compound appears to have a selective effect on monocyte chemotaxis (Dawson, 1980 ; Meacock et al, 1982 ; Goetzl & Valone, 1982), a cell type with well characterized accessory cell function for the immune system. The antitumour effects reported here, although demonstrating a relatively low potency of benoxaprofen, allow considerable speculation on a possible mechanism. Arguably it is unexpected that a compound which limits movement of cells to an inflammatory site should have such an antitumour effect. Whether 5-lipoxygenase inhibition, associated with cyclooxygenase inhibitory activity is responsible, or the effect on antigen presentation reported here will require further study. This latter effect could be the recognition of a new antiproliferative activity for the compound but the in vitro concentrations used would suggest that is not a major facet of benoxaprofen pharmacolgy.

REFERENCES

1. Dawson, W. (1980) : J. Rheumatol 7, Suppl 6:5-11.
2. Gauci, C.I. and Alexander P. (1975) : Cancer Letts 1:29-32.
3. Goetzl, E.L. (1980) : Immunology 40:709-719.
4. Goetzl, E.J. and Valone, F.H. (1982) : Arthritis and Rheumatism 25: 1486-1489.

5. Harvey J. and Osborne, D.J. (1983) : J. Pharmacol. Methods 9:147-155.
6. Harvey, J., Parish, H., Ho, P.P.K., Boot, J.R. and Dawson, W. (1983)
    J. Pharm. Pharmac. 35:35-45.
7. Malmsten, C.L., Palmblad, J., Uden, A.M. Radmark, O., Engstedt, L.
    and Samuelsson, B. (1980) : Acta Physiol. Scand. 110:449-451.
8. Meacock, S.C.R., Civil, G.W., Dawson, W. and Kitchen, E.A. (1982) :
    Eur. J. Rheumatol. and Inflamm. 5:51-60.
9. Showell, H.J., Naccache, P.H., Sha'afi, R.I. and Becker, E.L. (1980)
    Life Sciences 27:421-426.
10. Wilkinson, P.C. (1974) : In : Chemotaxis and Inflammation, Churchill
    Livingstone, Edinburgh and London.

Icosanoids and Cancer, edited by H. Thaler-Dao, et al. Raven Press, New York © 1984.

Natural Cytotoxic Cell Activity Enhanced by Leukotriene B_4: Modulation by Cyclooxygenase and Lipoxygenase Inhibitors

*Marek Rola-Pleszczynski, *Lyne Gagnon, and †Pierre Sirois

*Laboratoires *d'Immunologie et de †Pharmacologie, Département de Pédiatrie, Faculté de Médecine, Université de Sherbrooke, Sherbrooke, Québec, J1H 5N4 Canada*

Lymphoid cells with natural cytotoxic activity have been recognized for several years. They can lyse spontaneously tumor or virus-infected targets and are thought to play a role in cancer surveillance and resistance to virus infections (4,12). There are at least two, and possibly more, subsets of such cytotoxic cells: natural killer (NK) and natural cytotoxic (NC) cells. NK cells have been most extensively studied and are primarily active against target cells of the leukocyte class (v.g. the K562 cell line, in man). NC cells have been described in mice (22) and are primarily active against cells that form solid tumors. We have recently suggested the existence of such a subset in man, using the monoclonal antibody HNC-1A3(18).

The lytic mechanism(s) for natural cytotoxicity is not established, but at least two independents steps have been defined, namely target cell binding followed by lysis (11,5). In addition to direct effector-target cell interaction, possible involvement of a soluble mediator has been suggested (23). The activation of the lytic process may also require the release of fatty acids from the cell membrane. Phospholipid methylation was shown to be increased in NK cells following their contact with sensitive targets and NK activity to be reduced by inhibition of methyltransferase or by inhibitors of phospholipase A_2(6). These observations suggest that arachidonic acid metabolites may be required for NK cell activity. Among them, prostaglandins (PGs) have rather the opposite effect, exogenous PGE_2 suppressing NK function (7). We therefore explored the possibility that other products of arachidonic acid metabolism be involved in natural cytotoxic activity, and particularly products of lipoxygenation.

We have recently shown that leukotriene (LT)B$_4$ markedly augments natural cytotoxic activity against virus-infected target cells (16). We now present the extension of our work using various metabolic inhibitors of arachidonic acid metabolism as well as non-infected tumor target cells.

MATERIALS AND METHODS

Human peripheral blood mononuclear leukocytes (PBML) were obtained by density gradient centrifugation of heparinized venous blood on a Hypaque-Ficoll gradient. They represented 75-90% lymphocytes and 10-25% monocytes. After three washes, they were resuspended in appropriate concentrations in MEM medium supplemented with 10% fetal bovine serum.

Target cells for the cytotoxicity assay consisted of the human prostatic adenoma MA-160 cell line either uninfected or persistently infected with herpes simplex virus type 1 (HSV). These cells and their use have been previously described (13). In addition, the classical NK target cell line K562 was employed as described (18).

Cytotoxic activity of PBML was measured using a ^{51}Cr-release microassay as described (13). Target cells were labeled with ^{51}Cr (Na^{51}CrO$_4$, New England Nuclear), washed three times and distributed into microtiter wells at a concentration of 5 X 10^3 cells per well. In most experiments, PBML were then added to half of the wells at a concentration of 2.5 X 10^5 cells per well, giving an effector to target cell ratio of 50:1. Alternate wells contained medium alone. Cytotoxicity was assayed by measuring the ^{51}Cr content of culture supenatants. Cytotoxic activity was expressed as % specific ^{51}Cr release using the following formula:
% specific ^{51}Cr release = (R_E-R_S/R_T-R_S) X 100 where R_E represents experimental release, R_S, spontaneous release and R_T, total releasable ^{51}Cr.

To study the effect of LTB$_4$ as well as of the various lipoxygenase and cyclooxygenase inhibitors on the cytotoxic activity of PBML, appropriate concentrations of the products were prepared in medium MEM and added to additional sets of microtiter wells containing PBML-targets or medium-targets cultures. Cytotoxicity was expressed as above. LTB$_4$ was a generous gift from Dr J. Rokach, Merck-Frosst Laboratories. 3-amino-1-(m-(trifluoromethyl)-phenyl)-2-pyrazoline (BW755C) was kindly supplied by the Wellcome Research Laboratories. Indomethacin and nordihydroguaiaretic acid (NDGA) were from Sigma Chemicals (St-Louis, MO) and OKY-1581 was from ONO Pharmaceuticals (Japan).

RESULTS

When normal human PBML were incubated with increasing concentrations of LTB$_4$ during a 5-hr cytotoxicity assay, a very significant (p< 0.01) augmentation of their natural cytotoxic (NC) activity against HSV-infected targets was observed (Fig. 1).

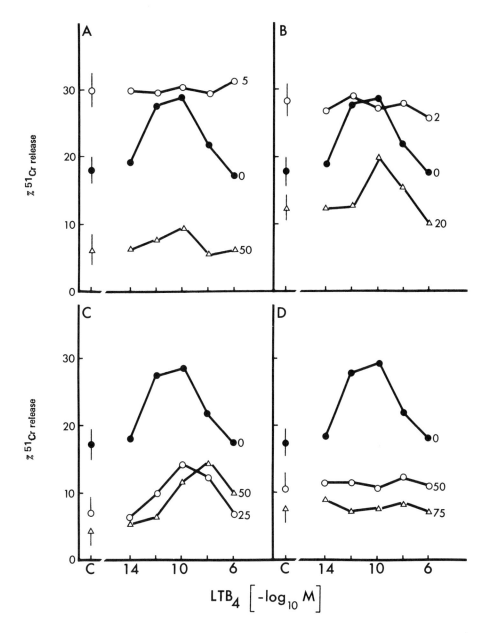

Fig. 1   Cytotoxicity of human PBML against HSV-1-infected target cells
in the absence (C) or the presence of increasing concentrations of LTB₄ (●). In addition, the following inhibitors
were used at noted concentrations (in ug/ml, except in panel
B:uM): Panel A: BW755C; B: indomethacin; C: NDGA and
D: OKY-1581.

Concomitantly, we studied the effects of four inhibitors of
arachidonic acid metabolism on NC activity in the absence or in the
presence of LTB₄. BW755C, an inhibitor of both cyclooxygenase and
lipoxygenase showed a bimodal effect. At low concentration (5 µg/ml)
it markedly enhanced NC activity and the addition of LTB₄ had no
further effect in this situation (Fig 1A). In contrast, a higher (50
µg/ml) concentration of BW755C inhibited NC activity. LTB₄ slightly,
but not significantly, increased this low level of NC activity. In a
rather similar fashion, indomethacin, a more selective inhibitor of
cyclooxygenase, enhanced NC function in the presence or absence of
LTB4 (Fig. 1B) at a low concentration (2µM). A higher concentration
(20µM) of indomethacin was rather inhibitory but nevertheless allowed
LTB₄ to stimulate significantly NC activity at 1×10^{-10}M.

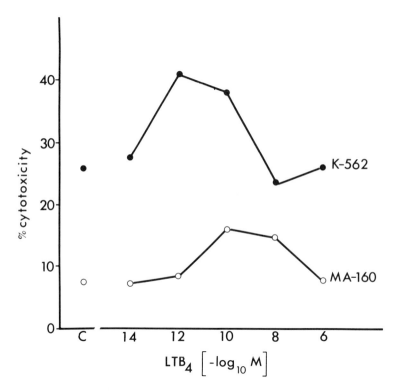

Fig. 2 Cytotoxicity of human PBML against uninfected MA-160 or K562
        target cells in the absence (C) or presence of increasing
        concentrations of LTB4.

In contrast, inhibition of lipoxygenation by NDGA resulted in a
marked reduction of NC activity (Fig 1C) which could however be
restimulated by exogenously added LTB₄. Surprisingly, the thromboxane
synthetase inhibitor OKY-1581 also significantly depressed NC activity
(Fig 1D). Unlike NDGA however, OKY-1581 did not allow exogenous LTB₄
to enhance cytotoxic activity.

In order to assess whether the NC augmenting potential of LTB_4 was restricted to cytotoxicity directed against virus-infected target cells, we also studied the effect of LTB_4 on cytotoxicity of human PBML against uninfected MA-160 cells as well as K562 target cells. As illustrated in Fig. 2, an enhancement similar to that reported previously with virus-infected targets was observed using these two uninfected tumor cell lines.

DISCUSSION

Recent studies have demonstrated that leukotrienes (LTs), in addition to their myotropic properties, also strongly affect several leukocyte functions. For instance, LTB_4 was shown to stimulate neutrophil aggregation (1), chemokinesis (2,9), chemotaxis (9,3), degranulation (3,21), hexose transport (1) and cation fluxes (8). In addition, we have recently demonstrated that LTB_4 can induce human T lymphocytes to exert a suppressor cell activity with the cooperation and mediation of adherent cells and cyclooxygenase products (14,19). LTB_4 was also shown to suppress LIF production (10). On the other hand, LTB_4 can strongly augment natural cytotoxicity of human peripheral blood lymphocytes against herpes simplex virus-infected target cells (15,16), a process which appears to be dependent on the lipoxygenase pathway (16). Our findings were corroborated by the observations of Seaman (20) who recently reported that NDGA and higher doses of BW755C reversibly inhibit NK activity. We also demonstrated that the NC-enhancing properties of LTB_4 were shared to a significant extent by the parent molecule LTA_4, but only weakly by LTD_4, while 5-HETE 12-HETE and stereoisomers of LTB_4, were inactive (17). In this paper, we presented the extension of our studies by showing that LTB_4 augments natural cytotoxicity of uninfected as well as virus-infected target cells. LTB_4 also enhances killing of the typical NK-sensitive K562 target cell line, thus suggesting that a common step may be involved in the lytic process even though distinct effector cell populations are involved in the respective killing of MA-160 and K562 target cells (18). Ongoing studies are aimed at elucidating this phenomenon.

On the other hand, our studies also provide a new approach for examining the mechanism of natural cytolysis and suggest that lipoxygenase products may play a key role in this activity. It is unlikely that LTB_4 is by itself a mediator of cell lysis, because target cells are not killed in the presence of LTB_4 alone. It would appear however that lipoxygenation of arachidonic acid or the addition of LTB_4 may facilitate the release of other mediators of cell lysis, such as the NK cytotoxic factor (NKCF,23).

Previous evidence and our more recent findings lead us to hypothesize that a delicate balance may normally exist between the various pathways of arachidonic acid metabolism in regulating natural cytotoxicity (Fig. 3). Products of cyclooxygenation, principally PGs, are inhibitory and blocking this pathway by indomethacin and low doses of BW755C enhances NC activity. In contrast lipoxygenation is required for NC function and blocking by NDGA, diethylcarbamazine (DEC; data not shown) or higher doses of BW755C reduces NC activity. LTB_4 may be the lipoxygenation product required to allow NC function

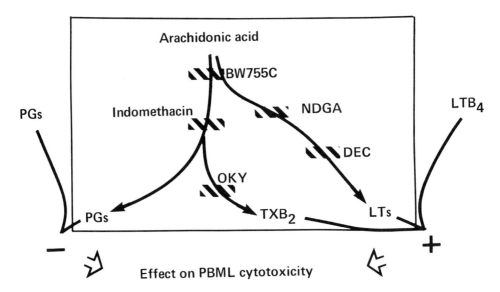

Fig. 3   Suggested effects of products of arachidonic acid metabolism
         and of some inhibitors on human natural cytotoxic activity.

to be initiated or maintained, but we have no direct proof for this
presently. Of interest, and quite to our surprise, the thromboxane
synthetase pathway also appears to be important for NC function.
Further studies will be needed to help explain this initial
observation.

     In conclusion, the compelling evidence for a major role of
arachidonic acid metabolites in NC function must be born in mind when
inhibitors of these metabolic pathways are developped and used for
their anti-inflammatory potential.

REFERENCES

1.   Bass, D.A., Thomas, M.J., Goetzl, E.J., DeChatelet, L.R. and
     McCall, C.E. (1981).
     Biochem. Biophys. Res. Comm. 100:1-7.

2.   Ford-Hutchinson, A.W., Bray, M.A., Doig, M.V., Shipley, M.E. and
     Smith, M.J.H. (1980).
     Nature 286:264-265.

3.   Goetzl, E.J. and Pickett, W.C. (1980).
     J. Immunol. 125:1789-1791.

4.   Herberman, R.B., Djeu, J.Y., Kay, H. D., Ortaldo, J.R., Riccardi,
     C., Bonnard, G.D., Holden, H.T., Fagnani, R., Santoni, A. and
     Puccetti, P. (1979).
     Immunol. Rev. 44:43-70.

5. Hiserodt, J.C., Britvan, L.J. and Targan, S.R. (1982).
    J. Immunol. 129:1782.

6. Hoffman, t., Bougnoux, P., Hattori, T., Chang, Z-L and Herberman,
    R.B. (1982).
    In: NK cells and other effector cells. Edited by R.B.
    Herberman. Academic Press, New York, p. 955.

7. Koren, H.S., Anderson, S.J., Fischer, D.G., Copeland, C.S. and
    Jensen, P. (1981).
    J. Immunol. 127:2007-2013.

8. Naccache, P.H., Sha'afi, R.I., Borgeat, P. and Goetzl, E.J.
    (1981).
    J. Clin. Invest. 67:1584-1587.

9. Palmer, R.M.J., Stepney, R.J., Higgs, G.A.,, and Eakins, K.E.
    (1980).
    Prostaglandins 20:411-418.

10. Payan, D.G. and Goetzl, E.J. (1983).
    J. Immunol. 131:551-553.

11. Quan, P.C., Ishizaka, T. and Bloom B.R. (1982).
    J. Immunol 128:1786.

12. Roder, J.C. and Pross, H.F. (1982).
    J. Clin. Immunol. 2:249-263.

13. Rola-Pleszczynski, M. (1980).
    J. Immunol. 125:1475-1480.

14. Rola-Pleszczynski, M., Borgeat, P. and Sirois, P. (1982).
    Biochem. Biophys. Res. Comm. 108:1531-1537.

15. Rola-Pleszczynski, M., Gagnon, L. and Sirois, P. (1983).
    Fed. Proc. 42:437.

16. Rola-Pleszczynski, M., Gagnon, L. and Sirois, P. (1983).
    Biochem. Biophys. Res. Comm. 113:531-537.

17. Rola-Pleszczynski, M., Gagnon, L., Rudzinska, M., Borgeat, P. and
    Sirois, P. (1983).
    Prostagl. Leukotr. Med. 11: in press.

18. Rola-Pleszczynski, M. and Lieu, H. (1983).
    Cell. Immunol. in press.

19. Rola-Pleszczynski, M., and Sirois, P. (1983).
    In: Leukotrienes and other lipoxygenase products, Piper, P.J.,
    Editor, Wiley and Sons, London, pp 234-240.

20. Seaman, W.E. (1983).
    Fed. Proc. 42:1379.

21. Showell, H.J., Naccache, P.H., Borgeat, P., Picard, S.,
     Vallerand, P., Becker, E.L. and Sha'afi, R.I. (1982).
     J. Immunol. 128:811-816.

22. Stutman, O., Lattime, E.C. and Figarella,, E.F. (1981).
     Fed. Proc. 40:2699.

23. Wright, S.C., Weitzen, M.L., Kahle, R., Granger, G.A. and
     Bonavida, B. (1983).
     J. Immunol. 130:2479.

Icosanoids and Cancer, edited by H. Thaler-Dao, et al. Raven Press, New York © 1984.

Studies on the Balance of Prostacyclin and Thromboxane A$_2$ in Patients with Malignant Tumours of the Breast and Uterus

*C. Benedetto, *M. Barbero, *M. Corrias, *E. Petitti,
*M. Massobrio, **S. Nigam, **R. Becker, **J. Hammerstein,
and †T. F. Slater

*Istituto di Ginecologia e Ostetricia, Cattedra A, 10126 Torino, Italy; **Institut für Gynäkologische Endokrinologie, Sterilitat und Familienplanung Klinikum Steglitz, Freie Universität Berlin, Berlin, Federal Republic of Germany; and †Department of Biochemistry, Brunel University, Uxbridge, Middlesex, United Kingdom

Prostaglandins are synthesized by virtually every type of cell, including neoplastic cells (2). The significance of their role in neoplastic transformation, tumour growth and metastasis is still unclear mainly because of the conflicting results obtained by the study of different prostaglandins and inhibitors of prostaglandin synthesis in various tumours (12). It seems likely that the thesis of "prostaglandins" in general causing either stimulation of tumour growth or tumour regression is inappropriate, and studies on the relationships between prostaglandins and cancer should focus on the roles of specific products of arachidonic acid metabolism in tumour physiology (13).

It is well known that thromboxane A$_2$ (TXA$_2$), the major metabolite of arachidonic acid in the platelets (17), stimulates platelet aggregation, whereas prostacyclin (PGI$_2$), the main product of arachidonic acid metabolism in isolated vascular tissue (15), is the most potent endogenous inhibitor of platelet aggregation yet discovered (14,16). As a consequence it has been suggested that PGI$_2$ and TXA$_2$ play an antagonistic and pivotal role in the control of vascular and platelet homeostasis (6).

Based upon the assumption that platelet-tumour cell and/or platelet-tumour cell-vessel wall interactions play an important role in tumour cell metastasis, Honn and coworkers (9,11) proposed that primary tumour cells, vesicles shed by the tumour cells and/or circulating tumour cells disrupt the intravascular balance between PGI$_2$ and TXA$_2$ in favour of platelet aggregation. They suggested that PGI$_2$ functions as an antimetastatic agent by inhibiting the attachment of tumour cells and/or tumour cell-platelet thrombi to the vascular endothelium (10). According to this hypothesis it has been found that the production of PGI_2 by variant cell lines of the mFS6 fibrosarcoma varies _inversely_ with their metastatic potential, while the production of TXA_2 by these same variants correlates _positively_ with their metastatic potential (7).

Studies on humans have demonstrated that malignant tumours of the breast produce substantial amounts of PGI_2 (3); moreover, high levels of 6-keto-$PGF_{1\alpha}$ (the stable metabolite of PGI_2) are present in the plasma of female patients with tumours of the genital tract (1). In these patients the concentration of 6-keto-$PGF_{1\alpha}$ declines after operation and/or radiotherapy if the tumour responds to treatment (1). Bennett and coworkers (3) suggested that some of the prostaglandin-like materials formed within breast tumours can be released into the bloodstream and can presumably affect blood elements and vessels. Such changes produced by prostaglandins in platelet aggregation and blood vessels might contribute to the development of metastases.

In view of the above possibilities we decided to investigate and evaluate: (a) the peripheral plasma levels of 6-keto-$PGF_{1\alpha}$ and TXB_2 in patients with breast cancer and malignant tumours of the uterus, both before and after surgical treatment; (b) the production of PGI_2 and TXB_2 by vessels draining and not-draining benign and malignant tumours of the human breast; and (c) the platelet sensitivity to PGI_2. The results so obtained have been correlated with the size and clinical extension of the tumour, cellular surrounding and histological type of the tumour, tumour cell embolism, lymphocytic reaction and axillary lymph node metastases, and the content of steroid receptors in the tumours.

The plasma levels of 6-keto-$PGF_{1\alpha}$ and TXB_2 were determined by radioimmunoassay after extraction and separation of the prostanoids by high pressure liquid chromatography according to Nigam et al (18). Randomly selected samples were taken to verify the values obtained by radioimmunoassay, using gas chromatography/mass spectrometry.

The production of PGI_2 by the samples of blood vessels, isolated during surgical operations, was evaluated with a bioassay based on the capability of PGI_2 to inhibit platelet aggregation induced by 1 µM ADP according to Bunting et al (5). 6-keto-$PGF_{1\alpha}$ and TXB_2 were also measured by direct radioimmunoassay in the incubation medium of the same blood vessels. The platelet sensitivity to PGI_2 in the plasma was determined according to Sinzinger et al (19).

Our preliminary results indicate that plasma levels of 6-keto-$PGF_{1\alpha}$ and TXB_2 in patients with breast cancer are higher than in controls and do not change during the follow-up period after the surgical operation, irrespective of the type and stage of the tumour

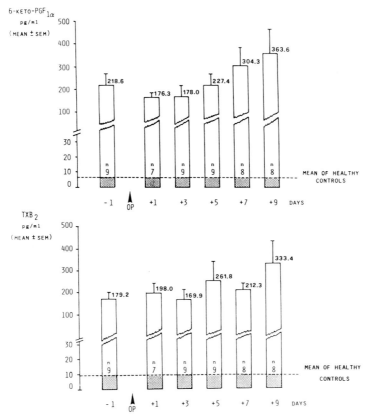

Fig. 1. The levels of 6-keto-PGF$_{1\alpha}$ and TXB$_2$ in peripheral plasma of patients with breast cancer before and after operation (OP).

(Fig. 1). This applies also to the balance between 6-keto-PGF$_{1\alpha}$ and TXB$_2$.

In contrast, there is a marked decrease in the plasma levels of 6-keto-PGF$_{1\alpha}$ in patients with adenocarcinomas of the endometrium during the period after operation, whilst the corresponding levels of TXB$_2$ remain unchanged (Fig. 2A). Such changes result in a considerable post-operative reduction of the ratio between 6-keto-PGF$_{1\alpha}$ and TXB$_2$ (Fig. 2B).

The vessels draining malignant tumours of the human breast apparently produce more PGI$_2$ than vessels not-draining the tumours of the same patients, or vessels taken from patients with benign tumours (Fig. 3). This feature appears to be inversely correlated with the presence of metastases in the axillary lymph nodes and with the clinical extension of the primary tumour; no correlation could be established with the degree of inflammatory reaction or with the lympho-vascular emboli of tumour cells. No conclusion can be reached with data so

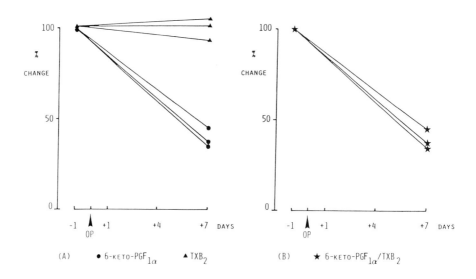

Fig. 2. Post-operative changes in the plasma levels of 6-keto-PGF$_{1\alpha}$ and TXB$_2$ (A) and in the ratio of 6-keto-PGF$_{1\alpha}$/TXB$_2$ (B) in patients with adenocarcinoma of the endometrium.

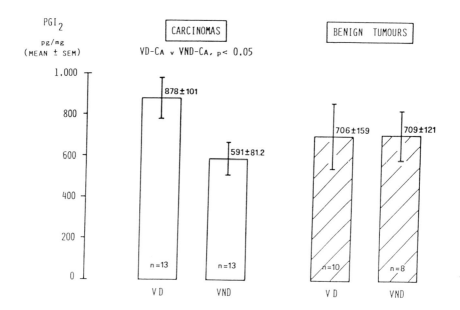

Fig. 3. The production of PGI$_2$ by vessels draining (VD) and not-draining (VND) malignant and benign tumours of the human breast.

far available concerning any relationship between PGI_2 production
by the vessels and the histological type and hormonal dependence
of the tumour. The levels of 6–keto–$PGF_{1\alpha}$ in the incubation media
of the same vessels draining the malignant tumours are higher than
those of TXB_2, whereas in corresponding samples obtained from vessels
draining benign tumours the levels of 6–keto–$PGF_{1\alpha}$ and TXB_2 are
similar.

The platelet sensitivity to PGI_2, expressed as the dose of the
synthetic standard necessary to suppress by half the aggregation
induced by ADP (ID_{50}), shows a significant increase in patients
with carcinomas of the breast and to a lesser extent in those with
benign tumours of the mammary gland, compared to healthy controls
(Fig. 4). In addition, the difference in platelet sensitivity between
patients with benign and malignant tumours is noteworthy and statistically significant.

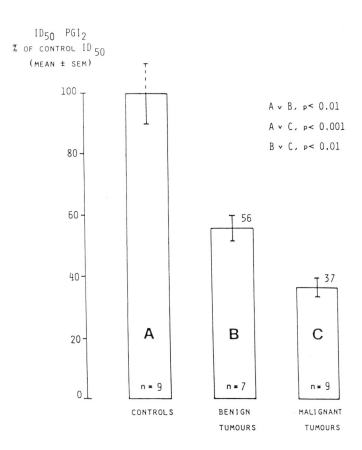

Fig. 4. Platelet sensitivity to PGI_2 in patients with benign and
malignant tumours of the breast compared to healthy controls.

Our data on peripheral plasma levels of 6-keto-PGF$_{1\alpha}$ and TXB$_2$ indicate that the presence of a malignant tumour of the breast is associated with an increase of both 6-keto-PGF$_{1\alpha}$ and TXB$_2$ compared to healthy controls; the surgical removal of the tumour does not seem to change the concentrations of 6-keto-PGF$_{1\alpha}$ and TXB$_2$. This finding suggests that breast cancer tissue may either produce substances that have a long-standing stimulatory effect on the production of PGI$_2$ and TXA$_2$ at other sites, or induce a prolonged general pathophysiological response. The pattern of change of 6-keto-PGF$_{1\alpha}$ in patients with adenocarcinomas of the endometrium is different and in agreement with the results of Alam et al (1), while TXB$_2$ shows the same behaviour as in patients with breast cancer. The latter observation could be explained as a result of the altered platelet functions (4) which can last for several months after the initial alteration occurred (20).

The data on the blood vessels draining the malignant tumours and on platelet sensitivity to PGI$_2$ in patients with breast cancer are consistent with the suggestion that some substances formed within the tumours and released into the bloodstream might affect blood elements and vessels. In addition, the finding that the production of PGI$_2$ by these vessels is inversely correlated with the presence of metastases to axillary lymph nodes and the clinical extension of the tumour is in agreement with the hypothesis of Honn et al (10) that PGI$_2$ might counteract the dissemination of the tumour.

The results on platelet sensitivity to PGI$_2$ do not confirm the observation made by Gisinger et al (8) in patients with colonic cancer. The possibility that different types of tumours could have a diverse or even opposite effect on vascular and platelet homeostasis remains to be investigated.

ACKNOWLEDGMENTS

We are grateful to the National Foundation for Cancer Research for financial support. The expert technical help of Dr. L. Rey, Dr. A.M. Tavella, C. Brühahn, A. Becker and V. Hasse is gratefully acknowledged. We express our thanks to Professor M.U. Dianzani for helpful advice. We are also most grateful to Dr. J. Salmon and Dr. S. Bunting of the Wellcome Research Laboratories (Beckenham, U.K.),for generously providing antisera and expert advice, and to Dr. J. Pike (Upjohn Company, Kalamazoo, Michigan, U.S.A.) for a generous gift of prostacyclin.

REFERENCES

1. Alam, M., Jogee, M., Macgregor, W.G., Dowdell, J.W., Elder, M.G. and Myatt, L. (1982): *Br. J. Cancer.* 45: 384 - 389.

2. Bennett, A. (1979):*Practical application of Prostaglandins and their Synthesis Inhibitors*, edited by S.M.M. Karim, Chap. 9. M.T.P. Press, Lancaster.

3. Bennett, A., Berstock, D.A., Carroll, M.A., Stamford,I.F.and Wilson, A.J. (1983): *Advances in Prostaglandins and Thromboxane Research*, edited by B. Samuelsson, R. Paoletti and P. Ramwell, Vol 12,pp. 299-302. Raven Press, New York.

4. Briel, R.C. and Lippert, T.H. (1981): *Eur. J. Obstet. Gynec. Reprod. Biol.* 12: 19 - 23.

5. Bunting, S., Moncada , S., Reed, P., Salmon, J.A. and Vane, J.R. (1978): *Prostaglandins*15: 565 - 573.

6. Bunting, S., Moncada, S. and Vane, J.R. (1983): In: *Br. Med.Bulletin "Prostacyclin, Thromboxane and Leukotrienes"*, edited by S. Moncada, pp. 271 - 276.

7. Donati, M.B., Borowska, A., Bottazzi, B., Dejana, E., Giavazzi, R., Rotilio, D. and Mantovani, A. (1982): In: *Abstract Book "V International Conference on Prostaglandins"* Florence, p. 136. Raven Press, New York.

8. Gisinger, C., Kefalides, A. and Sinzinger, H. (1982): In: *Abstract Book "V International Conference on Prostaglandins"* Florence,p. 201. Raven Press, New York.

9. Honn, K.V. (1982): In: *Prostaglandins and Cancer*, edited by T.J.Powles, R.S. Bockman, K.V. Honn and P.W. Ramwell, pp. 733 - 752. Alan R. Liss., New York.

10. Honn, K.V., Busse, W.D. and Sloane, B.F. (1983): *Biochem. Pharmacol.*, 32: 1 - 11.

11. Honn, K.V., Cicone, B. and Skoff, A. (1981): *Science*, 212: 1270-1272.

12. Karmali, R.A. (1980): *Prostaglandins and Medicine* , 5: 11 - 28.

13. Liu, S.C. and Knazek, R.A. (1982): *Prostagland. Leuk. Med.*,8: 191-198.

14. Moncada, S.and Vane, J.R. (1977): In: *Biochemical Aspects of Prostaglandins and Thromboxanes* , edited by N. Kharasch and J. Friend, p. 155. Academic Press, New York.

15. Moncada, S. and Vane, J.R. (1979): *Fed. Proc.*, 38: 66 - 71.

16. Mullane, K.M., Dusting, G.J., Salmon, J.A., Moncada, S. and Vane,J.R. (1979): *Eur. J. Pharmac.*,54: 217 - 228.

17. Needleman, P., Moncada, S., Bunting, S., Vane, J.R., Hamberg, M. and Samuelsson, B. (1976): *Nature*, 261: 558 - 560.

18. Nigam, S., Becker, R., Hammerstein, J., Benedetto, C. and Slater,T.F. (1983): *Acta Endocrinologica*, Stockholm, Abstract 296.

19. Sinzinger, H., Schernthaner, G. and Kaliman, J. (1981): *Prostaglandins*, 22: 773 - 781.

20. Svcezeklik, A., Gryglewski, R.J., Musial, J., Grodzenska, L., Serwonska, M. and Marcinkiewicz, E. (1978): *Thrombos. Haemostas.*,40: 66-74.

Icosanoids and Cancer, edited by H. Thaler-Dao, et al. Raven Press, New York © 1984.

Electron Paramagnetic Resonance and Fluorescence Titrations of Ovine Prostaglandin H Synthase with Hemin[1]

H. H. Ruf, D. Schuhn, and W. Nastainczyk

Physiological Chemistry, University of Saarland, D-6650 Homburg/Saar, Federal Republic of Germany

Prostaglandin H (PGH) synthase catalyses the oxidation of arachidonic acid to PGH_2 which is the initial step in the biosynthesis of prostaglandins, prostacyclin and thromboxanes (7). The purified enzyme is a polypeptide of about 70 kDalton requiring heme for the reconstitution of enzymatic activity (1,2,3,5). Heme binding has been measured by the increase of the Soret-band at about 410 nm upon the addition of hemin. The binding of 1 hemin/polypeptide (5) or 2 hemins/ polypeptide (3) have been concluded from the data. The number of hemins/ polypeptide required for the reconstitution of enzymatic activity, is still more controversial: less than 0.5 (2) (for the bovine enzyme) 1 (5) or 2 (3) have been reported.

Since the nature of the prosthetic group of the enzyme is essential for elucidation of the reaction mechanism we investigated the interaction of hemin with purified ovine PGH synthase by two alternative spectroscopic methods, namely fluorescence and electron paramagnetic resonance (EPR).

EXPERIMENTAL

PGH synthase (EC 1.14.99.1) was isolated from ram seminal vesicles according to Roth et al. (5) as apoprotein, a polypeptide of 72 kD. Protein was determined according to Lowry using bovine serum albumin as standard.

Fluorescence was measured with a SLM 8000 S fluorimeter at 22° C using cuvettes of 3x3 mm.

EPR spectra were recorded with a Varian E-9 spectrometer at 90K with the instrument settings: 9.18 GHz microwave frequency, 40 mW microwave power, 2,5 mT modulation amplitude and gain of 10000. Optical spectra of the EPR samples were recorded with an Aminco DW2 according to (6).

---

[1] This work was supported by Deutsche Forschungsgemeinschaft, Sonderforschungsbereich 38 – Membranforschung, project L3 and L4.

RESULTS

Electron Paramagnetic Resonance (EPR)

PGH synthase as isolated contained less than 0.05 heme/polypeptide as judged from optical and EPR spectra. Spurious EPR signals at g=4.3, characteristic of rhombic non-heme ferric iron, did not correlate with enzymatic activity and were not further investigated.

EPR signals around g=6, indicative of high spin ferric heme, with concomitant Soret-bands at 410 nm were observed only after the addition of hemin (fig.1). The high spin signals clearly evolved in a biphasic manner (fig.3.). Up to 1 hemin/polypeptide produced a signal at g=6.7 and 5.3 (rhombicity 9% according to Peisach et al. (4)) (fig.2). Under this condition the Soret-band was observed at 410 nm. At higher concentrations of hemin a signal at g=6.3 and 5.8 (rhombicity 3%) with a shoulder at g=7.2 appeared, very similar to the signal of hemin bound to bovine serum albumin. The Soret-band concomitantly shifted from 410 nm to lower wavelengths (to 404 nm with 6.1 hemins/polypeptide).

When this sample was subsequently titrated with KCN, an inhibitor of PGH synthase, the signal at g=6.7 and 5.3 disappeared first. The signal at g=6.3 and 5.8 disappeared only at higher KCN concentrations (data not shown).

These data indicated one heme binding site with a rather high rhombicity and with a high susceptibility of bound heme for KCN. There were additional heme binding sites with lower affinity for heme, lower rhombicity and lower susceptibility to KCN.

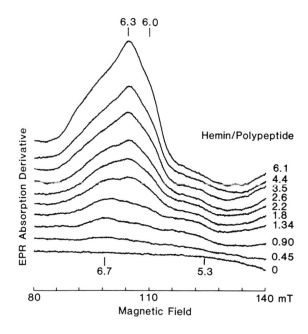

FIG. 1. EPR titration of PGH synthase with hemin which was added from a 5 or 10 mM solution in DMSO to a 44 µM solution of the apoprotein. The numbers at the vertical bars represent g-values.

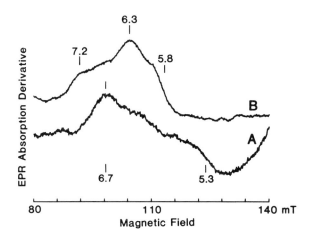

FIG. 2. Computed EPR difference spectra from the titration in fig. 1. Trace A represents the fourfold difference between the spectra with 0.9 and 0 hemin/polypeptide and trace B the twofold difference between 6.1 and 4.4 hemin/polypeptide, respectively.

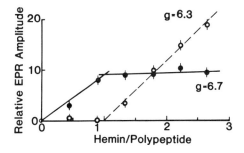

FIG. 3. Dependence of the amplitudes of the EPR signals at g = 6.3 and g = 6.7 on added hemin.

Fluorescence

PGH synthase apoprotein showed strong intrinsic fluorescence with an uncorrected emission maximum at 337 nm due to its tryptophan residues. Addition of hemin quenched this fluorescence in a biphasic manner (fig. 4). The first hemin quenched more effectively than subsequently added hemin. This behaviour indicated one heme binding site at the enzyme with stronger energy transfer from tryptophan(s) to hemin.

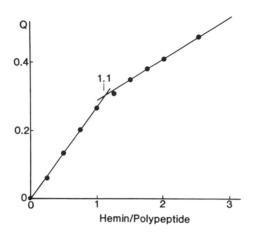

FIG. 4. Quenching of tryptophan fluorescence of PGH synthase by hemin which was added from a 100 mM solution in DMSO to a 1.8 μM solution of the apoprotein (quenching $Q = I_0/I - 1$ with I_0 intensity without hemin and I intensity with hemin, respectively).

CONCLUSIONS

We presented evidence that PGH synthase apoprotein binds one hemin at a specific site. This site induced a high rhombicity of 9% on the bound hemin presumably by coordination of the iron to an axial ligand. This hemin quenched tryptophan fluorescence more effectively indicating close contact to the tryptophan residue(s). Since one hemin/polypeptide maintains full enzymatic activity as reported recently (5) it is tempting to speculate that this specifically bound heme is the prosthetic group of PGH synthase.

Additional hemins were bound at non-specific hydrophobic sites with lower rhombicity of the ESR signal, less effective fluorescence quenching and Soret-bands below 410 nm. Such sites could be provided by the protein or by micelles of the protein with residual detergent. Presumably these sites are not effective in catalysis.

REFERENCES

1. Hemler, M., Lands, W.E.M., and Smith, W.L. (1976):
   J. Biol. Chem., 251:5575-5579.
2. Ogino, N., Ohki, S., Yamamoto, S., and Hayaishi, O. (1978):
   J. Biol. Chem., 253:5061-5068.
3. van der Ouderaa, F.J., Buytenhek, M., Slikkerveer, F.J., and
   van Dorp, D.A., (1979): Biochim. Biophys. Acta., 572:29-42.
4. Peisach, J., Blumberg, W.E., Ogawa, S., Rachmilewitz, E.A., and
   Oltzik, R. (1971): J. Biol. Chem., 246:3342-3355.
5. Roth, G.J., Machuga, E.T., and Strittmatter, P. (1981):
   J. Biol. Chem., 256:10018-10022.
6. Ruf, H.H., Wende, P., and Ullrich, V. (1979): J. Inorg. Biochem.,
   11:189-204.
7. Samuelsson, B., Goldyne, M., Granström, E., Hamberg, M.,
   Hammarström, S., and Malmsten, C. (1978): Ann. Rev. Biochem.,

Icosanoids and Cancer, edited by H. Thaler-Dao,
et al. Raven Press, New York © 1984.

Spectral Properties of the Enzyme Substrate Complex of Prostaglandin Hydroperoxidase and Prostaglandin G_2

W. Nastainczyk, H. H. Ruf, and D. Schuhn

Physiological Chemistry, University of Saarland, D-6650 Homburg/Saar, Federal Republic of Germany

SUMMARY

Arachidonic acid and PGG_2 react with prostaglandin H synthase in ram vesicular gland microsomes as well as with purified PGH synthase by formation of optical difference spectra with maxima at 430, 525 and 555 nm and minima at 410, 490 and 630 nm. In the absolute spectrum addition of PGG_2 to purified PGH synthase (containing 0.5 heme per polypeptide) causes a small decrease of the Soret band and a shift from 410 to 411 nm. The transient spectral complex decays at -12°C within 4 min. The decomposition is accompanied by inactivation of the enzyme and heme destruction. This complex is interpreted as an oxidized enzyme intermediate at the active site of the PG hydroperoxidase, presumably an oxo-ferryl complex.

INTRODUCTION

PG hydroperoxidase-catalysed conversion of PGG_2 to PGH_2 is associated with the formation of a potent oxidant (6, 8). As to the nature of this oxidant several hypothesis were published presuming an oxidizing radical species or singlet molecular oxygen (8). Recently, we have demonstrated the formation of singlet molecular oxygen by PGG_2 in microsomes from sheep vesicular gland or with purified PGH synthase (1). For the first step of this reaction we have proposed the formation of an oxo-ferryl complex (FeO) of PG hydroperoxidase, which may also be the oxidizing species in co-oxidation reactions of the enzyme (6). According to the postulated oxo-ferryl complex the formation of an unstable spectral enzyme complex has been observed in the reaction of PG hydroperoxidase with PGG_2 (9, 10).

To further characterize the spectral intermediate of PG hydroperoxidase we investigated the spectra resulting from addition of PGG_2 to the enzyme at low temperatures.

METHODS

Arachidonic acid was from Sigma. PGG_2 was prepared according to (5), sheep vesicular glands were obtained from the local slaughterhouse im-

mediately frozen in dry ice and stored at -80°C. Ram vesicular gland microsomes were prepared and PGH synthase was purified according to (11),
except that the buffers for the enzyme preparation did not contain NADH.
Protein determination was carried out as described by Lowry et al. (7).

Spectra were recorded at an Aminco DW2 or a Shimadzu UV-300 spectro-
photometer using 10 mm cuvettes (1 ml) provided with a temperature-con-
trolled holder (-20 to 37°C).

Ram vesicular gland microsomes or PGH synthase were suspended in Tris-
HCl buffer, pH 8.1 with 30 % glycerol. The incubation mixtures of the
PGH synthase contained equal amounts of hemin because of the heme requirement for enzyme activity. After addition of equal amounts of solvent to the reference cuvette the spectra were recorded immediately.

RESULTS AND DISCUSSION

Reactions of PGG_2 and arachidonic acid with purified PG hydroperoxidase as well as ram vesicular gland microsomes can be monitored by low-
temperature difference spectroscopy. When PGG_2 was added to the sample
cuvette at -20°C a difference spectrum with peaks at 430, 525 and 555 nm
and minima at 410, 490 and 630 nm emerged (Fig.1) Removal of oxygen by
gassing with nitrogen had no influence on the formation of the spectrum.
Purified PG hydroperoxidase or ram vesicular gland microsomes gave quali-
tatively similar spectra with PGG_2 as well as with arachidonic acid as

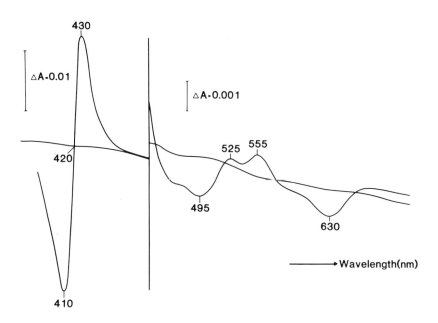

FIG. 1. Difference spectrum of purified PGH synthase with PGG_2
The two cuvettes contained 2.5 µM PGH synthase and 2.5 µM heme in Tris-
HCl buffer, pH 8.1 with 30 % glycerol. After balancing the baseline, the
reaction was started by addition of 10 µM PGG_2 (in acetone). The spectrum
was scanned immediately at 10 nm/s. Reaction temperature was -15°C.

substrate but the spectral intermediate complex of the purified enzyme
was more stable than in microsomal suspensions.

In the presence of 10 to 100 nmol PGG_2/nmol PGH synthase the Soret
peak at 430 nm disappeared within 4 min at $-12°C$ whereas the trough at
410 nm increased about 3-fold. Subsequent addition of PGG_2 after the
Soret band had vanished was not followed by a new complex formation but
by a further increase of the trough at 411 nm. Under such experimental
conditions inactivation of the enzyme and destruction of heme has been
observed as measured by oxygen consumption (3) and dipyridyl complex
formation of Fe^{3+}-protoporphyrin (4), respectively. The enzymatic activity could not be restored by addition of hemin to the cuvette. However,
when only small amounts of PGG_2 were added to PGH synthase solutions
(1 to 10 nmol PGG_2/nmol enzyme) the spectral change was reversible and
by further addition of PGG_2 the spectral intermediate could be reformed
several times. This demonstrated that the enzyme intermediate was not
a product of heme destruction. The amplitude of the difference spectrum
was dependent on the amount of microsomal protein and isolated PGH synthase but not on the free hemin concentration.

Under anaerobiosis the PGG_2-induced difference spectrum of the enzyme
complex did not change in magnitude and shape compared to the experiments
in the presence of dioxygen. This means that O_2 is not required for the
formation of the enzyme intermediate complex. But O_2 was required for
the formation of the enzyme complex with arachidonic acid both with ram

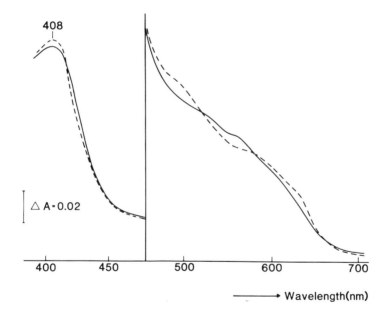

FIG. 2.   Absolute spectra from purified PGH synthase with PGG_2

The two cuvettes contained 20 μM (2 μM for the Soret region) PGH synthase in Tris-HCl buffer, pH 8.1 with 30 % glycerol. After addition of 15 μM
(2 μM for the Soret region) heme to the sample cuvette the absolute spectrum of PGH synthase was recorded (- - -). The reaction was started by
addition of 20 μM PGG_2 to the sample cuvette. Reaction temperature $-15°C$.
(——) absolute spectrum of the enzyme intermediate.

vesicular gland microsomes or purified PGH synthase. In the absolute spectrum addition of PGG_2 to a solution of purified PGH synthase was accompanied by a decrease of the Soret band and a red-shift from 410 to 411 nm (Fig. 2).

The amount of the enzyme which was converted to the intermediate could not be determined yet. So the observed absolute spectrum was a composite spectrum which does not allow the direct comparison with the documented spectra of the oxidized intermediates of peroxidase and catalase (Compound I and II) (2). Further studies, with other spectroscopic methods, will allow this comparison. But other facts, like the formation of $^1O_2$ (1), the transfer of an oxygen atom to a substrate molecule (6) and the formation of the spectral intermediate complex also by iodosobenzene (1) support the hypothesis that a transient FeO-species was involved in the catalytic mechanism of PG hydroperoxidase. This FeO-species could also be the unknown oxidizing species of the co-oxidation reactions of the enzyme.

ACKNOWLEDGMENTS

This work was supported by Deutsche Forschungsgemeinschaft, grants SFB 38- L 4 and DFG grant Na 127/2-1.

REFERENCES

1. Cadenas, E., Sies, H., Graf, H. and Ullrich, V. (1983): Hoppe Seyler's Z. Physiol.Chem., 364: 519-528.

2. Chance, B. (1952): Arch.Biochem.Biophys., 41: 404-415

3. Egan, R.W., Gale, P.H., and Kuehl, F.A., Jr. (1979): J.Biol.Chem., 254: 3295-3302.

4. Falke, J.E., editor (1964): Porphyrins and Metallporphyrins, pp. 181-182. Elsevier, Amsterdam.

5. Graff, G., Stephensson, J.M., Glass, D.B., Haddox, M.K., and Goldberg, N.D. (1978): J.Biol.Chem, 253: 7662-7676.

6. Kuehl, F.A., Humes, J.L., Ham, E.A., Egan, R.W., Dougherty, H.W. (1980): In: Prostaglandin and Thromboxan Research: Inflammation: The Role of Peroxidase-Derived Products, edited by Samuelsson, B., Ramwell, P.W. and Paoletti, R., pp.77-86, Raven Press, New York.

7. Lowry, O.H., Rosebrough, N.J., Farr, A.L., and Randall, R.J. (1951): J.Biol.Chem., 193: 265-275.

8. Marnett, J., and Reed, A.G. (1979): Biochemistry, 18: 2923-2929.

9. Nastainczyk, W., Cadenas, E., Sies, H., and Ullrich, V. (1983): In: Oxygen Radicals in Chemistry and Biology: Third Internat.Conference: Mechanism of Arachidonic acid-stimulated Singlet Oxygen Formation by Prostaglandin-Endoperoxide Synthase, edited by Bors, W., Saran, M., and Tait, D., pp. in press, De Gruyter & Co., New York.

10. O'Brien, P.J., and Rahimtula, A.D. (1981): Progr. Lipid Research 20: 295-298.

11. Roth, G.J., Machuga, E.T., and Strittmatter, P. (1981): J.Biol.Chem. 256: 10018-10022.

Icosanoids and Cancer, edited by H. Thaler-Dao, et al. Raven Press, New York © 1984.

Dependence of Lipid Peroxidation in Isolated Rat Hepatocytes on Glutathione Contents

E. Hietanen, J.-C. Béréziat, T. Heinonen, and H. Bartsch

International Agency for Research on Cancer, F-69372 Lyon, Cédex 08, France

Free radical-mediated reactions have recently gained increasing interest as a possible mechanism of chemical carcinogenesis and tissue toxicity. Free radical formation has been detected directly in tissues with the aid of ESR (electron spin resonance) signals during the activation of chemical carcinogens ; furthermore scavengers of free radicals have been shown to inhibit tumorigenesis (8, 12). Yet the direct evidence for a relationship between free radicals and cancer is lacking.

Free radicals may be formed from chemicals (4, 14) which in turn activate oxygen (1, 2) and further initiate lipid peroxidation (5, 6). Chemicals forming free radicals, activated oxygen species and lipid peroxidation products all cause chemiluminescence ; therefore this detection method might prove to be an efficient way to monitor free radical mediated oxidative reactions, in addition to other parameters measuring lipid peroxidation.

We have therefore studied in isolated hepatocytes the role of glutathione in the regulation of chemically-induced lipid peroxidation and the ralationship between lipid peroxidation and chemiluminescence following exposure to various chemicals.

MATERIALS AND METHODS

Hepatocytes were isolated from adult male BD6 rats (9) using collagenase digestion. Cell viability was tested by trypan blue exclusion. Hepatocytes were suspended (o.5-5x10^{6}cells/ml) in Krebs Ringer solution containing 25 mM HEPES: buffer, and the incubations (15 ml) were performed in a Rotavapor under air at 37°C. In experiments where glutathione was depleted, diethylmaleate (DEM) at a 2 mM final concentration was added 30 minutes before the addition of other ingredients. The final concentrations of other chemicals are shown in the tables. Carbon tetrachloride was added as such whereas other chemicals were dissolved in distilled water or saline. After various incubation times, aliquots of the hepatocyte suspension were taken and lipid peroxidation, glutathione (GSH) content and bio-and chemiluminescence were measured.

259

Lipid peroxidation was measured spectrophotometrically by malondi-aldehyde (MDA) production (13); glutathione (GSH) content (after preci-pitation of proteins) was determined as non-protein sulfhydryl groups (10). The chemiluminescence was measured in a LKB-1251 luminometer using 0.5 ml of a hepatocyte suspension (2.5×10^6 cells/ml) and adding the necessary reagents in 50 µl.

RESULTS

In isolated hepatocytes, Fe^{2+} enhanced lipid peroxidation was without effect on the glutathione content (Table 1).

TABLE 1. Effects of $FeCl_2$ on glutathione and lipid peroxidation in isolated hepatocytes

Incubation time (min.)	GSH Content ($nmol/10^6$cells)			Malondialdehyde ($nmol/10^6$cells)		
	$FeCl_2$ (final conc.)			$FeCl_2$ (final conc.)		
	Control	0.1 mM	0.5 mM	Control	0.1 mM	0.5 mM
0	37.0	–	–	–	–	–
5	26.9	29.7	31.3	0.80	3.28	4.38
15	26.3	29.4	28.1	0.88	7.80	8.90
30	25.0	28.4	27.5	1.47	6.54	9.23
60	23.1	25.0	21.9	1.81	7.76	9.63

When CCl_4 was incubated with hepatocytes alone, no change in the GSH content was seen and lipid peroxidation was not increased (Table 2). Even when GSH was depleted by diethylmaleate no increase in the lipid peroxidation was detected. However, when both diethylmaleate and CCl_4 were added to hepatocytes, lipid peroxidation was strongly increased (Table 2). The incubation of CCl_4 with $FeCl_2$ did not change the GSH content but lipid peroxidation was increased to the same extent as seen with $FeCl_2$ alone (Table 2).

TABLE 2 A, B. The effects of CCl_4 on the glutathione content (A) and lipid peroxidation (B) alone and after glutathione depletion

A.

Ingredients	Incubation time (min.)				
	0	5	15	30	60
	GSH content ($nmol/10^6$cells)				
Control	41.9	46.8	44.4	42.5	42.5
Diethylmaleate (DEM, 2 mM)	–	10.3	11.3	12.2	15.0
CCl_4 (5 mM)	–	41.9	39.7	38.8	33.8
DEM+CCl_4 (2 mM+5 mM)	–	11.4	9.4	10.6	12.2
CCl_4+$FeCl_2$ (5 mM+0.5 mM)	–	34.4	32.5	27.8	30.1

B.

	Ingredients			
Control	DEM (2 mM)	CCl_4 (5 mM)	DEM+CCl_4 (2 mM+5 mM)	CCl_4+$FeCl_2$ (5 mM+0.5 mM)
Lipid peroxidation (nmol malondialdehyde/10^6cells per 20 min.)				
0.60	0.58	0.56	17.40	8.0

CCl$_4$ at 1 mM final concentration enhanced lipid peroxidation (3.5-fold higher MDA production) after the depletion of GSH by DEM, but no increase in chemiluminescence was found. Cupric chloride (1 mM) or ethanol (100 mM) did not have any effects on MDA production or chemiluminescence when GSH was not depleted. Both FeCl$_2$ and FeCl$_3$ initiated chemiluminescence and MDA production. Paraquat (2.5 and 5 mM) caused chemiluminescence, but no increased MDA production.

DISCUSSION

Lipid peroxidation of unsaturated fatty acids is a complex series of reactions, which can be initiated by activated oxygen species or free radicals from xenobiotics and results in different end products (6). Thus by measuring aldehyde, alkene or diene formation or by detecting the bioluminescence of various excitated peroxy-radicals, lipid peroxidation can be monitored (4,5). Depending on the causative reactions, sometimes (but not always) the various methods to measure lipid peroxidation yielded uniform results (11,15). CCl$_4$ is known to be metabolized to a free radical which induces lipid peroxidation that can be detected by chemiluminescence (7). After administration of CCl$_4$ to rodents in vivo an increased bioluminescence was found (as compared to untreated controls) in liver homogenates: in vitro addition of GSH terminated the bioluminescence (7).

In our study when CCl$_4$ was added to hepatocytes in vitro, the lipid peroxidation (measured by MDA) was greatly dependent on the GSH content. This data confirm the important role of free radical trapping agents in controlling lipid peroxidation. Paraquat did not increase MDA production in microsomal assays despite an increased chemiluminescence.

In accordance with our data obtained in isolated hepatocytes, paraquat did not increase MDA production in microsomal assays despite an increased chemiluminescence (4). When paraquat was infused into the liver, no increase in the whole organ chemiluminescence was found, in contrast to the lungs where paraquat infusions induced both chemiluminescence and MDA production (1,3).

In our study in isolated hepatocytes, Fe^{2+} caused lipid peroxidation without requiring GSH depletion. This depletion was necessary for the CCl$_4$-induced lipid peroxidation, which can be explained by the trapping of the free CCl$_4$-derived radical, thus preventing the initiation of fatty peroxidation.

REFERENCES

1. Aldrich, T.K., Fisher, A.B., Cadenas, E., and Chance, B. (1983): J. Lab. Clin. Med., 101: 66-73.
2. Boveris, A., Cadenas, E., Reiter, R., Filipkowski, M., Nakase, Y., and Chance, B. (1980): Proc. Natl. Acad. Sci. USA 77: 347-351.
3. Cadenas, E., Arad, I.D., Fisher, A.B., Boveris, A., and Chance, B. (1980): Biochem. J., 192: 303-309.
4. Cadenas, E., Brigelius, R., and Sies, H. (1983): Biochem. Pharmacol. 32: 147-150.
5. Cadenas, E., Muller, A., Brigelius, R., Esterbauer, H., and Sies, H. (1983): Biochem. J., 214: 479-487.
6. Cadenas, E., Wefers, H., and Sies, H. (1981): Eur. J. Biochem., 119: 531-536.
7. Di Luzio, N.R., and Stege, T.E. (1977): Life Sci., 21: 1457-1464.

8. Emmanuel, N.N. (1982): In: Free Radicals and Cancer, edited by R.A. Floyd, pp. 245–319. Marcel Dekker, New York.
9. Moldéus, P., Hogberg, J., and Orrenius, S. (1978): In: Methods in Enzymology, edited by S. Fleischer and L. Packer, vol. 52. pp. 60–71. Academic Press, New York.
10. Saville, B. (1958): Analyst, 83: 670–672.
11. Smith, M.T., Thor, H., Hartzell, P., and Orrenius, S. (1982): Biochem. Pharmacol., 31: 19–26.
12. Ts'o, P.O., Caspary, W.J., and Lrentzen, R.J., (1977): In: Free Radicals in Biology, edited by W.A. Pryor, vol. 3, pp. 251–303.
13. Uchiyama, M., and Mihar, M. (1978): Anal. Biochem., 86: 271–278.
14. Wefers, H., and Sies, H. (1983): Arch. Biochem. Biophys., 224: 568–578.
15. Wright, J.R., Rumbaugh, R.C., Colby, H.D., and Miles, P.R. (1979): Arch. Biochem. Biophys., 192: 344–351.

Icosanoids and Cancer, edited by H. Thaler-Dao, et al. Raven Press, New York © 1984.

Serum Selenium and Gynecological Cancer: Effect of Selenium Supplementation on Plasma Malondialdehyde and Serum Glutathione Peroxidase

*A. Kauppila, *H. Sundström, **H. Korpela, **L. Viinikka, and †E. Yrjänheikki

*Departments of *Obstetrics and Gynecology, and **Clinical Chemistry, University of Oulu, SF-90220 Oulu 22; and †Oulu Regional Institute of Occupational Health, SF-90150 Oulu 15, Finland*

Evidence from animal experiments (12,16) and human epidemiological studies (7,21) indicates an association between deficient selenium intake and carcinogenesis. In animal studies, selenium supplementation has decreased the number and growth rate of carcinogen-induced malignant tumors (4, 6). The soil in Finland is selenium-poor and hence the nutritional selenium intake of Finnish people has been low (20). We have found low serum levels of selenium in Finnish patients with uterine (18) or ovarian cancer (19), and have observed that short-term selenium supplementation changed the serum activity of antioxidative glutathione peroxidase (GSH-Px) and the plasma concentration of malondialdehyde (MDA; indicative of lipid peroxidation) in ovarian carcinoma (H. Sundström, manuscript in preparation). In this report we briefly summarize our results from these studies.

SUBJECTS AND METHODS

From 1978 to 1981, the serum concentration of selenium was measured in patients with cervical, endometrial or ovarian cancer, and in their age-, weight- and place of residence-matched controls (Table 1). The mean ages of patients with cervical, endometrial or ovarian cancer were 60.3, 60.1 and 56.6 years, respectively. Serum GSH-Px activities and plasma MDA concentrations were measured in 19 patients with ovarian cancer during 1981-1982, in connection with combination cytotoxic chemotherapy with adriamycin (40 mg/m2), cyclophosphamide (500 mg/m2) and cis-platinum (50 mg/m2) or ftorafur (800 mg/m2). Blood samples were collected before, during and after cytostat infusion lasting about 10 hours. Twelve of these patients also received 96 ug of organic selenium (Selena, Lääketukku, Finland) daily for 10 days, starting 7 days before the cytotoxic chemotherapy.

Serum selenium concentrations (18), GSH-Px activities (5) and plasma MDA concentrations (22) have been measured by methods described elsewhere. In the statistical analysis of the results, the paired t test, random block design variance analysis with the Bonferrone t test, and the Wilcoxon rank signed test were employed.

TABLE 1. Mean (±SE) concentrations of serum selenium (umol/l) in patients with cervical, endometrial or ovarian cancer, and in their age-, weight- and place of residence-matched control women.

Site of cancer	N	Cancer patients	N	Control subjects	P
Cervix	37	0.82 ± 0.04	37	1.32 ± 0.05	< .001
Endometrium	64	1.01 ± 0.05	64	1.29 ± 0.05	< .001
Ovary	40	0.93 ± 0.04	40	1.22 ± 0.03	< .001

N = number of patients

RESULTS

Patients with cervical, endometrial or ovarian cancer had significantly lowered serum concentrations of selenium (Table 1). In ovarian but not in uterine cancer, old patients, and patients with advanced malignancy had lowered serum levels of selenium whereas in control subjects serum selenium did not depend on age.

Short-term selenium supplementation increased the serum concentration of selenium from 1.18 ± 0.04 SE to 1.41 ± 0.06 umol/l (p < .01). Cytotoxic chemotherapy decreased the activity of serum GSH-Px at the 6th hour (p < .01) but did not alter plasma MDA significantly (Table 2). Selenium supplementation inhibited the GSH-Px suppression induced by cytostats, and decreased the plasma level of MDA (p < .01).

TABLE 2. Mean (±SE) activity of serum glutathione peroxidase and the concentration of plasma malondialdehyde in ovarian cancer patients during and after one-day combination cytotoxic chemotherapy with or without preceding selenium supplementation.

Selenium supplement	N	Before therapy	6 h	24 h	48 h
			after the start of cytostats		
Glutathione peroxidase (u/l)					
No	19	394 ± 17	355 ± 14	379 ± 14	388 ± 17
Yes	12	389 ± 15	376 ± 16	394 ± 16	415 ± 26
Malondialdehyde (nmol/l)					
No	19	1.11±0.08	1.02±0.07	1.17±0.09	1.15±0.10
Yes	12	0.93±0.09	0.83±0.08	0.90±0.08	0.98±0.08

* p < .01

DISCUSSION

Our finding of low serum selenium concentrations in uterine and ovarian cancer agrees with many (1,10,15) but not all previous results (3,10). The intake of nutritional selenium in Finland is dependent on the amount of imported cereals. During the past few years it has been greater than at the end of the last decade. Hence, the concentration of serum selenium in 1981-1982 (text) was higher than in 1978-1981 (Table 1)

Selenium deficiency increases lipid peroxidation (14), which, in turn, may induce disturbances in cell membranes, in the generation of prostanoids (2), and in DNA function (11). Selenium is an essential component of GSH-Px and it participates in the elimination of H_2O_2 and other hydroperoxides (2,17). Its anticancer effect may also be attributable to other cellular functions, possibly DNA-synthetic activities (11).

Our short-term selenium supplementation appeared to induce beneficial biochemical responses. Organic selenium rapidly increased the serum level of selenium, as also seen in other studies (9), and it decreased the plasma concentration of MDA by nearly 20 %. This changed MDA is a sign of reduced lipid peroxidation which, in turn, suggests protection against carcinogenic oxidative damage of cellular membranes. In animals, adriamycin increased the MDA concentration in cardiac muscle, and administration of antioxidants suppressed MDA formation and the appearance of subacute cardiac changes (13). Selenium supplementation may thus also diminish the risk of cardiac injury in patients receiving cytotoxic chemotherapy. Prevention of GSH-Px suppression by selenium during cytotoxic therapy can also be regarded as a positive effect of this supplementary therapy.

The clinical and biochemical effects of exogenous selenium in human cancer patients are insufficiently known. Our preliminary results indicate the necessity of larger and longer-lasting clinical trials employing clinical and biochemical parameters of response.

ACKNOWLEDGEMENTS

The investigations have been supported by Yrjö Jahnsson Foundation, and Finnish Foundation for Cancer Research.

REFERENCES

1. Calautti, P., Moschini, N., and Stievano, B.M. (1980): Scand. J. Haematol., 24:63-66.
2. Editorial (1983): Lancet, 1:685.
3. Goodwin, W.J., Lane, H.W., Bradford, K., Marshall, M.W., Griffin, A.C., Geopfert, H., and Jesse, R.H. (1983): Cancer, 51:110-115.

4. Griffin, A.C. (1979): Adv. Cancer Res., 29:419-442.
5. Günzler, W.A., Kremers, H., and Flohe, L. (1974): Z. Klin. Chem. Klin. Biochem., 12:44-448.
6. Jacobs, M.M. (1980): Prev. Med., 9:362-367.
7. Jansson, B., Seibert, B., and Speer, J.F. (1975): Cancer, 36:2373-2384.
8. Levander, O.A. (1982): Ann. NY Acad. Sci., 393:70-82.
9. Levander, O.A., Alfthan, G., Arvilommi, H., Gref, C.G., Huttunen, J.K., Kataja, M., Koivistoinen, P., and Pikkarainen, J. (1983): Am. J. Clin. Nutr., 37:887-897.
10. McConnel, K.P., Broghamer, W.L., Blotky, K.J., and Hurt, O.J. (1975): J. Nutr., 105:1026-1031.
11. Medina, D., Lane, H.W., and Tracey, C.M. (1983): Cancer Res., 43:2460-2464.
12. Medina, D., and Shepherd, F. (1980): Cancer Lett., 8: 241-245.
13. Myers, C., McGuire, W., and Young, R. (1976): Cancer Treat. Rep., 60:961-962.
14. Schamberger, R.J. (1972): J. Natl. Cancer Inst., 8:1941-1947.
15. Schamberger, R.J., Rukovena, E., and Longfield, A.K. (1973): J. Natl. Cancer Inst., 50:863-870.
16. Schrauzer, G.N., White, D.A., and Schneider, C.J. (1978): Bioinorg. Chem., 8:387-396.
17. Sunde, R.A., and Hoekstra, W.G. (1980): Nutr. Rev., 8: 265-273.
18. Sundström, H., Yrjänheikki, E., and Kauppila, A.: Int. J. Gynaecol. Obstet. In press.
19. Sundström, H., Yrjänheikki, E., and Kauppila, A.: Carcinogenesis. Submitted.
20. Varo, P., and Koivistoinen, P. (1981): Int. J. Vit. Nutr. Res., 51:79-84.
21. Willet, W.C., Morris, J.S., Pressel, S., Taylor, J.O., Stampter, M.J., Rosner, B., Schneider, K., and Hames, C.G. (1983): Lancet, 1:130-134.
22. Yagi, K. (1976): Biochem. Med., 15:212-216.

Icosanoids and Cancer, edited by H. Thaler-Dao, et al. Raven Press, New York © 1984.

Prostaglandins and Interleukin 1 Produced by Phagocytic Cells of the Thymic Reticulum in Culture Are Able to Regulate Thymocyte Proliferation

*M. Papiernik, **F. Homo-Delarche, and **D. Duval

**U7 INSERM and *U25 INSERM, Hôpital Necker, 75015 Paris, France

Many investigations have been carried out to study the character-istics and the roles of cells of the monocyte-macrophage lineage or related cells with dendritic morphology present in lymphoid organs. Various types of phagocytic and dendritic cells have been described in peripheral lymphoid tissues, where they represent the main constituant of spleen and lymph node stroma (3). Cells comparable to macrophages, dendritic or interdigitating cells of the peripheral organs have also been observed in the thymus in vivo and can be isolated in vitro from thymic tissue. Papiernik and coworkers have recently described a tech-nique leading to the proliferation of phagocytic cells of the thymic reticulum in culture (P-TR-C) (5). Despite their phagocytic properties in vitro, these cells contain very few lysosomes and their morphology is closer to interdigitating cells described in the thymus in vivo, than to the conventional macrophage. Moreover, these cells are able to induce the proliferation of syngeneic thymocytes, which were highly enriched in thymic medullary cells (5). In the present work, we demons-trate that P-TR-C are able to produce different factors involved in the regulation of thymocyte proliferation, i.e. interleukin 1 (IL 1) and prostaglandins (PGs).

MATERIALS AND METHODS

Mice

DBA/2 (H-2^d) 5-6 week old female mice were used in all experi-ments.

Culture of P-TR-C

The technique used to obtain P-TR-C has been extensively described before (5). In brief, primary monolayer cultures were established from thymic stroma. P-TR-C proliferated on these monolayers and were releas-ed into the culture medium as non adherent cells with a hairy aspect. P-TR-C were replated in multiwell tissue culture plates (2.5 x 10^5

cells/ml) where they became adherent in a few hours. Cells were kept in control medium (RPMI 1640, supplemented with 1 % penicillin and strep-tomycin and 10 % FCS) for 2 x 2 days. The medium was then replaced by fresh medium with or without the drugs to be tested.

Determination of PG production

Extraction of prostaglandins from the culture medium was performed according to a modification of the Frölich's technique (7). Pgs were then measured by radioimmunoassay (RIA).

IL 1 assay

IL 1 was tested by the biological assay described by Gery et al. (2), using the ability of IL 1 to induce the proliferation of thymocy-tes in the presence of Con A.

The absence of IL 2 activity in P-TR-C supernatants was verified using an IL 2-dependent cell line (CTLL 2).

RESULTS AND DISCUSSION

Determination of PGs production by RIA

We have measured the four types of Pgs (PGE_2, $PGF_{2\alpha}$, 6 keto $PGF_{1\alpha}$ and TXB_2), which have been described in the supernatants of monocyte-macrophage lineage cells (8).

The total levels of PG secreted may vary from one culture to an-other (5000-10.000 pg/ml/24 h): we thus expressed the secretion of each PG as a percentage of the total amounts of PGs produced in each experi-ment. The major compound released into the culture medium appears to be TXB_2, which represents almost 40 % of the total secretion. PGE_2 and 6 keto $PGF_{1\alpha}$ both represent around 25 % of the secretion, whereas $PGF_{2\alpha}$ is a minor component representing only 10 % of the total secre-tion. In addition, the proportion of the various PGs secreted remained almost constant during the course of a given culture (up to 6 days).

Effect of indomethacin on PG production by P-TR-C

We have studied the effect of IM on the secretion of the various types of PGs. The cells were first incubated in the absence of drug for 24 h in order to determine basal levels of PG secretion. The medium was renewed and replaced by 1 ml of fresh medium with or without (control) $10^{-6}M$ IM. The culture medium was then renewed every day or every two days and replaced by fresh medium + IM. As shown in Figure 1, the action of IM was markedly different according to the prostaglandin tes-ted. After 24 h incubation in the presence of the drug, there was a marked inhibition of PGE_2 and 6 keto $PGF_{1\alpha}$ production, whereas the secretion of $PGF_{2\alpha}$ and TXB_2 was not affected. A slight inhibition of $PGF_{2\alpha}$ production was only observed after longer incubation (up to 5 days) in the presence of the drug. Similar differences in the pattern of modulation of PG production have been described in other types of cells (1, 4) and remain to be explained.

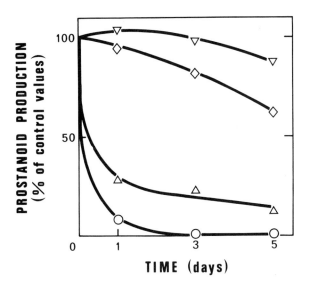

TIME (days)

FIG.1. Effect of IM (10^{-6}M, 5 days) on PG production by P-TR-C.
PGE_2 (0), 6 Keto $PGF_{1\alpha}$ ($\triangle$), $PGF_{2\alpha}$ ($\diamond$) and TXB_2 ($\triangledown$).

Antagonistic effects of IL 1 and PGE_2 produced by P-TR-C on thymocyte proliferation

As shown in Table 1, thymocytes alone stimulated by Con A had a very poor proliferative response. When thymocytes were cultured with

Table 1. Effect of PGE_2 on the proliferation of thymocytes induced by Con A in the presence of IL 1-containing P-TR-C supernatant (a)

Nature of P-TR-C stimulation	PGE level (pg/ml)	Thymocyte response to Con A (cpm) % of P-TR-C supernatant added			
		25	12	6	3
	PGE produced				
None	1056	1082	2589	2567	2252
LPS	2679	1433	2353	2745	2318
LPS + IM(b)	285	5889	13753	11252	6076
	PGE added(c)				
LPS + IM(b)	2500	2233	2749	2347	1535

(a) Thymocytes (8 x 10^5/well) were stimulated by Con A for 72 h in the presence of serial dilutions of P-TR-C supernatants.
(b) IM (10^{-5}M).
(c) The same PGE_2 concentration as that produced by P-TR-C stimulated by lipopolysaccharide (LPS) was added exogenously to the supernatant.

Con A in the presence of supernatants from P-TR-C or from P-TR-C co-cultured with LPS, the background level of the response was slightly enhanced but was not dependent upon the supernatant concentration.

According to the well documented effects of type E PG in immune response (8), we suspected PGE_2 to have an inhibitory effect in this model. Indeed, the supernatant from P-TR-C stimulated by LPS in the presence of IM was able to induce a dose-dependent proliferation of thymocytes co-cultured with Con A. As already shown P-TR-C are able to secrete PGE_2 spontaneously, and this production is enhanced by LPS (Table 1). Then, LPS-stimulated P-TR-C supernatants contained an IL 1 activity which could only be revealed when the secretion of PGE_2 was blocked by IM, as confirmed by RIA. Conversely, exogenous PGE_2 added to supernatant containing an IL 1 activity and in which endogenous PGE_2 secretion had been blocked by IM, inhibited the proliferation of thymocytes in response to Con A (Table 1).

The target of PG inhibition may be either the IL 1 producers (P-TR-C), the IL 1 target cells (thymocytes) or both. To determine whether P-TR-C IL 1 secretion are sensitive to PGE_2, the supernatant from P-TR-C stimulated by LPS was dialyzed to remove PGs and then tested for IL 1 activity. The disappearance of PGE_2 from these supernatants was confirmed by RIA. The IL 1 biological activity could be recovered in P-TR-C supernatants (in the absence of indomethacin), when PGE_2 has been removed by dialysis, thus suggesting that PGE_2 does not inhibit IL 1 secretion by P-TR-C, but rather blocks thymocyte proliferation (6). These results show that P-TR-C produce two factors IL 1 and PGE_2, which have antagonistic effects on thymocyte proliferation. Moreover, antiinflammatory agents are able to modulate PGs secretion, which is one of the factors of the thymic microenvironment involved in the control of lymphocyte proliferation.

REFERENCES

1. FISHER, A., DURANDY, A., MAMAS, S., McCAL, E., DRAY, F., and GRISCELLI, C. (1982) Clin Exp Immunol 49: 377-385.
2. GERY, I., GERSHON, R.K., and WASKSMAN, B. (1972) J Exp Med 136: 128-142.
3. HOEFSMIT, E.C.M. (1975) In: Mononuclear Phagocytes in Immunity, Infection and Pathology, edited by R. VAN FURTH, pp. 129-146. Blackwell Scientific Publications, London.
4. KELLY, J.P., JOHNSON, M.C. and PARKER, C.W. (1979) J Immunol 122: 1563-1571.
5. PAPIERNIK, M., NABARRA, B., SAVINO, W., PONTOUX, C., and BARBEY, S. (1983) Eur J Immunol 13: 147-155.
6. PAPIERNIK, M., and HOMO-DELARCHE, F. (1983) Eur J Immunol 13: 689-692.
7. SALMON, J.A., and FLOWER, R.J. (1979) In: Hormones in Blood, edited by C.M. GRAY and V.M.T. JAMES, Academic Press, New York, 2: 237-245.
8. STENSON, W.F., and PARKER, G.W. (1980) J Immunol 125: 1-5.

Icosanoids and Cancer, edited by H. Thaler-Dao, et al. Raven Press, New York © 1984.

Influence of Non-Esterified Fatty Acids on the Activity of Lymphocytes and Macrophages of Two Lines of Mice Genetically Selected for Their Low or High Response to Phytohaemagglutinin

*S. Gauthier-Rahman, *M. Liacopoulos-Briot, **G. Vallette, †C. Stiffel, *J. Parlebas, **N. Christeff, and **E. A. Nunez

*U.20 INSERM, CNRS LA 143, Hôpital Broussais, 75014 Paris; **U.224 INSERM, CNRS ERA 881, Faculté Xavier Bichat, 75018 Paris; and †U.125 INSERM, CNRS ER 70, Institut Curie, 75005 Paris, France

Numerous studies have shown that non esterified fatty acids (NEFAs) have an effect on cell mediated and humoral immune responses that may be inhibitory (8, 12) or stimulatory (5). The activation of T lymphocytes by mitogens elicits a full range of lymphocyte immune functions (4) and is widely used as a measure of cell mediated immunity (4). With a view to analyze the relationship between NEFAs and cell mediated immune responses, two lines of mice genetically selected for the high (Hi/PHA) or low (Lo/PHA) response of their T lymphocytes to phytohaemagglutinin (PHA) (14) were employed. The nature and the concentration of NEFAs in their spleen cells, the effect of different fatty acids on the PHA response and on the migration of spleen and induced peritoneal exudate cells were studied in the two lines.

MATERIAL AND METHODS

Animals. These experiments were performed in 2 to 7 months old Hi/PHA and Lo/PHA mice from F 23 to F 25 generations of our own breeding colonies.

Reagents. NEFAs were obtained from Sigma Chemical Co, St-Louis, USA ; PHA was from Wellcome Research Laboratories, Beckenham, England ; Tritiated methyl thymidine ^{3}H TdR, 1 Ci/mmol was obtained from CEA, Saclay, France.

Methods. Spleens of adult male mice were used for preparation of 105 000g cytosols as described (1) and their fatty acid concentration determined by gas chromatography as in (17). The response to PHA was measured by incorporation of ^{3}H TdR in spleen cells (14) after 2 days of culture in serum-free medium in presence or not of different concentrations of fatty acids. The migration of spleen and induced peritoneal cells (PEC) from agarose microdroplets was studied with a novel photoelectric procedure as in (3) in presence or not of different concentrations of fatty acids during culture over three days.

RESULTS

NEFA CONCENTRATIONS IN CYTOSOLS OF SPLEEN CELLS OF Hi/PHA AND Lo/PHA
MICE.

The levels of saturated, mono, di and tri unsaturated fatty acids were
but little different in the two lines. In contrast, the concentration of
polyunsaturated fatty acids (PUFAs) in Lo/PHA was twice that in Hi/PHA
(Table 1).

Table 1 - Endogenous NEFA concentrations in spleen cytosols of Hi/PHA
         and Lo/PHA male mice (µg/mg protein ± se).

Line of mice	Total NEFAs	Saturated	Mono, di, tri, ene	Polyene*
Hi/PHA	21 + 5	7.5 + 1.5	11.5 + 3	0.6 + 0.3
Lo/PHA	23 + 6.5	8 + 2	13 + 4.5	1.5 + 0.3

* $0.01 < P < 0.05$

EFFECT OF NEFAs ON THE PHA RESPONSE OF SPLEEN CELLS OF Hi/PHA AND Lo/PHA
MALE MICE.

Fig. 1 shows that the incorporation of [3]HTdR by spleen T lymphocytes was
clearly inhibited in both lines by the polyunsaturated docosahexaenoic
acid (C22:6). This inhibition was dose-dependent and greater in Lo/PHA
than in Hi/PHA mice. Thus 1.8 µg/10[6]cells of C22:6 were required for 50%
inhibition in Hi/PHA cells whereas only 0.36 µg/ 10[6]cells were sufficient for the same effect in Lo/PHA. Similar results were obtained with
arachidonic acid (C20:4). In contrast, the saturated palmitic acid
(C16:0) was without effect on [3]HTdR incorporation in Hi/PHA and was
only inhibitory at high concentrations (10 µg/ 10[6]cells) in Lo/PHA.
Lo/PHA cells thus appear to be more sensitive to the inhibitory effect
of PUFAs.

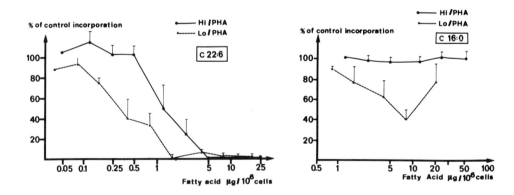

Figure 1 : Effect of NEFAs on PHA induced [3]HTdR uptake in Hi/PHA and
           Lo/PHA spleen cells.

EFFECT OF NEFAs ON THE MIGRATION OF SPLEEN AND INDUCED PERITONEAL
EXUDATE CELLS (PEC) OF Hi/PHA OR Lo/PHA MICE.

The migration of normal spleen (about 80% lymphocytes) and Freund
incomplete adjuvant induced peritoneal exudate cells (about 80% macrophages) was differentially inhibited in the two lines of mice in
presence of exogenous PUFAs (C20:4 and C22:6) in dose and time dependent manner. After 15 hours of culture, a biphasic effect was observed
on spleen cells of both lines, with stimulation of migration at low
concentrations of 0.05 - 0.5 µg/ml (low zone) and increasingly greater
inhibition at concentrations of 25 µg/ml onwards (high zone). After
48 hours of culture, inhibition in the high zone increased up to 80% or
more in both lines whereas the stimulatory effect in the low zone
lessened especially in Lo/PHA mice. By 72 hr, significant inhibition of
Lo/PHA (20% or more) was observed in the low zone, but this was absent
in Hi/PHA. Peritoneal exudate cells especially of Lo/PHA were even more
sensitive to inhibition by low concentrations of PUFAs than spleen cells
(Table 2). Twenty per cent inhibition of Lo/PHA PEC was obtained with
about 12 times lower concentrations of PUFAs as compared to Hi/PHA, this
ratio being 2 for spleen. In contrast, the saturated fatty acid C16:0
was without significant inhibitory effect on the migration of spleen and
PEC of both lines except at the highest concentration tested
(100 µg/ml).

Table 2 : The effect of C20:4 and C22:6 on the migration of spleen
and peritoneal exudate cells of Lo/PHA and Hi/PHA mice.

| FATTY ACIDS | Fatty acid concentrations (µg/ml) required for 20 % Migration Inhibition on Day 3 | | | | | |
| | Peritoneal exudate | | | Spleen | | |
	Lo/PHA	Hi/PHA	Ratio $\frac{Hi}{Lo}$	Lo/PHA	Hi/PHA	Ratio $\frac{Hi}{Lo}$
C20 : 4	0.63	7.6	12	3.8	6.3	1.66
C22 : 6	0.5	5.7	11.5	6.3	13.8	2.2

DISCUSSION AND CONCLUSION

Two lines of mice genetically selected for their low (Lo/PHA) or high
(Hi/PHA) response to PHA were studied with a view to clarify the rôle of
NEFAs in cell mediated immune phenomena. The ratio of the PHA response
of Hi/PHA to Lo/PHA is 44:1 for lymph node cells and 12:1 for spleen
cells (15). The greater reactivity to PHA of Hi/PHA mice is accompanied
by greater cell mediated immune reactions such as MLR (6) and GVH (7).
Analysis of NEFAs extracted from spleen cytosols of the two lines showed
that Lo/PHA cytosols have a two fold higher concentration of PUFAs than
Hi/PHA. The higher content of PUFAs in Lo/PHA spleen cells was found to
be associated with a greater sensitivity of Lo/PHA cells to the
inhibitory effect of low doses of exogenous PUFAs in studies involving
[3]HTdR incorporation in response to PHA, and during migration of spleen
and PEC from agarose microdroplets. The time - dependent nature of the
inhibition of migration by low concentrations of PUFAs in Lo/PHA mice
suggests a faster rate of incorporation and/or a different catabolic
fate for PUFAs in Lo/PHA mice. Macrophage migration and [3]HTdR incorpo-

ration were inhibited by both C20:4, precursor of prostaglandins, prostacyclin and other oxygenated derivatives as well as by C22:6.
whose metabolic fate is still unknown.
These findings are in agreement with what is already known of the association of normal lymphocyte and macrophage function with lipids. Thus
stimulation of lymphocytes by PHA is followed by increased lipid
metabolism (10) increased turnover of membrane phospholipids (9) and
preferential incorporation of PUFAs into plasma membrane (11). Similarly
cell mediated immune responses were found to generate unsaturated fatty
acids in mice and guinea-pig lymphocytes (2). Even in the absence of
other phagocytic or pharmacologic stimulation, exogenously supplied C20:4
was shown to be rapidly incorporated into cell membrane phospholipids and
metabolized by resting mouse macrophages (13). Changes in cell membrane
composition influence its fluidity (16) and could thereby modify cell
migration.
The higher content of PUFAs in Lo/PHA cytosols together with differences
in rate of incorporation and/or metabolism of PUFAs as suggested above,
could afford a partial explanation of the differential inhibition observed in the two lines.

ACKNOWLEDGMENTS

This work was supported by grants from CNRS (Immunopharmacology), the
Fondation pour la Recherche Médicale and University PARIS VII.

REFERENCES

1. Clerc-Hofmann, F., Vallette, G., Secco-Millet, C., Christeff,N.,
    Benassayag, C., Nunez, E.A. (1983) C.R. Acad. Sci. 296 : 53-58
2. Cyong, J. and Okada, H. (1976) Immunology 30 : 763-767
3. Gauthier-Rahman, S., Morlat, J.L., Lecas, G., Bouin, M. (1982),
    J. Immunol. Methods 53 : 77-89
4. Hume, D.A. and Weidemann, M.J. (1980) in : Mitogenic lymphocyte
    transformation. Elsevier/North Holland, New-York
5. Kelly, J.P. and Parker, C.W. (1979) J. Immunol. 122 : 1556-1562
6. Liacopoulos-Briot, M., Stiffel, C., Lambert, F., Decreusefond,C.
    (1981) Cell. Immunol. 44 : 29-38
7. Liacopoulos-Briot, M., Stiffel, C., Lambert, F. and Decreusefond,C.
    (1981) Cell. Immunol. 62 : 448-455
8. Merten, J. and Hughes, D. (1975) Int. Arch. Allergy Appl. Immunol.
    48 : 203-210
9. Resch, K., Ferber, E., Odenthal, J. and Fisher, H. (1971) Eur.J.
    Immunol. 1 : 162-165
10. Resch, K. and Ferber, E. (1972) Eur. J. Bioch. 27 : 152-161
11. Rode, H.N., Szamel, M., Schneider, S., Resch, K. (1982) Bioch.
    Biophys. Acta 688 : 66-74
12. Santiago-Delpin, E.A., Roman-Franco, A.A., Colon, Z.A. (1982) J.
    Exp. Med. 155 : 535-547
13. Scott, W.A., Pawlowski,N.A., Andreach, M., Cohn, Z.A. (1982) J.
    Exp. Med. 155 : 535-547
14. Stiffel, C., Liacopoulos-Briot, M., Decreusefond, C. and Lambert,F.
    (1977) Eur. J. Immunol. 7 : 291-297
15. Stiffel, C., Liacopoulos-Briot, M., Decreusefond, C., Lambert,F.
    (1983) Cell. Immunol. 77 : 77-91
16. Toyoshima, S. and Osawa, T. (1975) J. Biol. Chem. 250 : 1655-1660
17. Vallette, G., Benassayag, C., Savu, L., Delorme, J., Doumas, J.,
    Maume, G. and Maume, B.F. (1980) Biochem. J. 187 : 851-856

Icosanoids and Cancer, edited by H. Thaler-Dao, et al. Raven Press, New York © 1984.

Antineoplastic Prostaglandin: Antitumor Effect of PGA and PGJ Derivatives

Masanori Fukushima and Taketoshi Kato

Aichi Cancer Center, Department of Internal Medicine and Laboratory of Chemotherapy, Chikusa-ku, Nagoya 464 Japan

Prostaglandin E and A series have been demonstrated to inhibit cell proliferation in various cell lines in vitro and in vivo during the past decade. Block of cell growth by PGE was observed for the first time as a coupled event of cell differentiation induced by PGE (5). In 1976 Santoro et al. described potential antitumor effect of PGE on B16 melanoma in vitro and also in vivo (6). In the following year these investigators introduced a potent antitumor PGE analog which acts longer time than the mother compound (7). In 1979 Honn et al. first described the evidence that PGA has stronger inhibitory activity of DNA synthesis than PGE (3). We have recently described marked inhibition of cell proliferation and DNA synthesis by PGD_2 (1), and have found that PGD_2 dehydrate, 9-deoxy-Δ^9-PGD_2 (PGJ_2), has three times stronger activity than the mother compound (2). We also observed stronger effect of PGA_2 than PGE_2 in the same experimental condition. From these facts we can conclude that the cyclopentenone ring structure is an essential moiety to exert cytotoxicity, and probably the antitumor agents are actually cyclopentenone PGs, the dehydrate of PGD_2 or PGE_2, that is PGJ_2 or PGA_2, respectively. Our major interest is to investigate the possibility to develop new antineoplastic species from PG derivatives. In this communication we present some recent results of new PGA and PGJ derivatives which is far active than other PG derivatives reported in the past.

METHODS

Cell growth inhibitory activity of PG was determined as described previously (1). L1210 mouse leukemia culture cells were used for this assay. Cells (1 x 10^5 cells/ml) were plated and after 4 days culture in the presence of serial concentration of PG, the cell number was counted. From the dose response curve, concentration required for 50% inhibition of cell growth (IC50 value) was determined. PGs dissolved in 99.5% ethanol were added to obtain final concentrations indicated.

Antitumor activity in vivo was determined using Ehrlich ascites tumor bearing mice. Ehrlich ascites tumor cells (1 x 10^5 cells/mouse) were inoculated intraperitoneally into ICR mice weighing 24 $\pm$ 2 g. PGs were given i.p. once daily from day 1 to 5, and the survival time was observed. The percentage increase in life span (ILS) was calculated from the formula :(mean survival time of treated group/mean survival time of control group) x 100 -100.

RESULTS AND DISCUSSION

In order to screen antitumor activity of PGE_2, PGA_2, PGD_2, and PGJ_2, we designed animal experiments using Ehrlich ascites tumor bearing mice which is a primary screening system for antineoplastic agents. Among PGs examined, only cyclopentenone PGs, PGA_2 and PGJ_2 prolonged the survival time of the tumor bearing mice as shown in TABLE 1. Strikingly, PGJ_2 produced 17% of long survivor at the dose of 30 mg/kg/day. Twenty mg/kg/day of PGs showed no significant antitumor effect. Antitumor activity in vivo well corresponded with in vitro activity expressed as IC50. PGA_2 and PGJ_2 are at least two times more effective than the parent molecule in vitro (TABLE 1).

TABLE 1.   Antitumor activity of PGE_2, PGA_2, PGD_2 and PGJ_2 in vitro and in vivo.

PG	in vitro activity IC50 value	in vivo activity		
		dose[a]	survival	ILS 60-day survivor
	µg/ml	mg/kg/day	days	%
PGE_2	4-7	30	16.5 ± 2.2	-3.5 0/6
PGA_2	1-2	30	23.7 ± 5.8	38.4 0/6
PGD_2	2-4	30	16.6 ± 1.9	-3.0 0/6
PGJ_2	0.5-1	30	26.0 ± 2.5	52.0 1/6
none	-	-	17.1 ± 1.8	0 0/10

a/ 5 days consecutive treatment.

From this experiment it was shown that considerably high dose of PG was required to obtain antitumor activity in vivo. This treatment was well tolerated and the only side effect observed was transient diarrhea. The grade of diarrhea was apparently different among these PGs and inverse correlation was observed between antitumor activity and diarrhea inducible activity. The weakest was PGJ_2 and the strongest was PGE_2 for diarrhea induction (2). Therefore the action mechanism of cell growth inhibition seems to be different from other PG effect. As for this issue at present the only evidences demonstrated are that cell growth inhibition is caused by DNA synthesis inhibition (1,3) via cAMP independent mechanisms (8). These facts indicate that antitumor activity of PG can be dissociated from other pharmacological effect such as smooth muscle contracting activity.

On the basis of several lines of evidences mentioned above, we selected PGA and PGJ as the candidates of parent molecule to develop more effective derivatives. Here we propose the name of antineoplastic PG for cyclopentenone PG such as PGA, PGJ and its derivatives.

From chemical aspects, we tried the introduction of a double bond at C_7 to potentiate the alkylating activity of cyclopentenone moiety of PGA. We synthesized Δ^7-PGA_1 and 12-epi-Δ^7-PGA_1 and examined antitumor activity as described above. Δ^{12}-PGJ_2 was also examined, since this compound also has a double bond adjacent to the ketone group of the cyclopentenone ring. Structure of these new synthetic PG derivatives are shown in FIG.1.

Recently we have found that PGD_2 is converted to Δ^{12}-PGJ_2 in human plasma (4). We described earlier that PGD_2 changed to PGJ_2 in aqueous solution during incubation at 37° (2), so we thought that PGD_2 might be converted to PGJ_2 in plasma in the same way as PGE_2 to PGA_2. However, we detected Δ^{12}-PGJ_2 instead of PGJ_2 after the incubation of PGD_2 in human plasma, and we also found that PGJ_2 is converted rapidly to this new metabolite. Thus Δ^{12}-PGJ$_2$ is suggested to be a naturally occurring PG in human tissues.

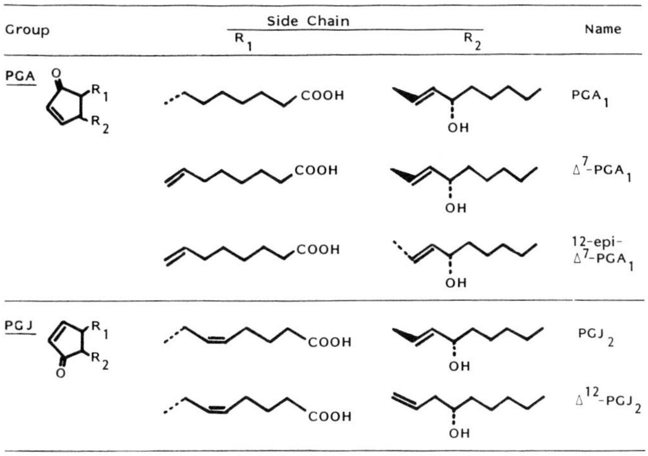

FIG. 1. STRUCTURE OF ANTINEOPLASTIC PROSTAGLANDIN

TABLE 2. Antitumor activity of Δ^7-PGA$_1$, 12-epi-Δ^7-PGA$_1$, and Δ^{12}-PGJ$_2$ in vitro and in vivo.

Agent	in vitro activity IC50 value	in vivo activity		
		dose	survival days	ILS %	60-day survivor
	μg/ml	mg/kg/day			
Δ^7-PGA$_1$	0.2-0.4	20$^{a/}$	25.7 $\pm$ 5.3	37.4	1/6
12-Epi-Δ^7-PGA$_1$	0.2-0.4	20$^{a/}$	33.0 $\pm$ 9.8	76.5	1/6
			(18.7 $\pm$ 1.4)	0	(0/10)
Δ^{12}-PGJ$_2$	0.5-1.0	20$^{b/}$	32.2 $\pm$ 6.0	103.8	1/6
			(15.8 $\pm$ 1.5)	0	(0/6)

Numbers in parenthes indicate mean survival time of control group.
a/Five-days consecutive treatment. b/Three-days consecutive treatment.

As shown in TABLE 2, Δ^7-PGA$_1$ showed a potent cell growth inhibitory activity and the IC50 value was approximately 0.3 μg/ml. Cytotoxic activity of these derivatives is more than ten times stronger than that of the parent molecule, and are comparable to an established antineoplastic agent such as mitomycin C (IC50 :0.1-0.3 μg/ml) under the same experimental conditions. Unexpectedly, the 12-epi type was as active as the natural compound. Thus the stereochemistry of the R$_2$ side chain is not required to exert cytotoxicity. Further studies on requirements for antitumor activity are described in the forthcoming paper. In vitro activity of Δ^{12}-PGJ$_2$ was almost the same as that of PGJ$_2$ suggesting that PGJ$_2$ is in part con- to Δ^{12}-PGJ$_2$ in the media which contains 10% fetal calf serum.

Again corresponding with the in vitro results, these antineoplastic PGs showed potent antitumor activity in vivo also. The effective dose was over 20 mg/kg/day for these compounds. Seventeen percent of mice lived more than 60 days without loss of weight by consecutive administration of these compounds. At this dose 12-epi-Δ^7-PGA$_1$ and Δ^{12}-PGJ$_2$ did not induce diarrhea, while Δ^7-PGA$_1$ induced marked diarrhea. Furthermore a single injection of 100 mg/kg/day 12-epi-Δ'-PGA$_1$ resulted in 72.1% ILS with 33% of 60-day survivor indicating a comparable activity to 200 mg/kg /day injection of cyclophosphamide which showed 103.8% ILS with 50% 0f 60-day survivor.

Thus we could develop several PG derivatives which have comparable antitumor activity in vivo to clinically useful antineoplastic agent such as cyclophosphamide. The limiting toxicity dose, maximum tolerated dose and antitumor spectrum are now under investigation.

ACKNOWLEDGEMENT

This work was supported in part by Grants-in-aid for Cancer Research from the Ministry of Education, Science and Culture, and by the subsidy from the Ishida Foundation (Nagoya). We thank Drs. S. Kurozumi (Teijin Ltd. Tokyo), H. Amemiya (Fuji Chemical Industries Ltd., Toyama), and Y. Arai (Ono Pharmaceutical Co. Ltd., Osaka) for their kind supply of synthetic PG and its derivatives.

REFERENCES

1. Fukushima, M., Kato, T., Ueda, R., Ota, K., Narumiya, S., and Hayaishi, O. (1982): Biochem. Biophys. Res. Commun.,105;956-964.

2. Fukushima, M., Kato, T., Ota, K., Arai, Y., Narumiya, S., and Hayaishi, O. (1982): Biochem. Biophys. Res. Commun.,109; 626-633.

3. Honn, K.V., Dunn, J.R., Morgan, L.R., Bienkowski, M., and Marnett, L. J. (1979): Biochem. Biophys. Res. Commun.,87;795-801.

4. Kikawa, Y., Narumiya, S., Fukushima, M., Wakatsuka, H., and Hayaishi, O. (1984): Proc. Natl. Acad. Sci. USA,(in press).

5. Prasad, K.N. (1972): Nature New Biol.,236;49-52.

6. Santoro, M.G., Philpott, G.W., and Jaffe, B.M. (1976):Nature,263;777-779.

7. Santoro, M.C., Philpott, C.W., and Jaffe, B.M. (1977): Cancer Res.,37; 3774-3779.

8. Wiley, M.H., Feingold, K.R., Grunfeld, C., Quesney-Huneeus, V., and Wu, J.M. (1983): J. Biol. Chem.,258;491-496.

Icosanoids and Cancer, edited by H. Thaler-Dao,
et al. Raven Press, New York © 1984.

Relevance of Cellular Interactions in PGE$_2$-Mediated Natural Killer Cell Inhibition

Christoph Gisinger, Christoph C. Zielinski, and Martha M. Eibl

*2nd Department of Medicine, Vienna Medical Hospital and Institute of Immunology,
University of Vienna, A-1090 Vienna, Austria*

Natural killer (NK) cells have been demonstrated to be involved in
the immune surveillance of tumor development (11). Although the
control of NK activity by various substances, e.g. interferon (4),
interleukin 2 (3) or prostaglandins (1) has been clearly shown in both
rodents and man, little is known about the cellular interactions
mediating the effects of these substances upon NK cells. Reports of
NK activity are only sparse: thus, in some reports monocytes and
polymorphonuclear cells (12,6) have been shown to suppress NK
activity in various sustems, and the role of T cells remained unclear,
although the interdependence of T cell population in NK-interferon
interactions has been demonstrated recently (8,14). We have investigated the role of T-cells in the production of prostaglandins (PGE$_2$) and
in the PGE$_2$-mediated inhibition of NK activity.

Methods:
Blood was obtained from a total of 40 healthy volunteers. Isolation of
peripheral blood mononuclear cells (PBMC) and the depletion of T cells
((PBMC)-T) was performed as described earlier (2). 5×10^7 PBMC or
(PBMC)-T were suspended in 5 ml RPMI 1640 (Gibco; Grand Island, N.Y.)
supplemented with 10% FCS and incubated in plastic petri dishes at
37°C in a CO$_2$-incubator for 18 hours. The supernatants were aspirated,
spun at 500 g for 10 minutes and stored at -20°C until further use.
Natural killer cell (NK) assays: The cell line K 562 (9) was used as
target cell population. Target cells were labeled with 200 µCi ^{51}Cr
(Behringwerke AG; Marburg, W.-Germany) and adjusted to a concentration
of 1.25×10^5/ml. All assays were carried out in triplicate in
microtiter plates in a total volume of 0.2 ml in effector:target cell
(E:T) ratios of 100:1, 50:1 and 25:1. The plates were centrifuged at 30 g
at 20°C for 5 minutes, incubated at 37°C in a CO$_2$ incubator for 8 hours
and spun again at 500 g and 4°C for 10 minutes. 100 µl of the
supernatant were aspirated and counted in a gamma spectrometer.
Specific lysis was calculated according to previous descriptions (6).
Maximum lysis was obtained by incubation of ^{51}Cr-labelled target cells
with 0.1% sodium lauryl sulfate (Sigma; St. Luis, MO). In NK assays
in which the influence of supernatants of various origins upon NK
activity was to be studied, effector cells were suspended entirely in the
undiluted supernatant under investigation. Synthetic PGE$_2$ (Dinoprostone;
Upjohn; Crawley, W. - Sussex) was added to the NK assays in concentrations
of 10^{-4}M and 10^{-5}M. Indomethacin (Sigma) was added in concentrations

of 10^{-4} and 10^{-6}M to the PBMC or (PBMC)-T the supernatants of which were used for further experiments.

Assays for prostaglandins: the supernatants were extracted and analysed by a radioimmunoassay (Prostaglandin E$_2$ ^{3}H-Ria-kit; Seragen Inc, Boston, MA) using an antibody to PGE$_2$ and a ^{3}H-PGE$_2$-tracer and expressed as as µg/ml. In addition thin-layer-chromatography showed PGE$_2$, PGE$_1$ and PGD$_2$ to be the main metabolites (results not shown), rat fundus strip bioassay was used to assess the biologic activity of prostaglandins gained by the described method. Statistics: the mean $\pm$ standard error (SEM) and the median of the data were calculated. Statistical analyses were performed by student's-t-test for independent data and for paired samples.

Results:

Influence of PBMC supernatants upon NK activity: supernatants derived from PBMC incubated overnight suppressed NK activity significantly in E:T ratios of 50:1 and 25:1 (p<0.005).

The inhibitory activity of PBMC supernatants was abolished by the addition of 10^{-6}M indomethacin at the start of the incubation period. Supernatants of PBMC were analysed for the content of PGs in a blinded fashion. Radioimmunoassay data showed that PBMC supernatants contained high amounts of PGE$_2$ (26.6 ± 4.1µg/ml). In contrast, supernatants to which indomethacin had been added at the initiation of the PBMC incubation contained very little or no PGE$_2$ (4.9 ± 0.7 µg/ml). In order to investigate the involvement of T cells in the regulation of PGE$_2$ production by PBMC, (PBMC)-T were incubated overnight. The supernatants derived from (PBMC)-T populations inhibited NK activity significantly and to a similar degree as did supernatants derived from PBMC. Inhibitory activity of the former supernatants was reversible by the addition of 10^{-6}M indomethacin (Table 1). In correlation to these findings, the production of PGE$_2$ by (PBMC)-T was similar to PBMC(32 ± 5.3 µg/ml.)

		E:T=50:1	E:T=25:1
NK PBMC	(%lysis)	59.3 ± 4.9	54.9 ± 4.8
	+ PBMC-supern.	41.1 ± 2.8	34.2 ± 4.0
	+PBMC-supern. + Indom.	52.7 ± 4.8	50.4 ± 5.6
	+(PBMC)-T-supern.	44.1 ± 3.6	34.5 ± 4.4
	+(PBMC)-T-supern.+Indom.	50.0 ± 5.7	47.6 ± 6.9

Table 1: NK activity of PBMC and its inhibition by various supernatants

Inhibition of the NK activity of (PBMC)-T populations: In order to further investigate the role of T cells in the regulation of PGE$_2$ activity upon NK cells, the influence of supernatants of PBMC and (PBMC)-T populations was studied in an assay system which was designed to assess the importance of the immediate presence of T cells for PG-mediated regulation of NK activity. While NK activity of (PBMC)-T populations did not differ significantly (p>0.1 from NK activity of PBMC(E:T 50:1 46.8 ± 5.8% lysis; 25:1±44.4 5.1% lysis), no inhibition of NK activity of (PBMC)-T was achieved by supernatants of either PBMC(E:T 50:1 41.8 ± 5.9%, 25:1 37.2 ± 6.6% lysis)-or (PBMC)-T origin. Moreover, the addition of 10^{-6}M indomethacin did not alter the pattern of NK activity by (PBMC)-T populations. A further analysis percentage of inhibition of NK activity was made (table 2).

E:T	$\underline{NK}_{PBMC}$ + supern. cont. PGE_2	$\underline{NK}_{(PBMC)-T}$ + supern. cont. PGE_2
50:1	31.2	5.6
25:1	30.8 (%inh. NK)	10.5 (%inh. NK)

Table 2: A comparison of inhibition of NK activity of PBMC and (PBMC)-T induced by PGE_2-containing supernatants (i.e. of PBMC and (PBMC)-T origin). The medians of the percentages of NK inhib. are shown.

Direct addition of synthetic PGE_2 to NK assays of PBMC or (PBMC)-T populations corroborated the results obtained with supernatants derived from PBMC and (PBMC)-T (table 3).

	$\underline{NK}_{PBMC}$	$\underline{NK}_{(PBMC)-T}$
10^{-4}M PGE_2	56.1 ± 11.2	22.0 ± 6.9
10^{-5}M PGE_2	51.9 ± 8.3	11.6 ± 5.6

Table 3: Percentage of inhibition of NK cell activity of PBMC and (PBMC)-T after addition of various concentrations of synthetic PGE_2. The data are shown as $\bar{x} \pm$ SEM.

Discussion:

In the present paper we report that PGE_2 has been produced by PBMC both in the presence and in the absence of T cells. The main cell type producing PGs in the peripherial blood is known to be the monocyte (7), and it is probable that activation of this cell population by adherence to plastic surfaces led to the described effect in correspondence to other systems in which various stimuli have been used to elicit similar effects (13). It is obvious, however, that the step of PGE_2 release was independent of T cells. In contrast, NK activity was inhibited by PGE_2-containing supernatants or by synthetic PGE_2 only when T cells were present in the effector cell population. NK cells in humans have been described to consist of a variety of different (5), but at least two (10,15) subpopulations. Whether the regulation of NK activity requires the interaction of two distinct subsets is not yet determined. If this would be the case, rosetting with sheep erythrocytes might have removed a subpopulation of NK cells which was to a large extent inhibitable by the action of PGE_2. However the minimal difference of NK activity of (PBMC)-T versus PBMC is contradictory to such a possibility. PGE_2 in a concentration of 10^{-5}M did not inhibit NK activity in the absence of T cells; the slight inhibition observed with a concentration of 10^{-4}M PGE_2 could be due to an effect mediated by small numbers of contaminating T cells or by direct influence upon an NK effector cell.

Conclusion:

a) PGE_2 was produced by incubation of PBMC in plastic petri dishes overnight. b) The production of PGE_2 was independent of the presence of T cells c) The PGE_2-containing supernatants were able to inhibit NK activity of PBMC, but not of (PBMC)-T d) Similar results were obtained by the addition of synthetic PGE_2. Thus T cells did not have any influence upon the production of PGE_2; but PGE_2-mediated inhibition of NK activity occurred only in the presence of T cells.

Acknowledgments:
This study was supported by a grant of the "Fonds zur Förderung der wissenschaftlichen Forschung" project Nr 4620

References:
1) Brunda, M.J., Heberman, R.B., Holden, H.T. (1980): J. Immunol. 124:2682.
2) Eibl, M., Zielinski, C.C., Ahmad, R., Steurer, F., Rockenschaub,A. (1980): Clin. Exp. Immunol. 41:176.
3) Henney, C.S., Kuribayashi, K., Kern, D.E., Gillis, S. (1981): Nature 291:335.
4) Heberman, R.B., Ortaldo, J.R., Bonnard, G.D. (1979): Nature 277:221.
5) Hercend, T., Reinherz, E.L., Meurer, R., Schlossman, S.F., Ritz, J. (1983): Nature 301:158.
6) Koren, H.S., Anderson, S.J., Fischer, D.G., Copeland, C.S., Jensen, P.J. (1981): J. Immunol. 127:2007.
7) Kurland, J.I., Bockman, R.(1978): J. Exp. Med. 147:952.
8) Minato, N., Reid, L., Cantor, H. Lengyel, P., Bloom, B.R. (1980): J. Exp. Med. 152:124.
9) Ortaldo, J.R., Oldham, R.K., Cannon, G.C., Heberman, R.B. (1977): J. Natl. Cancer Inst. 59:77.
10) Ortaldo, J.R.,Sharrow, S.O., Timonen, T. Heberman, R.B.(1981): J. Immunol. 127:2401.
11) Roder, J.C., Haliotis, T. (1980): Immunology Today 1:96.
12) Seaman, W.E.,Gindhart, T.D., Blackman, M.A., Dalal, B., Talal, N., Werb,Z. (1982):J.CLin. Invest. 69:876.
13) Stenson, W.F., Parker, C.W.(1980): J. Immunol. 125:1.
14) Torres, B.A.,Farrar, W.L., Johnson, H.M. (1982):J.Immunol. 128:2217.
15) Zarling, J.M., Clouse, K.A., Biddison, W.E., Kung, P.C.(1981): J. Immunol. 127:2575.

Subject Index

Subject Index[1]

---

[1]British and American spellings are used in the text. For consistency, this index uses American spellings only.